Children in Pain

Joseph P. Bush
Stephen W. Harkins
Editors

Children in Pain
Clinical and Research Issues From a Developmental Perspective

Foreword by Lonnie Zeltzer
Afterword by Barbara G. Melamed

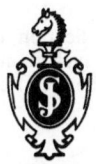

Springer-Verlag
New York Berlin Heidelberg London Paris
Tokyo Hong Kong Barcelona Budapest

Joseph P. Bush
Department of Psychology
Virginia Commonwealth University
806 West Franklin Street
Richmond, VA 23284-2018
USA

Stephen W. Harkins
Department of Gerontology
Virginia Commonwealth University
MCV Station
Richmond, VA 23298
USA

There are 8 illustrations in this volume.

Library of Congress Cataloging-in-Publication Data
Children in pain : clinical and research issues from a developmental
  perspective / edited by Joseph P. Bush and Stephen W. Harkins.
      p.   cm.
   Includes bibliographical references and index.

paper)
   1. Pain in children.   I. Bush, Joseph Paul.   II. Harkins, Stephen
W.
   [DNLM: 1. Child Development.   2. Pain — in infancy & childhood.
3. Pain — psychology.   WL 704 C536]
RJ365.C47 1991
618.92 — dc20   90-10452

Printed on acid-free paper.

ISBN-13: 978-1-4684-6415-3   e-ISBN-13: 978-1-4684-6413-9
DOI: 10.1007/978-1-4684-6413-9

© 1991 Springer-Verlag New York Inc.

Softcover reprint of the hardcover 1st edition 1991

Typeset by Bytheway Typesetting Services, Norwich, NY.

9 8 7 6 5 4 3 2 1

This book is dedicated to my father and mother,
Bartholomew and Lorraine Bush,
and to my friend and colleague, Mario Saravia.
— JPB

This book is also dedicated to Emily and Janice.
— SWH

Foreword

The early history of medicine focused on treatment of symptoms that were often seen as the disease itself (e.g., bloodletting) or some punishment for a wrongdoing (e.g., "the pox"). The beginning of the 19th century saw a zeal for investigating the etiologies of symptoms in order to uncover the diseases that they represented. Symptoms were seen as clues to the diagnosis of a disease but were often ignored in the quest for the pathophysiology of the illness. In fact, it was sometimes frowned upon to treat the symptoms because their elimination might mask the patient's actual medical condition. For example, treating pain was especially dangerous if its etiology was not precisely known, because acute pain was a signal that something was wrong with the body (e.g., appendicitis). Even when the reason for the pain was known (bleeding into the joint of a hemophiliac), there was concern that treatment of the pain might reduce or delay adequate treatment for the underlying disease. Thus, there was a shift in medicine that overtly or covertly frowned on the amelioration of symptoms, such as pain, as less important and less worthy of attention compared with the quest for diagnosis.

Pain began to become a subject of interest in a variety of ways. For example, experimental psychologists such as Ernest Hilgard and Fred Evans were primarily interested in hypnosis, and pain responses and experiences in the laboratory were examined in relation to hypnotizability. There were psychologists and anatomists such as Ronald Melzack and Patrick Wall who were interested in theories and mechanisms in pain transmission and pain control and proposed the famous "gate theory." Clinicians such as John Bonica were interested in helping people cope with the experience of pain and developed one of the first, and probably still the most famous, interdisciplinary pain clinics. Meanwhile, basic scientists such as John Liebeskind, a physiological psychologist, were learning about pain inhibitory systems and, in particular, the important role of the periaqueductal gray area of the brain as a site rich in opioid receptors. His laboratory has been studying the phenomenon of stress-induced analgesia and the role of pain in reducing tumor surveillance (specifically, cytotoxic natural killer cell [NK] activity). With all of these exciting developments in the study of pain phenomena (and certainly I have left out many other notable individuals and major findings), the concept that pain in children might be different from that in adults and that it should be studied in its own right has been a very recent event.

The developing interest in pain came from the clinical concerns of pediatric nurses who were often the members of the medical staff left with the responsibility of managing a child's pain in the hospital. Orders for analgesic medication were often left rather ambiguous and written as PRN (pro re nata), which meant that the nurses caring for the hospitalized child had to assess the level of the child's pain and then make decisions about the use of pharmacologic agents. This responsibility and dilemma propelled nurses into the research arena, specifically that of developing tools for pain assessment in children, especially young ones. The published studies by nurses of pain assessment (initially appearing in the nursing journals read primarily by the members of that profession or as chapters in nursing textbooks) initially highlighted the clinical problem of pain in children. Psychologists and child psychiatrists were often called to consult on child patients whose "source" of pain could not be identified or on adolescent patients with known conditions likely to cause pain (e.g., sickle cell disease) who complained of pain longer than what otherwise might be "expected." The question asked of the consultant was often, "Is this pain real?" These clinical dilemmas brought psychologists and child psychiatrists into the arena of the investigation of pediatric pain. Studies were designed to evaluate cognitive-behavioral strategies that would help children cope with pain. A few pediatricians even became interested in the problem and began to document not only the undertreatment of pain in children but also the lack of knowledge that physicians had regarding pain evaluation and treatment in children. Developmental psychologists began to apply their expertise to learn about pain assessment in infants, and anesthesiologists began to publish their findings on the deleterious biologic consequences of inadequate pain management during surgery and in the postoperative period in babies who were born prematurely. In particular, this latter series of studies documented the capacity for nociception even in preterms, which previously had been considered inconceivable because of the immaturity (incomplete myelination) of these small infants' central nervous systems. Also it was expected that their limited cognitive abilities would render them immune to the "experience" (emotional suffering) of pain so that even if they felt pain, it would not have any lasting sequelae (i.e., because they would not remember early painful experiences such as circumcisions anyway). Pediatric pain management services began to emerge in a few hospitals and each had its own unique character, depending on the level of hospital or other financial support and the primary discipline of its staff (e.g., anesthesiologist-oriented with high frequency of epidural catheter analgesia and other regional blocks, or psychologist-oriented with heavy emphasis on cognitive-behavioral interventions and family therapy). What united these professionals from many disciplines was their sincere interest in reducing the suffering of children and their excitement about what they were doing, both clinically and in research. This enthusiasm was certainly evident at the first international conference on pediatric pain held in Seattle a few years ago. It was this same enthusiasm and desire to call attention to the problem of pain in children and to highlight how much we still do not understand that led, I believe, to a number of recent textbooks, monographs, and special issues of journals devoted to the subject of pediatric pain.

When Dr. Joseph Bush first approached me to write a foreword to his new book on pediatric pain, my first response was that there had not been enough time for new developments in the field since the last texts for there to be yet another text on pediatric pain. However, he agreed to let me read the preprint of the text and what I found was a totally new, refreshing approach to the discussion of pain in children. What distinguished it from other texts in the field was a continuous thread throughout the book highlighting the developmental trajectory of childhood as the window through which one must view pain in children. It discusses theories about pain experiences and pain behaviors from this developmental perspective and reviews the literature from within this context. The opening chapter by Drs. Bush and Harkins quite clearly sets the tone for the rest of the book and poses many of the dilemmas with which those of us who treat children in pain and who are involved in pain research are struggling. The second chapter by Dr. Lizette Peterson and associates lays out the major developmental issues that guide the reader through the remaining chapters. In fact, I found myself considering issues that she had raised as I read each of the other chapters. While all chapters were excellent, I found the chapter by Dr. Donald K. Routh and Marjorie D. Sanfilippo on acute pain particularly refreshing because he not only provided a most comprehensive review of the literature but also did this while pointing out in a sensitive manner the dilemmas and alternative explanations raised by the findings. All chapters are well written and approach their topic areas within a developmental framework. Drs. Bush and Harkins have brought together an excellent group of psychologists/scientists who not only write well but also truly understand children and pain from a child's view.

This book is unique in that the developmental trajectory is maintained throughout the book and it is the first book on childhood pain written from a purely developmental and clinical psychology perspective. Speaking as a pediatrician, I find the absence of psychological jargon refreshing and thus would recommend this book to not only psychologists and child psychiatrists but also nursing and other medical specialists (e.g., pediatricians, anesthesiologists) as well. It clearly raises the important issues in childhood pain and points out the critical questions to be addressed by future research.

LONNIE ZELTZER

Preface

This volume presents the current state of knowledge in psychosocial aspects of pain in children. Contributions from leading scientists and practitioners are integrated within a developmental perspective, providing an introduction to the conceptual and methodological tools essential to the understanding of new work in this area. More than a comprehensive survey of major new work in pediatric pain, then, the authors present an understandable explanation of the directions in which work and thinking in this area are moving, and why. A consistent and persuasive argument is made that models of pain, assessment and intervention techniques, and research designs must be sophisticated in terms of an appreciation for developmental considerations.

This book was written for individuals interested in clinical applications and for practitioners interested in understanding the basic ideas of this important and burgeoning area that increasingly crosses over disciplinary boundaries. Pediatricians, dentists, nurses, anesthesiologists, physical therapists, pharmacologists, psychiatrists, health educators and many others deal of necessity with the psychological aspects of pain in children. An important goal of this book has been to increase the accessibility of psychological knowledge, methods and perspectives to individuals inside and outside of the discipline of psychology.

Warm thanks are extended to everyone who encouraged and tolerated my efforts in conceiving and preparing this book, especially my wife, Catherine Radecki-Bush. Thanks also to my current and past graduate students, who have helped me develop and articulate my ideas as well as contributing their own, particularly Kareen Gholl, Jeff Gillman, Marlene Maron, Roger Rape, Vickie Reid, Deborah Schroeder, Angie Smith, and especially Randi Ross and Julie Ciocco, who also spent many hours helping edit the manuscript.

JOSEPH P. BUSH

Contents

Contributors

BARBARA L. ANDERSEN, PHD   Department of Psychology, Ohio State University, Columbus, OH 43210-1222, USA

DANIEL J. BURBACH, PHD   Riverhill Psychological Associates, 21 E. Waldo Boulevard, Manitowoc, WI 54220, USA

JOSEPH P. BUSH, PHD   Department of Psychology, Virginia Commonwealth University, Richmond, VA 23284-2018, USA

KENNETH D. CRAIG, PHD   Department of Psychology, University of British Columbia, Vancouver, BC, V6T 1Y7, Canada

JANET FARMER, MS   Graduate student in Clinical Psychology at the University of Missouri, Columbia, MO 65211, USA

VIVIAN GEDALY-DUFF, DNSc   Department of Family Nursing, School of Nursing, Oregon Health Sciences University, Portland, OR 97201-3098, USA

JEFFREY B. GILLMAN, PHD   Department of Psychology, Children's Hospital, Columbus, OH 43205, USA

RUTH V.E. GRUNAU PHD   British Columbia Children's Hospital, Vancouver, BC, V6H 3V4, Canada

CYNTHIA HARBECK, PHD   Department of Psychology, Children's Hospital, Columbus, OH 43205, USA

STEPHEN W. HARKINS, PHD   Department of Gerontology, Virginia Commonwealth University, Richmond, VA 23298, USA

NANCY L. HOAG, PHD   Department of Psychiatry, Guthrie Clinic, Guthrie Square, Sayre PA 18840, USA

KAY HODGES, PHD   Department of Psychology, Eastern Michigan University, Ypsilanti, MI 48197, USA

PAUL KAROLY, PHD   Department of Psychology, Arizona State University, Tempe, AZ 85287, USA

SHARON L. MANNE, PHD   Department of Psychiatry, Sloan-Kettering Memorial Cancer Center, New York, NY 10721, USA

MARLENE MARON, PHD   Postdoctoral Fellow at Harvard Medical School, Cambridge, MA 02138, USA

BRUCE J. MASEK, PHD   Department of Psychiatry, Children's Hospital, Boston, MA 02115, USA

PATRICIA A. MCGRATH, PHD   Child Health Research Unit, Children's Hospital of Western Ontario, London, Ontario, N6C 2V5, Canada

PATRICK J. MCGRATH, PHD   Department of Psychology, Dalhousie University, Halifax, Nova Scotia, B3H 4JI, Canada

BARBARA G. MELAMED, PHD   Ferkauf Graduate School of Psychology, Albert Einstein College of Medicine at Yeshiva University, Bronx, NY 10461, USA

LARRY L. MULLINS, PHD   Department of Psychiatry and Behavioral Sciences, University of Oklahoma Health Sciences Center, Oklahoma City, OK 73190, USA

LIZETTE PETERSON, PHD   Department of Psychology, University of Missouri, Columbia, MO 65211, USA

SUSAN PISTERMAN, PHD   Department of Psychology, Children's Hospital of Eastern Ontario, Ottawa, Ontario, K1H 8L1, Canada

DONALD K. ROUTH, PHD   Department of Psychology, University of Miami, Coral Gables, FL 33124, USA

MARJORIE D. SANFILIPPO   Doctoral candidate in Clinical Psychology at the University of Miami, Coral Gables, FL 33124, USA

LAWRENCE J. SIEGEL, PHD   Ferkauf Graduate School of Psychology, Albert Einstein College of Medicine at Yeshiva University, Bronx, NY 10461, USA

KAREN E. SMITH, PHD   Department of Pediatrics, Division of Pediatric Psychology, University of Texas Medical Branch, Galveston, TX 77550, USA

JAMES W. VARNI, PHD   Behavioral Pediatrics Program, Orthopaedic Hospital, Los Angeles, CA 90007, USA

MARIE ANNE B. VIEYRA, PHD   Behavioral Medicine Program, North Shore Children's Hospital, Salem, MA 01970, USA

GARY A. WALCO, PHD   Schneider Children's Hospital, Long Island Jewish Medical Center, New Hyde Park, NY 11042, USA

LONNIE ZELTZER, MD   Department of Pediatrics, University of California, Los Angeles, Los Angeles, CA 90024-1752, USA

MICHELLE ZINK Graduate student in Clinical Psychology at the University of Missouri, Columbia, MO 65211, USA

1
Conceptual Foundations: Pain and Child Development

Joseph P. Bush and Stephen W. Harkins

Improving the adequacy of pain management in children receiving medical services is a compelling clinical and research goal that crosses disciplinary boundaries. The importance of adequate pain management in children is derived both from humanitarian concerns and from enhancement of the child's medical/functional status. Largely unexplored at this time is a third issue: what are the long-term effects of early medical/illness pain experiences on the child? Recent research findings have been highly critical of the apparently prevalent undermanagement of pain in children, and are beginning to indicate ways in which improvements may be made. Increasingly, this work is pointing to the importance of developmental considerations in understanding and providing appropriate clinical responses to children in pain.

There are intriguing difficulties inherent in the task of pain assessment. The experience of pain is subjective, for which no unique physiological correlates have been found. Difficulties in discerning another's pain are exacerbated in a number of ways. First, one's pain expression and subjective pain experience are likely to be influenced by the awareness that another person is attending to one's pain and may make a decision or other response based upon his/her own perception. Thus, there is an observer reactivity problem arising from the aversive nature of pain and the belief that its being perceived and acknowledged by another may imply a responsibility for that person to make some caring or helping response. This, in turn, represents the second difficulty: the objectivity of one who attempts to assess pain in another is likely to be compromised by any response imperatives that may be explicitly or tacitly associated with recognizing that the other is in pain (Craig & Grunau, in chapter 7). This factor may be particularly significant when the other is a child. Motives to help or to avoid the necessity of making certain responses may predispose one to over- or underestimate a child's pain. The influence of the personal beliefs of health professionals on their assessments of children's pain are particularly salient when objective clinical measures are not used. Because of the difficulty and unfamiliarity of pediatric pain measures, they are underutilized in medical settings, often resulting in inadequate pain management (Beyer & Byers, 1985; Craig, Grunau, & Branson, 1987).

Children's cognitive grasp of pain as an abstract concept encompassing a variety of subjective experiences and having certain shared meanings between people is developmentally incomplete. The institutional context of the medical setting and the legitimate and referent authority of the health professional may support an assessment of the child's pain that is in conflict with the child's subjective experience. The absence of consensual validation of the child's pain as reality may lead to a further disparity between the child's subjective experience and the assumptions and perceptions of caregivers, exacerbating communication problems and contributing to poor pain management and potential alienation of the child's trust in medical care.

It is almost a truism that there is a need for greater integration of empirical, theoretical, and clinical work with respect to the understanding and management of pain in children. Furthermore, the disparate literatures of a number of scientific/professional disciplines are involved, including pediatrics, psychology (health, child clinical, and developmental), nursing, anesthesiology, child psychiatry, pharmacology, and dentistry. Difficulties in assimilating these burgeoning literatures are compounded by the importance of integrating as well one's own subjective pain experiences and empathic response capabilities. Currently there is a flurry of work, particularly an amassing of empirical data, in the area of pain generally and with regard to stress and coping. Clearly, then, there is a need to organize new findings and to integrate them with theories and clinical practices involving children.

Recent work in the development of coping styles and abilities in children is particularly relevant to pediatric pain. For some time, researchers have been applying cognitive developmental schemes to children's understanding of pain as a concept, and of the reasons for painful procedures. In addition, evidence for stylistic coping predispositions, recognized for some time in adults, is also emerging for children (Peterson & Toler, 1986). Coping may be thought of as serving the basic motive of control (Rothbaum, Weisz, & Snyder, 1982), i.e., as a fundamental process in the self-regulation of experience. Thus, coping should function to minimize aversive or unwanted experience, as well as to maintain the perception of a sufficient level of expected ongoing control over experience. Perceptions of reduced control or intensified aversive experience, then, should stimulate increased coping behavior. To the extent that pain is perceived as indicating a breakdown of this fundamental sense of having sufficient control over one's experience, increased coping (or catastrophizing) behavior is to be expected. These behaviors may be adaptive or maladaptive (e.g., avoiding needed treatment) from a medical management perspective, and may in fact be motivated not so much by pain as by low perceptions of control. This conceptualization explains the effectiveness of interventions that increase perceptions of control in aversive medical treatment situations (e.g., Kavanaugh, 1983), as well as suggesting that there may be developmentally specific vulnerabilities for learning to expect low levels of control in certain contexts.

Pain in Children: Language and Concepts

Difficulties in integrating the findings of different researchers and the reports of clinicians have arisen due to inconsistencies in the language and organizing concepts used to discuss pain. Such difficulties are compounded when concepts that encompass objective and subjective aspects are applied across the human life span, due to the elusive but profound differences in the nature of experience in the adult, adolescent, child, and infant. It is thus important to understand the various explicit and implicit assumptions, orientations, and uses of language one is likely to encounter in the scientific and professional literatures.

Pain Concepts and Definitions

Jay (1985) provided a general definition of pain that is representative of most current scholarly thinking. She described pain as an interaction of overt, covert, and physiological responses, which may be stimulated by tissue insult and which may be produced and maintained by other antecedent and consequent conditions. Most investigators and clinicians make a number of important distinctions between acute and chronic pain. Acute pain is not only more time-limited than chronic pain, but is rarely seen as primarily psychogenic (though acute pain responses are certainly psychologically inflected). Acute pain is seen as more frightening and anxiety-provoking, and as serving a signal function to indicate the need to engage in protective or reparative behavior. Chronic pain is not conceptualized in terms of adaptive value, and is generally associated with prolonged disability and psychological difficulties (e.g., frustration, anger, depression) rather than alarm. The psychological impact of chronic pain on the individual is likely to be greater than that of acute pain (Jay, Elliott, & Varni, 1986), and to include responses associated with antecedent or consequent stimulus situations, family systems problems, or the expression of underlying individual psychopathology. A further categorization proposed by Varni (1984) differentiates procedural pain (most often associated with medical procedures such as debridement), disease pain, pain associated with traumatic injury, and an ambiguous set of painful conditions not associated with identifiable disease or physical trauma nor clearly psychogenic (e.g., some headaches and abdominal pain). This last category is particularly challenging in children (see Hodges & Burbach, in chapter 10; Vieyra, Hoag, & Masek, in chapter 14), confounding the traditional practice of prescribing pharmacological treatment for somatogenic and behavioral or psychopharmacological treatment for psychogenic pain (McGrath, 1987a).

As noted by Gillman and Mullins (chapter 5) and by Walco and Varni (chapter 12), the simplistic downward extension of these categories, formulated on the basis of work with adults, is extremely problematic. Chronic pain in particular, as presented above, is probably not a very useful rubric with children (Jay, 1985), though pain meeting at least the temporal aspects of this definition certainly occurs in children (Walco & Varni, in chapter 12). Children are more likely than adults to experience recurrent pain (Apley, 1976; McGrath, 1987a), which shares characteristics of acute and chronic. Recurrent pain may include procedural (e.g., repeated bone marrow aspirations in a leukemic child), disease (e.g., recurring painful episodes in a child suffering from sickle-cell anemia), and pain of ambiguous etiology (recurrent abdominal pain, migraine headaches) types.

Semantic complexities in defining pain are especially evident when considering pain in infants. Are developmental differences (neurological, cognitive, learning history) between infants and older people so profound that it is improper to speak of pain in infants? Until recently, it was commonplace for health professionals to assert that infants do not experience or remember pain (Bush, 1990; Craig et al., 1987; Routh & Sanfilippo, in chapter 15), thus avoiding the sometimes considerable clinical difficulties in managing pain in this vulnerable, nonverbal population. Although such a viewpoint is now less common, little is understood about pain phenomena in infants. Research has established that behavioral and physiological responses suggestive of distress and avoidance occur in the neonate following tissue insult (Manne & Andersen, in chapter 13), and that such responses show a meaningful developmental progression throughout infancy (Craig & Grunau, in chapter 7). Studies of infant facial expressions in response to ostensibly painful stimuli have detected consistent structural similarities with adult facial pain expressions (Craig et al., 1987; Craig & Grunau, in chapter 7), supporting the notion of a superordinate pain construct across the life span.

Pain measurement is difficult due to the multidimensional nature of the human pain experience. The sense of pain is not a unitary function; it subsumes many component processes that may vary with type of pain (Melzack, 1973). Several of these dimensions, however, can be separately evaluated in adults and older children using standardized measures of pain quantity and quality. In particular, researchers have made considerable progress in the separate measurement of the nociceptive or sensory intensity aspects of a painful event versus its immediate dysphoric characteristics. These sensory and affective components of pain are separable in older children (McGrath, in chapter 4) and adults (Harkins, Price, & Martelli, 1986; Price, Harkins, & Baker, 1987). The recognition that the affective but not the sensory component of pain is influenced by its perceived meaning (Price, 1988) and personality (Harkins et al., 1986) has obvious implications for treatment of adults. The verbally mediated assessment tools for evaluation of pain sensory intensity, immediate unpleasantness, meaning of the pain to the individual, and pain-related suffering are clearly useful in young children but may be limited to those children who have mastered several complex cognitive-linguistic developmental tasks.

Thus, pain intensity and suffering appear less amenable to separate assessment in children, probably because children are less able to utilize linguistic discriminations to differentiate the complexities of subjective experiences. Numerous investigators and clinicians have noted that, as one considers increasingly younger children, pain and its specific negative affects appear more and more inextricably confounded (LeBaron & Zeltzer, 1984). Furthermore, it is difficult to separate negative responses to any specific pain from emotions associated with hospitalization, illness, and physical confinement (Beyer & Byers, 1985). It has been argued that it may be most useful to work with a superordinate "distress" construct with young children, encompassing pain and anxiety (Jay et al., 1986; Routh & Sanfilippo, in chapter 15). Clearly, indices of behavioral distress in young children should be expected to reflect the aggregate of aversive responses across sources (McGrath, 1987b; Ross & Ross, 1988; Manne & Andersen, in chapter 13).

Questions regarding the complexities of pain, negative affect, suffering, behavioral distress, and perceived meaning are of interest from a developmental perspective, in addition to their bearing on clinical assessment and intervention issues. An implicit model seemingly underlying many current conceptualizations of pain suggests a general distress factor in infants and very young children. This "general distress" response might be aroused by a variety of environmental, physiological, and psychological events, though differentiation of activation thresholds and behavioral manifestations probably begins extremely early. A general distress response has obvious adaptive value, both signaling the child's discomfort to its caretakers and stimulating self-regulatory (coping) behaviors to reduce distress (see Craig & Grunau, in chapter 7; Routh & Sanfilippo, in chapter 15).

This model is consistent with the diminishing ability of assessment techniques to differentiate pain from other sources of suffering and negative affect with decreasing age of the child (Ross & Ross, 1988), as well as with the consistency in facial pain expression observed across infants (Craig & Grunau, in chapter 7). Ross and Ross (1984), based on data from interviews of 994 5- to 12-year-old California schoolchildren, noted a consistent tendency for children to provide unidimensional definitions of pain that emphasize general discomfort. Clinicians as well as researchers have noted the tendency of young children to globalize pain (Apley, 1976; Siegel & Smith, in chapter 6). Research on the development of children's pain concepts and other pain-related cognitions also indicates increasing globality in younger children's responses, consistent with the general progression toward increasing differentiation of perception and specificity of responding in both cognitive and emotional development (see Peterson, Harbeck, Farmer, & Zink, in chapter 2). This was supported by Gaffney and Dunne (1986), whose scoring of sentence completion tasks by 680 children revealed a significant and direct relation between the variety of themes used to define pain, and chronological age between 5 and 14 years.

Some preliminary support for this model was also revealed in a factor analytic study of children's pain, which suggested further complexity beyond a first general factor. Gillman and Bush (1991) administered a broad spectrum of sensory, affective, evaluative, and cognitive self-report pain items to 83 6- to 13-year-olds representing two chronic (juvenile rheumatoid arthritis and inflammatory bowel disease) and one acute procedural (phlebotomy) populations. Principal factors analysis revealed four factors that accounted for 67.7% of the variance in the total sample. The first factor, including verbal as well as nonverbal items representing a wide array of domains (sensory, affective, evaluative), was labeled by the authors "general misery," and accounted for 22.8% of the total variance. Results also indicated that levels of this general misery factor varied considerably among subjects, but did not differentiate patient groups, further supporting its interpretation as a nonspecific factor. More specific subsequent factors, on the other hand, accounted for less overall variance but contributed much more to differentiating patient groups in a discriminant analysis. More research is clearly needed to validate and extend these early findings.

Developmentally, the experience of pain is seen as increasing in both generality and specificity. On the one hand, learning and experience may assimilate or condition an increasing variety of stimuli to pain schemas/responses. That is, individuals may show pain responses to a wider array of stimuli, over the course of development. On the other hand, individuals may learn to discriminate painful from merely distressing stimuli, and may increasingly differentiate and modulate their pain responses according to specific stimulus situation characteristics. These changes might be accounted for by learning associated both with pain experiences and through exposure to pain behaviors in others. Research evidence indicates that the expression (if not the subjective experience, as well) of pain is modulated by behavioral factors even in neonates. Grunau and Craig (1987) found that infants' facial expressions following heel lance varied with their behavioral state, and not just with tissue insult variables. They interpreted these findings as indicating that the state of the organism (its level of behavioral arousal) affects pain expression, even developmentally prior to opportunities for learning pain responses. This view may suggest that pain is innately a higher level process that is dependent upon a number of subsidiary processes that are in turn subject to developmental modification.

One extremely important process that undergoes developmental change and that fundamentally influences pain experience and expression, is the individual's coping with, and level of control over (ability to self-regulate), aversive experience. A fundamental developmental task of childhood involves the acquisition of competencies contributing to increasing self-regulatory abilities, among which the minimization of pain and suffering is clearly prominent (Craig & Grunau, in chapter 7; Peterson et al., in chapter 2). We are just beginning to understand the role of cognitive development, and of cognitive coping style, in these self-regulatory abilities that are involved in the experience of pain. Key roles are indicated for the ability to understand the cause of painful sensory experience and for the ability to interpret or reframe the meaning of painful sensory experience as nonthreatening to one's self-regulatory control, in determining the quality (including the perceived painfulness) of that experience. Certainly it is now unambiguous that the perceived meaning of pain has a major impact on suffering in adults (Price, 1988). The ability to attribute and modify the meanings of pain and the suffering associated with nociceptive events is critical in the child's pain behavior. When exposure to pain models, learning the social-cultural meanings associated with pain, and various reinforcement contingency histories are taken into account, it is not surprising that there is increasing variability in the distress and suffering components of pain experience, with increasing age (Routh & Sanfilippo, in chapter 15).

Related Constructs

Assessment of children in pain often entails drawing conclusions regarding the abnormality or maladaptive consequences of pain responses. Related constructs, "excess disability" and "abnormal illness behavior," have yet to be adequately defined with reference to children. As with adults, similar levels of pain frequently result in different levels of disability in different children. As noted by McGrath and Pisterman (chapter 9), such determinations must consider school, learning, and social-emotional developmental agenda in ways that are very different from adults. In addition, assessment in cases involving chronic pain, as well in epidemiological research, may require evaluation of the effects of pain on the quality of children's lives. An excellent review of quality of life research in adult oncology patients and an agenda for extending this work to pediatric populations has been prepared by Mulhearn and his colleagues (Mulhearn et al., 1989).

It is difficult to separate the effects of pain from some efforts to control it. Resting, for example, may be construed as "down time" (i.e., unproductive, not engaged in school or work), or as therapeutic and enabling. Similarly, complaining may be seen as out-of-control distress behavior, or as seeking interpersonal assistance. There is considerable unclarity in the use of the term *coping*. Some conceptualizations place coping on a continuum with defense mechanisms as attempts to deal with perceived threat, differentiated primarily on the basis of accessibility to consciousness and distortion of reality. In common usage, coping is often used to refer to healthy, successful responses to stressful events. These definitions have proven unsatisfactory, the latter because it confuses the behavior with its effects, and the former largely because it relies upon such vague criteria. A more precise and useful definition of coping, particularly with respect to pain, emphasizes the motive of restoring a desired level of perceived control over undesirable circumstances (Craig & Best, 1977; Rothbaum et al., 1982). Research (reviewed by Siegel & Smith, in chapter 6) has indicated that both actual and perceived control over painful events is associated with decreased aversiveness for the individual, as well as increased tolerance. Coping behavior may thus be outwardly directed and problem-focused (e.g., taking aspirin in response to a headache) or inwardly directed and emotion-focused (e.g., telling oneself that the pain of a dental anesthetic injection will be over shortly and will prevent more intense subsequent pain), or may be classified in a variety of other ways (Lazarus, 1977). Such coping behavior may or may not prove to be effective or may even have severely maladaptive consequences. Understanding the coping motive underlying apparently disordered behavior in a disruptive child patient may help health care practitioners to respond more appropriately in difficult treatment situations.

Coping behaviors, serving the goal of increasing perceived control, are critical determinants of the experience of pain. More successful coping is defined by success in restoring perceived control, which in turn results in a less aversive experience. Developmental processes and learning experiences have a profound effect on coping abilities and expectations, as described by Siegel and Smith (chapter 6). The cognitive dimension of coping is influenced by the ability to understand the reasons for painful medical procedures, by having the ability to understand the notion of limited duration, and by the ability to communicate with others sufficiently well to obtain information. Included in this is the appraisal of threat and of one's resources for responding to it (Craig & Best, 1977; Siegel & Smith, in chapter 6). The behavioral dimension includes particular coping behaviors such as relaxing, and positive or distracting self-talk. The psychosocial dimension includes social skills such as the ability to elicit interpersonal support from others as well as learning the expected role behaviors of patients and people in pain. The child's level of self-efficacy expectations appears to be particularly important; a child who expects to be able to restore a sufficient level of control when faced with pain is likely to engage in coping behaviors expected to serve that goal. Research is beginning to indicate the value of interventions that enhance self-efficacy and perceived control in children undergoing painful procedures, ranging from play and instructional sessions to patient-controlled analgesia (Maron & Bush, in chapter 11; McGrath, in chapter 4; Routh & Sanfilippo, in chapter 15; Siegel & Smith, in chapter 6). Researchers have found that, as children develop, they tend to engage in more cognitive coping (Curry & Russ, 1985; Siegel & Smith, in chapter 6), though developmental changes in more overt behavioral coping are less apparent.

Essential Developmental Concepts

Cognitive Development

The dominant theoretical perspective in work applying cognitive developmental ideas and findings to problems in pediatric pain over the past decade has been Piaget's genetic epistemology (Piaget, 1965). Although no longer at the cutting edge among investigators of cognitive development, Piaget's work has been shown to have heuristic and practical value in terms of both its methods and its insights into the subjective experience of the child. Piaget's "revised clinical method" utilizes a partly standardized approach to the study of the individual child, in which the emphasis is not so much on the child's answer to questions as on the reasoning process that leads to the answer. Thus, the child is presented with a challenging stimulus or dilemma, such as a pendulum that swings through an arc of varying length as a weight is moved up or down its arm, or a question such as "where does pain come from?" Predetermined initial questions are followed by a more individualized follow-up, intended to reveal the premises and rules of logic used by the child in comprehending the stimuli.

A number of useful ideas that have emerged from Piagetian theory are frequently encountered in the pediatric pain literature (Bush, 1990). One of the most fundamental of these is the notion that children of all ages do reason and comprehend according to more-or-less internally consistent principles that are generally unlikely to be explicit to themselves or to their adult audiences. Piaget argues that knowledge is constructed out of propositional elements known as schemes. These schemes are actively constructed and integrated by the developing child in his/her constantly ongoing effort to maintain a cognitive map of the world, or a set of blueprints for operating in the world. Such successive construction, deconstruction, and reconstruction to attain a more adequate knowledge/map is a fundamental process of biological adaptation that is highly developed in humans. Furthermore, since the child operates according to his/her own self-constructed maps, his/her behavior can be well understood by an adult only through the sometimes difficult process of learning about and then "entering into" the child's logical system. It is here that the work of researchers applying Piagetian notions to children in pain has been so valuable (Bush, 1987).

Piaget believed that children's reasoning develops through four broad stages (sensorimotor, preoperational, concrete operations, and formal operations), each characterized by qualitatively different types of logic. This is one of the most problematic aspects of his theory; first, because of heterogeneity within stages and homogeneity across stages (i.e., ambiguity of stage transitions) and second, because of findings indicating that young children apparently use logic that should be beyond their current abilities, when examined under optimal conditions. Thus, for example, overly simple application of Piagetian stage-specific expectations regarding how a child will reason about a particular subject (such as a painful medical procedure) may be misleading to the extent that particular experiences support islands of cognitive precocity. Harbeck and Peterson (in review; Peterson et al., in chapter 2), in fact, found that chronological age was superior to scores on a Piagetian conservation-identity task in predicting the cognitive maturity of the responses of preschoolers, first and third graders, and college freshmen to a series of questions about pain. Nevertheless, it is reasonable to expect that children within a given stage are likely to understand and to think in a manner generally characteristic of that stage. To the extent that this is true, this can be of considerable value to individuals attempting to communicate with and to understand the behavior of children in pain (Craig & Grunau, in chapter 7; Manne & Andersen, in chapter 13). Research has provided some support for a Piagetian developmental progression in children's verbal definitions of illness (Bibace & Walsh, 1980) and of pain (Gaffney & Dunne, 1986). Gedaly-Duff (chapter 8) provides a number of highly illustrative examples of children's pain responses that would be grossly misunderstood according to typical adult logic, but that may be recognized and responded to much more appropriately when understood using Piagetian concepts.

Piagetian constructs are particularly useful in efforts to understand children's responses to painful medical procedures. Children at certain developmental stages may be especially vulnerable to certain types of distortion or misunderstanding regarding the reasons for or consequences of pain experienced at the hands of medical professionals (Maron & Bush, in chapter 11; McGrath & Pisterman, in chapter 9). For instance, the Piagetian notion of immanent causality has been used to explain the tendency of preoperational children to misconstrue pain as punishment for wrongdoing (Jay, 1985) or as malicious behavior on the part of the medical professional. Although others (Ross & Ross, 1984) have found little evidence of children perceiving pain as punishment, the more general point (that the meanings attributed to pain vary with cognitive developmental level and affect the suffering associated with painful experiences) is compelling (Maddux, Roberts, Sledden, & Wright, 1986; Maron & Bush, in chapter 11; Siegel & Smith, in chapter 6; Vieyra, Hoag & Masek, in chapter 14). Furthermore, interviews with children have indicated that preschoolers have little comprehension of the motives underlying the behaviors of physicians while interacting with their patients, even when the children recognize the typical topography of these behaviors (Haight, Black, & DiMatteo, 1985). Children's acquisition of concrete operations (usually around 7 years of age) seems to be associated with increased ability to understand cause-and-effect relationships as well as (gradually) more complex, multivariate patterns of causation (Peterson et al., in chapter 2; Siegel & Smith, in chapter 6). This is likely to bring about a significant increase in cooperativeness during painful medical procedures, because of the corresponding increase in their ability to understand realistically the reasons behind the procedures (Craig et al., 1987; Jay et al., 1986;

Siegel & Smith, in chapter 6). It has also been noted (Jay et al., 1986; Maron & Bush, in chapter 11) that young children are particularly likely to experience heightened distress associated with pain when visible stigmata are involved, particularly when these appear gruesome such as in burn treatment.

Important contributions to the understanding of the role of cognitive development in children's responses to pain are also emerging from more recent theoretical formulations associated with information processing models. Peterson et al., (in chapter 2), for example, explore the implications of information models of memory development for understanding young children's limited ability to utilize their past experiences in coping with a current painful experience. There are also developmental changes in children's linguistic abilities and vocabularies relative to pain, medical procedures, physiological and psychological processes, and coping responses. Such changes affect the child's reasoning about painful experiences (Craig & Grunau, in chapter 7; Peterson et al., in chapter 2) as well as communication with health professionals (Maron & Bush, in chapter 11). It may be anticipated that an increase in the application of information processing models will be seen in future work in pediatric pain.

Coping and Control

Just as the perceived meaning of pain is a developmentally inflected process that influences suffering, so too is perceived coping capacity. Both of these appraisals will determine the individual's sense of control and of the controllability of pain. Pain that is appraised as trivial, as well justified in terms of some consequent benefit, as extremely time-limited, or as well within one's capacity to tolerate it, is not likely to upset one's sense of control. Coping maneuvers may be engaged to alter any of these or other dimensions of appraisal, so as to preserve a sufficient level of perceived control. Clearly, many of these maneuvers involve reframing (reinterpretation or reattribution) or other processes that might be referred to collectively as rationalization. It is in fact difficult for most adults to imagine enduring any substantially aversive experience without engaging in rationalization. Equally clearly, the sophistication of one's ability to rationalize normally increases as a function of cognitive developmental level.

Rothbaum et al., (1982) used the term *primary control coping* to refer to efforts to alter objective conditions (e.g., rest and relax a sore muscle, take aspirin for a headache), whereas their term *secondary control coping* refers more to rationalization (i.e., cognitive maneuvers to maintain the perception of control). Band and Weisz (1988) reported evidence that secondary control coping is more dependent on highly developed cognitive processes than is primary control coping, at least in medical situations. They administered structured interviews to 73 first-to-seventh graders regarding their coping responses to several stressful situations. Relative to peer, school, and loss-related stressors, medical situations elicited significantly fewer primary control coping responses, and in older children these diminished while secondary control coping responses to medical stressors became more prevalent. The authors suggest two developmentally mediated interpretations for their findings. First, secondary control coping develops later than primary control coping because it is more subtle and therefore less amenable to observational learning. Second, primary control coping is generally the preferred mode of coping and secondary control is attempted only when primary fails or is appraised as likely to fail. Young children, then, are more likely to respond to medical stressors with primary control coping efforts such as escape, protest, or behavioral disruption in order to prevent the painful procedure from being completed. With experience, children learn that opportunities for primary control are minimal in medical situations (in fact, this may be overlearned) and that secondary control coping is more efficacious. Similar findings were reported with diabetic children (Band, 1990).

This model is also consistent with earlier findings reported by Brown, O'Keefe, Sanders, and Baker (1986), who administered questionnaires to 487 normal 8- to 18-year-olds regarding their spontaneous coping and catastrophizing responses to three situations: dental treatment, delivering an oral report, and a personal stressor. Positive self-talk was the most common response reported for the dental situation, and its frequency increased with age. The most common catastrophizing response to dental work was cognitively focusing on pain and negative affect, which was consistent across the age range studied. The ratio of coping to catastrophizing was worst in the dental situation, among the three stressors, though this ratio improved with age. These results suggest that responses during dental treatment are more limited to the cognitive realm than with other stressors, and that children become more successful at coping in this manner over the course of their school and teenage years. Although the positive self-talk responses were not designated by the authors as secondary control coping, the examples provided ("It's not so bad," "I can take this," and "Be brave") (p. 351) all involve cognitive maneuvers to enhance perceptions of control. Curry and Russ (1985) also found age-related increases in cognitive coping (efforts to maintain control through reframing), based on their observation and interviews with 30 8- to 10-year-olds undergoing dental treatment.

Researchers looking at other stressors have found that emotion-focused coping is poor in young children and improves with age (Compas, Malcarne, & Fondacaro, 1988), whereas problem-focused coping is fairly stable across childhood. Since emotion-focused coping also generally requires more cognitive than behavioral responding relative to problem-focused coping, these findings further support the notion that sophisticated secondary control coping is dependent upon rather highly developed cognitive processes. More research is needed to delineate this relationship, but it might be expected that efficacious secondary control coping with pain would begin to emerge during the later school years (concrete operations), and become well established in the teen years (formal operations).

Psychosocial Development

Closely tied to cognitive development in childhood are changes in interactions with others, in particular increases in the complexity of social situational influences on behavior. Responses to pain have been shown to be sensitive to socializing influences and to developmentally mediated changes in the interactional contexts in which pain behaviors are emitted. As children develop, they expect to exercise more self-control, rather than relying so much on parenting agents (Burke, Solotar, Silverman, & Israel, 1987). These changes are supported by social norms that dictate that mature individuals attempt to inhibit the expression of pain (Beyer & Byers, 1985), though these norms vary considerably among cultures and subcultures (Reid & Bush, 1990). Age-related increases in self-control have also been observed during procedures such as bone marrow aspirations (LeBaron & Zeltzer, 1984).

Many of the developmental changes in psychosocial influences on pain and pain responding, however, are related to changes in attempts to enhance control through interactions with others. Craig and Grunau (chapter 7) explain that pain responses in the infant are normally affectively dominated, but that the socialization of these responses begins early in infancy. Adaptive responding to aversive conditions at this age largely depends on effective communication with caregivers. Ross and Ross (1984), based on interviews of 994 normal 5- to 12-year-old California schoolchildren, found that over 99% reported that the most helpful factor in coping with pain was the availability of their parents. Increases in self-control in the face of aversive conditions should be associated with an age-related decrease in the solicitousness of parental responding to child distress behaviors. A number of authors (Craig & Grunau, in chapter 7; McGrath, in chapter 4; Peterson et al., in chapter 2; Routh & Sanfilippo, in chapter 15; Siegel & Smith, in chapter 6) have noted that excessive attention to pain complaints is likely to reinforce pain behavior and may worsen the child's suffering and associated disability. The definition of "excessive attention" is of course profoundly inflected by developmental status, although changes may be more qualitative than quantitative. Research using the Child Illness Reinforcement Scales revealed no main effect for age in 147 second-to-twelfth graders (Walker & Zeman, 1989).

Age-related changes in the responses of parenting agents to children in pain has received insufficient research attention. Burke and her colleagues (Burke et al., 1987) were unable to detect age trends in parental expectations for child self-control, using a broad-spectrum questionnaire. Bush (Bush &

Cockrell, 1987; Bush, Melamed, Sheras, & Greenbaum, 1986), based upon observational coding of videotaped mother-child interactions in a pediatric outpatient clinic immediately prior to physician examination, found few differences in what mothers actually did with their children as a function of age. Instead, these studies revealed more age-related patterns in reciprocity and dyadic behavioral sequence, as opposed to simple behavioral frequencies. For example, rates of child information-seeking and maternal information-providing were fairly stable in children ranging from 5 to 10 years of age, but became more desynchronized (i.e., more likely to occur nonreciprocally) in the older-child dyads. That is, older children engaged in information-seeking that involved less of their mothers' participation than did younger children, and mothers of older children continued to provide similar levels of informational input to their older children, even when the older youngsters did not seek this information from them. These findings suggest that children may begin to cope at more mature levels prior to their parents' expectations that they do so, whereas parenting behaviors may fail to keep pace with the children's developing coping competencies. This is consistent with the finding of Dunn-Geier, McGrath, Rourke, Latter, and D'Astous (1986) that the mothers of adolescents who were not coping well with chronic intractable benign pain tended more frequently to discourage coping behaviors than did mothers of better-coping youngsters. Jay (1985) argued that parents can best encourage their children's coping with pain by positively reinforcing and providing responsive support for specific coping behaviors, inhibiting their own distress, and avoiding reinforcing child distress behaviors. These results (Bush & Cockrell, 1987) also indicated that parenting behaviors that were more responsive to the child's current behavior were more effective than more "noncontingent" parenting (as suggested by Jay, 1985), and that parents whose parenting behavior was more specific and contingent in a particular area, such as information provision, tended to display more effective parenting behaviors in other ways as well.

Dysfunctional family systems may also impair the development of adaptive self-control capabilities for coping with pain. Family interaction patterns that have been associated with inculcating excessive pain responses in children include the overly solicitous family (Walker & Zeman, 1989; Peterson et al., in chapter 2), families in which the child is exposed to an adult who models pathological pain behavior (Bush, 1987; Osborne, Hatcher, & Richtsmeier, 1989; Hodges & Burbach, in chapter 10; McGrath, in chapter 4; Peterson et al., in chapter 2), and families in which intractable problems are avoided by the child's symptom presentation (Bush, 1990; Hodges & Burbach, in chapter 10; Maron & Bush, in chapter 11; Peterson et al., in chapter 2), or in which a parent—particularly a depressed parent—is emotionally overinvolved (enmeshed) with the affected child (McGrath & Pisterman, in chapter 9).

Beliefs, Affects, and Attitudes

A fundamental principle of cognitive psychology, based on attribution theory, is that individuals' explanations for their own behavior and the behavior of others has a causal influence on their future behavior and on affective and coping responses (Baucom, 1987; Perlman & Peplau, 1981). Attitudes may be defined as more-or-less durable sets of beliefs that usually encompass multiple attributions, associated with characteristic affective and coping sets, and that are focused on classes of behaviors, individuals, or other stimuli. These constructs are widely employed in the psychological literature on children in pain. Little is known, however, about the development and modifiability of children's beliefs and attitudes as related to their coping with pain (McGrath & Pisterman, in chapter 9).

Bush and Holmbeck (1987) reported the development of the Children's Health Care Attitudes Questionnaire (CHCAQ), an analogue-assisted measure of attitudes toward health care providers, settings, and procedures, which is suitable for children as young as 5 years. Three dimensions of attitudes (preference for approach-avoidance, expected effectiveness-ineffectiveness of health care, and like-dislike) were identified by factor analysis, consistent with Gochman and Saucier's (1982) finding that children's perceived susceptibility to illness is general across types of health problems. At least until adolescence, attributed ineffectiveness scores were positively correlated with age. This increase in skepticism about medical care may be due to the cognitive developmental trend toward abandoning magical thinking, i.e., the curative "ritual power" of physician role behaviors (Haight et al., 1985), which is only gradually replaced by understanding of the purposes of these behaviors. More avoidant attitudes were associated with higher painfulness ratings of a variety of medical procedures. Although results were inconclusive as to causality in this relationship (though bidirectional causality seems highly plausible), these findings suggest that painful medical experiences may exacerbate avoidant attitudes and possibly behavioral avoidance of health care. Avoidant attitudes were also associated with dislike for medical personnel, procedures, and settings, suggesting that physician-child relationship enhancement may also help to reduce avoidance of health care. Jay (1985) suggested that this relationship may be mediated by child anxiety, which she sees as inversely associated with the child's level of trust in the clinician.

Children learn sick-role behavior (Walker & Zeman, 1989; Peterson et al., in chapter 2), many pain behaviors, and norms for social interactions in medical settings. It seems likely that adverse emotional responses to pain are in large part innate, since it is vital to the survival of the infant that distress be effectively communicated to others as protection from possible tissue damage (Owens, 1984). Interactions with medical professionals constitute recurring instances in which both of these learning processes occur; innate responses are conditioned and role behaviors are socialized. Little is known about the influence of physician and parent behaviors in these contexts on this ongoing learning, though some research has investigated more immediate effects of these behaviors (Bush et al., 1986; Melamed & Bush, 1985; Weinstein, Getz, Ratener, & Domoto, 1982).

Sentence completion protocols collected from 680 Irish 5- to 14-year-olds by Gaffney and Dunne (1986) indicate that older children are more likely than younger ones to recognize "positive" aspects of pain and to incorporate a psychological component in their concepts of pain. Supported by learning and cognitive development, these changes enable the older child to accept painful procedures with less disequilibrium and to recognize the role of positive attitudes, accurate understanding, and affective state in pain tolerance. It could be the case that these cognitive/attitudinal changes, lying entirely within the domain of cognitive coping maneuvers supporting the perception of pain as "acceptable" or "controllable," accompany the development of the capacity to discriminate pain intensity from suffering. As Band and Weisz (1988) reported, children appear to engage in more secondary control coping in medical situations as a function of age; perhaps they not only develop the cognitive ability to do so but also learn that painful medical procedures are relatively unamenable to primary control efforts and that they are in fact able to control or change their feelings without being in control over the external situation (Peterson et al., in chapter 2).

Current Trends in Pediatric Pain

Problems and Progress

Analgesic and Anesthetic Medication

Evidence has begun to accumulate documenting past and current inadequacies in the clinical management of children's pain. Much inadequacy is attributable to the withholding of available analgesic and anesthetic agents (Bush, 1987; Craig et al., 1987; Eland & Anderson, 1977; Elliott & Jay, 1987; Sukhani, 1989; McGrath, in chapter 4), to the unfamiliarity of health care personnel with nonpharmacological techniques, and to our lesser understanding of pain in children than in adults (McGrath, 1987a). Many of these inadequacies have been addressed and to some extent ameliorated in recent years, but it is important to recognize and challenge the outdated beliefs and misperceptions that appear to have supported poor practice.

Contrary to beliefs prevalent in the past, evidence is conclusive that nociception occurs in the neonate (Craig & Grunau, in chapter 7). The necessary anatomical structures and functional capacities are present (Truog & Anand, 1989), and neurochemical responses occur to normally pain-inducing stimuli that are attenuated by anesthesia (Anand & Hickey, 1987; Fletcher, 1987). Early studies that had supported these former beliefs and more valid recent work documenting neonatal nociception are summarized elsewhere (Craig & Grunau, in chapter 7; Routh & Sanfilippo, in chapter 15). Furthermore, persistent behavioral responses to pain are also evident in the neonate, implying some memory of pain—also inconsistent with common past beliefs.

Nevertheless, practices based upon these now-discredited assumptions continue (American Academy of Pediatrics, 1987). For example, it is now less frequent but still not unusual for neonates to undergo protracted surgical procedures with no anesthesia whatsoever, though curare is typically administered to induce paralysis (Shearer, 1986). This practice has been condemned by pediatricians and anesthesiologists (American Academy of Pediatrics, 1987), who argue that safe anesthesia and analgesia are now possible in neonates (Purcell-Jones, Dormon, & Sumner, 1988; Sukhani, 1989), and that adequate interoperative pain relief should be provided to neonates according to the usual prudent criteria applied to adults. This is justified both on humanitarian grounds and for more thoroughly suppressing the stress response to surgery (Sukhani, 1989). Anesthesia should not be withheld solely on the basis of age or level of cortical development (American Academy of Pediatrics, 1987).

A recent survey of 362 neonatologists suggests that understanding of the importance of these changes is spreading, with 87% of respondents reporting recent changes in their pain management practices—almost all reported that they do use anesthesia during surgery with infants—and 100% averring that infants do feel pain (McLaughlin, Hull, & Cramer, 1991). Considerable variability was still present, however, in administration of postoperative analgesics. Respondents using fewer postoperative analgesics reported higher estimates of drug risks in this population and were more likely to rate neonates as feeling less pain than adults, relative to those who reported using more analgesics. These findings indicate the need for further exploration of the factors influencing decision-making in physicians and nurses responsible for patient pain management, and for providing accurate information regarding analgesic risks and pain responses in juvenile populations.

Difficulties in measuring pain in children lead health professionals to rely on personal beliefs regarding pain in children (Beyer & Byers, 1985), and on personal attitudes and misinformation regarding narcotics (Craig et al., 1987; Ross, Bush, & Crummette, 1991; Sukhani, 1989). The p.r.n. (as necessary) prescription of analgesics for postoperative pain management, still standard practice in most American hospitals, has been criticized as virtually guaranteeing very low drug delivery to child patients (Bush, Holmbeck, & Cockrell, 1989; Eland & Anderson, 1977; Gadish, Gonzalez & Hayes, 1988; Morrison & Vedro, 1989; McGrath, in chapter 4). Nurses systematically underestimate children's pain (Craig et al., 1987), overestimate the risks associated with narcotic analgesics (Eland & Anderson, 1977; Morrison & Vedro, 1989; Ross et al., 1991), and see pediatric pain management as a low-priority job responsibility for which they are inadequately trained (McCaffery, 1977).

A promising alternative to p.r.n. analgesia for children is patient-controlled analgesia (PCA). This technique employs a push-button device by means of which the patient self-administers a bolus of analgesic medication (typically morphine or another narcotic) through an infusion pump connected to an intravenous line (Graves, Foster, Batenhorst, Bennett, & Baumann, 1983). The dose and "lockout interval" between doses are determined by the physician and cannot be overridden by the patient. Bolus administration may be superimposed on continuous narcotic infusion, and PCA may be begun with a larger initiating bolus dose (McCaffery, 1977).

Evaluation of the efficacy of pain management achieved with children using PCA has been uniformly positive (Graves et al., 1983). Adequate to superior pain management (relative to traditional methods) was reported using PCA in ten 11- to 19-year-olds following nonemergency surgical procedures (Brown & Broadman, 1987), and in twenty 10- to 19-year-old girls following spinal surgery (Rauen & Ho, 1989). Positive results have also been found with younger children. Dodd, Wang, and Rauck (1988) reported that all eight of their 6- to 16-year-olds using PCA following abdominal or thoracic surgery enjoyed very good pain control. Similar results were reported by Means, Allen, Lookabill, and Krishna (1988) in 18 orthopedic surgery patients as young as 5 years old. Nevertheless, questions remain regarding the minimum age at which children generally become cognitively capable of learning to use the PCA pump appropriately (Gedaly-Duff, in chapter 8).

P.r.n.-administered intramuscular injections of narcotic analgesics have been found to be associated with a 5- to 6-hour pain cycle (Ferrante, Orav, Rocco, & Gallo, 1988), in which (a) the patient experiences increasing pain to a threshold at which a request is made to the nurse for an analgesic; (b) the nurse responds to the call and screens the patient's need for analgesic medication; (c) the nurse obtains and administers a bolus dose of the analgesic; (d) the patient experiences pain relief; (e) the patient becomes sedated; (f) the sedation wears off and the patient continues to enjoy pain relief; and (g) the patient's pain again increases, reinitiating the cycle. This cycle is not observed using PCA, in which much more frequent, smaller doses are self-administered by the patient when in his/her judgment they are needed, resulting in a significantly more stable level of medication in the bloodstream, a more consistent level of analgesia, and less sedation (Kane, Lehman, Dugger, Hansen, & Jackson, 1988).

PCA has also been shown to have rates of complications and negative side effects as low or lower than more traditional approaches (Brown & Broadman, 1987; Dodd et al., 1988; Rauen & Ho, 1989; Rodgers, Webb, Stergios, & Newman, 1988; McGrath, in chapter 4). Total amounts of narcotics used tend to be less than or similar to traditional methods, with PCA patients initially giving themselves more but then tapering off dose frequency (Rauen

& Ho, 1989; Rodgers et al., 1988; McGrath, in chapter 4). Respiratory depression and excessive sedation, in particular, appear to be more adequately prevented; first, through judicious selection of dosage level and lockout interval and, second, because of the hierarchical nature of narcotic effects (Graves et al., 1983). Analgesia occurs at lower plasma concentrations than does sedation, which in turn occurs at lower levels than respiratory depression. Since patients on PCA receive smaller and more constant dosages, their plasma concentrations are more likely to be concentrated above the level of analgesia and below the level of significant sedation. The patient would have to pass through the level of sedation, during which he/she is unlikely to press the PCA control button, prior to approaching levels usually associated with respiratory depression. Adults have been found to self-administer analgesics to a level of moderate pain relief rather than complete pain cessation, in order to maintain a clear sensorium (Graves et al., 1983). Supportive findings with children were reported by Rauen and Ho (1989) and by Rodgers et al. (1988), who found no evidence of excessive sedation in their PCA study samples.

Evidence has also indicated consistent preferences for PCA over p.r.n.-administered analgesic injections, among patients, parents, nurses, and physicians (Brown & Broadman, 1987; Dodd et al. 1988; Graves et al., 1983; Means et al., 1988; Rauen & Ho, 1989; Rodgers et al., 1988; McGrath, in chapter 4). Reasons for this preference include avoiding injections, decreased demand on nurse time for narcotic administration and documentation (Brown & Broadman, 1987), and enhanced patient control over analgesia and level of sedation.

More accurate and individualized titration of dosing with PCA, along with its elimination of the "pain cycle," may also be associated with enhanced postoperative recovery (Graves et al., 1983; Kleiman, Lipman, Hare, & MacDonald, 1987). Dodd et al. (1988), for example, reported accelerated return to normal activity levels in their eight PCA subjects. These findings, however, are largely anecdotal and require further investigation.

It is also theoretically reasonable to expect that PCA would be associated with enhanced learning and long-range psychological benefits relative to traditional approaches. If in fact PCA produces a greater perception of self-control over pain, as reported anecdotally by several investigators (Brown & Broadman, 1987; Rauen & Ho, 1989), then these patients should experience hospitalization as less traumatizing and aversive than patients who feel less in control. Greater freedom from the "pain cycle," from excessive sedation, and from intramuscular injections would all seem likely to contribute further to a more benign postsurgical experience in children. This, in turn, should be associated with lower levels of medical fears, less avoidant behavioral tendencies relative to medical care, more positive attitudes toward health care providers, and more positive control expectations in subsequent painful situations. These questions have not been addressed in research to-date on pediatric PCA.

Pain Assessment

Pain assessment has been hampered in the past by a number of difficulties. These have included vague or inconsistent definitions of pain and failure to make assumptions explicit, as well as difficulties in dealing with the subjective nature of pain phenomena (McGrath, Cunningham, Goodman, & Unruh, 1986; Karoly, in chapter 3). The field has been advanced by such refinements as separating perceived pain intensity from suffering, and focusing as specifically as possible on more particular constructs such as pain sensation, pain behavior, and pain complaints.

One particularly problematic assumption for pain measurement has been the dichotomizing of psychogenic and somatogenic pain. A request to provide differential diagnosis of psychogenic pain or of the psychogenic component in a patient's pain complaints often underlies referrals to consult/ liaison psychologists and psychiatrists. The oversimplification inherent in these referrals is compounded by the common practice of diagnosing pain as psychogenic based upon failure to detect an adequate somatogenic etiology (Bush, 1987; Elliott & Jay, 1987). This is often done, for example, in children with recurrent abdominal pain (Friedman, 1972), in which case the differential contribution of somatic and psychological factors is far from clear (Hodges & Burbach, in chapter 10). Such labeling may affect profoundly the treatment subsequently offered to the patient (McGrath, 1987a; Tarnowski, Gavaghan, & Wisniewski, 1989).

Specialized training and developmentally sensitive measurement techniques are needed to assess pain in children, and especially in infants (Truog & Anand, 1989; Craig & Grunau, in chapter 7). The best existing measures appear to be generally appropriate for acute but not for chronic pediatric pain (Craig et al., 1987), in which it is more likely to be needed. Most of these measures focus on the quality of the child's response to pain onset, and deal little if at all with tonic pain and with the coping responses (Craig & Grunau, in chapter 7). In the absence of well-accepted approaches to the measurement of chronic and intermittent pediatric pain, clinicians necessarily rely upon intuition and judgment (Beyer & Byers, 1985). Data have already been summarized documenting the apparent inadequacies that result from the contamination of these judgments by conflicting motives and misinformation, too often with unfortunate outcomes (McGrath et al., 1986; Shearer, 1986).

Progress has been made in the assessment of pain intensity in children by the introduction and psychometric validation of analogue scales, which at least in part circumvent younger children's verbal limitations (Beyer & Aradine, 1987; Bush, 1990; Ross & Ross, 1988; Wong & Baker, 1988; Karoly, in chapter 3). The Faces scale, for example, has been shown to have adequate test-retest reliability and interval scale measurement properties in children as young as first grade (Bieri, Reeve, Champion, Addicoat, & Ziegler, 1990). Likewise, the visual analogue scale has proven useful with children as young as 4 to 7 years or older (McGrath, 1987a; McGrath et al., 1986). Even with preschoolers, Belter and his colleagues have shown that a variety of analogue measures are valid and reliable at least for the gross differentiation of general pain intensity levels such as "none," "little," "severe" (Belter, McIntosh, Finch, & Saylor, 1988). On the other hand, word checklists have been shown to be useful in assessing pain in children approximately 8 years old or older (Gillman & Bush, 1991; Wilkie et al., 1990). Projective techniques, although they may be used to facilitate communication, have not been demonstrated to have sound psychometric properties in the assessment of pain in children (McGrath et al., 1986; Karoly, in chapter 3).

Interview and observational approaches have also begun to emerge that measure how children cope with chronic pain as well as with painful medical procedures (Bush, 1987; Curry & Russ, 1985; Jay et al., 1986; Karoly, in chapter 3; Manne & Andersen, in chapter 13; Siegel & Smith, in chapter 6). These methods are extremely sensitive to children's developmental status and are therefore both more difficult and more powerful than other less specific approaches. Modes of nonverbal pain expression, readily amenable to objective observation, are increasingly susceptible to amplification or inhibition and to extranociceptive influences with increasing age (Craig & Prkachin, 1983; Elliott & Jay, 1987; LeBaron & Zeltzer, 1984). Some of these influences, such as hospitalization and separation, physical stigmata and limitations on mobility, may in turn have different distress-producing potentials as a function of child developmental status (Beyer & Byers, 1985; Maron & Bush, in chapter 11). More research is needed on developmental changes in interview and observational pain protocols (McGrath et al., 1986). Models and instruments that comprehend the multivariate nature of pain phenomena are also being developed for use with children (Karoly, in chapter 3; McGrath & Pisterman, in chapter 9; Walco & Varni, in chapter 12).

Conclusions, Recommendations and Future Directions

Analgesic Drugs

The well-documented inadequacies in pediatric pain management attributable to suboptimal utilization of analgesic drugs clearly suggests an agenda for developing and evaluating new policies and delivery systems in this area. More intensive and up-to-date training of nurses and physicians in pediatric pain and in the pharmacological properties of narcotics is certainly needed (Anand & Hickey, 1988; Bush, Holmbeck, & Cockrell, 1989; Ross et al., 1991). Alternatives to p.r.n. prescription, such as PCA, should be evaluated extensively with pediatric populations. More research is also needed in the application of underutilized anesthetic techniques with children, such as regional anesthesia (Purcell-Jones et al., 1988; Sukhani, 1989; Truog &

Anand, 1989; McGrath, in chapter 4). Caudal and penile nerve blocks, for example, have been found to be safe and effective in small-scale clinical investigations with children undergoing genital surgery and circumcision (Dixon, Snyder, Holve, & Bromberger, 1984; Jensen, 1981; Lunn, 1979).

Given children's well-documented fear of injections (Cuthbert & Melamed, 1982; Rape, Bush, & Saravia, 1988; McGrath, in chapter 4), alternatives to injection as a method of analgesic delivery need to be thoroughly evaluated. Oral administration or utilization of indwelling intravenous lines should be preferred over giving the child another shot. For cases in which injection is indicated, promising modified procedures such as the needleless syringe (Saravia & Bush, 1991) or preparation of the injection site with topical lignocaine cream (Manne & Andersen, in chapter 13) or with a cooling agent (Eland, 1981) merit further investigation.

Some fundamental issues need to be considered with respect to the ethical or values dilemma associated by many with administering narcotics to children. The imperative of protecting children from unnecessary suffering weighs against the perception of narcotics as evil. It is clear that the values and beliefs of health professionals as well as of patients and their parents determine narcotic administration practices, along with clinical management considerations. Value-laden concerns about narcotics include risks of addiction and of predisposing patients to drug abuse. For example, it may be that administration of analgesics denies the patient an opportunity to learn to cope with pain without drugs. Dworkin (1986) advanced a parallel argument regarding the use of drugs for behavior management of children in dental situations, expressing concern that this might reinforce learning that drugs represent a preferred means of coping with any dysphoric experience.

On the other hand, the right of individuals to relief and protection from unnecessary pain and suffering is fundamental and in fact is arguably the primary justification for the existence of the medical professions. The fact that narcotics and certain other drugs are often abused does not diminish their value when used appropriately. This suggests that optimal learning implies not maximum avoidance of drug use, but rather the appropriate use of this powerful but dangerous tool. Research is needed on the physiological and cognitive processes involved in the development of opiate dependence in infants and children (McLaughlin et al., 1991), and in the modifiability of these processes through presentation of narcotics in concert with cognitive-behavioral interventions (Dworkin, 1986). As Craig and Grunau (chapter 7) explain, it may well be the case that a greater disposition to develop narcotic craving and eventual abuse is induced by undermanagement of patients' pain (leaving them suffering and anticipating the next dose as the only foreseen relief) than by provision of sufficient analgesic medication to maintain comfort. Adequate pain management has been associated by many authors as well with better patient compliance and less emotional trauma (Eland & Anderson, 1977; Maron & Bush, in chapter 11).

Specialized Training

In addition to more and better training in the use of pharmacological pain management methods with children, health professionals working with children in pain should learn an integrated, multiple-intervention approach that comprehends pain in its psychosocial as well as its physiological contexts. More basically, training should emphasize the need for a more empirical orientation according to which pain management interventions are more individualized, drawing on assessment data encompassing physiological, psychosocial, and developmental processes (Compas et al., 1988; Karoly, in chapter 3). Research amply supports the commonsense notion that different individuals have different coping strengths and styles, and it is more and more clear that interventions to enhance adjustment to highly aversive experiences such as pain should, whenever practicable, capitalize on these preferences (Manne & Andersen, in chapter 13; Maron & Bush, in chapter 11; Siegel & Smith, in chapter 6; Vieyra et al., in chapter 14).

Research in pediatric pain can contribute to this broader, more contextualized approach, by efforts to bridge the gap between laboratory and clinical investigative efforts. Following basic research into nociceptive processes, investigators should consider subjective pain phenomena and functional changes. Both paradigmatic (Karoly, in chapter 3) and empirically driven (Walco & Varni, in chapter 12) research efforts are needed (Peterson et al., in chapter 2). Considerable sophistication is needed in defining appropriate dependent variables for clinically applicable, scientifically interesting studies. For example, modulation of perceived pain intensity is an extremely limited construct for conceptualizing the efficacy of pain management interventions. Particularly in cases of chronic pain, other aspects of a desirable outcome include quality of life, functional status, developmental inflection, sense of control and of subjective well-being, and coping with subsequent painful events. The appropriate goal in many clinical situations may not be pain elimination, but rather an individualized definition of optimal management (Elliott & Jay, 1987). On the other hand, researchers must be careful to guard against uncontrolled inflation of experiment-wise false-positive error rate when employing large numbers of dependent variables (Jay et al., 1986; Peterson et al., in chapter 2).

Training should also de-emphasize interprofessional sectarian rivalries. Both clinical and research efforts, as well as the fundamental conceptualizing of problems in pediatric pain, must draw on multidisciplinary perspectives. Integrated intervention approaches are chronically underutilized and underinvestigated. There is, for example, a need for basic and applied research into synergistic interactions between pharmacological and behavioral pain management interventions, and comparing the relative efficacy of these interventions separately with well-defined clinical populations (Dworkin, 1986; Jay, Elliott, Katz, & Siegel, 1987).

These considerations suggest the potential value of establishing multidisciplinary pediatric pain clinics, especially in university medical centers, both to facilitate research of this nature and to coordinate the efforts of various disciplines (Anand & Hickey, 1988; Owens, 1984). Such centers would be well equipped to integrate new research information across disciplinary boundaries and to coordinate the specialized training needed to provide optimal care to children in pain (Craig et al., 1987). In addition to its research and training missions, the multidisciplinary pediatric pain clinic would function as an integrated center for the provision of collaborative team consultation services for children in pain (Gillman & Mullins, in chapter 5).

The Developmental Significance of Childhood Pain Experiences

Surprisingly little is known about the long-range impact on children of their early pain experiences, despite the prominent role suggested by learning theory formulations. Longitudinal research is needed to examine the effects of pain experiences in infancy and early childhood on coping responses to subsequent painful events and on attitudes and beliefs related to medical contacts. Such research is important not only so that the effects of painful medical procedures and conditions on children can be better understood, but also for its contribution to our basic understanding of how humans may learn to "feel" pain (Merskey, 1970). Some evidence has been reported that indicates that repeated pain experiences may sensitize children, lowering their threshold for future pain events (Walco & Varni, in chapter 12), predisposing them to make more catastrophizing cognitive attributions regarding pain (Eland & Anderson, 1977), or conditioning them to associate pain with certain varieties of interpersonal contact (Langland & Langland, 1988). Research has also indicated that children with recurrent abdominal pain are more likely than other children to suffer from chronic pain later in their lives, including nonabdominal pain (Hodges & Burbach, in chapter 10). A number of causal mechanisms may be hypothesized to underlie this relationship, though none have been proven, including overlearning of the pain role and pain responses as a means of coping with stress, reinforcement of pain behaviors, an underlying "pain prone" personality trait, and maintenance of pain behaviors by family system characteristics (Walker & Zeman, 1989; Peterson et al., in chapter 2).

There is also evidence that painful experiences are associated with short-term behavioral disruption in infants and children (American Academy of Pediatrics, 1987; Anand & Hickey, 1987; Craig & Grunau, in chapter 7). Since significant pain usually occurs in context with other stressors (e.g., hospitalization, serious illness, traumatic injury, etc.), it is indeed difficult to separate the unique contribution of pain to neurotic personality development or to other dysfunctional learning, or to the development of coping competencies and general "toughness" (Beyer & Byers, 1985; Maron &

Bush, in chapter 11). Evidence indicates that health beliefs, attitudes, and behavior patterns established in childhood are likely to persist (Maddux et al., 1986), as are conditioned fears such as fear of dental treatment (Routh & Sanfilippo, in chapter 15).

Also largely unexplored is the influence of treatment variables on the long-term psychosocial impact of childhood pain experiences. Some evidence does suggest that better management of painful experiences in childhood may be associated with better pain tolerance in adulthood (Beyer & Byers, 1985; Bush, 1990; McGuire & Dizard, 1982), but this is highly inferential. There is more evidence to support the notion that children's manner and degree of success in coping with painful experiences, which may of course be influenced by treatment variables, in turn influences their future coping with other painful experiences. Learning processes affect assessment both of the controllability of the painful event and of one's capacities for coping with it. Thus, successful early experiences in coping with pain may help to enhance future coping with related experiences (Curry & Russ, 1985). On the other hand, such generalization does not appear to occur automatically, at least in cases of intervention-assisted coping. Jay et al. (1987) reported substantial reductions in pain and distress following training cognitive-behavioral coping skills to leukemic children undergoing bone marrow aspirations, but were unable to find any evidence to support generalization of these skills to other procedures.

Siegel and Smith (chapter 6) argue that generalization of coping skills, and in fact the difference between a painful experience ultimately having positive or negative effects on the child's future coping, may be mediated by the child's development of self-efficacy. That is, children may learn that they are capable of performing certain coping responses, and furthermore that the performance of these responses renders the pain experience more controllable.

References

American Academy of Pediatrics (1987). Neonatal anesthesia. *Pediatrics, 80*(3), 446.

Anand, K. S., & Hickey, P. R. (1987). Pain and its effects in the human neonate and fetus. *New England Journal of Medicine, 317*(21), 1321–1329.

Anand, K. S., & Hickey, P. R. (1988). Pain in the neonate and fetus. *New England Journal of Medicine, 318*(21), 1399.

Apley, J. (1976). Pain in childhood. *Journal of Psychosomatic Research, 20,* 383–389.

Band, E. B. (1990). Children's coping with diabetes: Understanding the role of cognitive development. *Journal of Pediatric Psychology, 15*(1), 27–41.

Band, E. B., & Weisz, J. R. (1988). How to feel better when it feels bad: Children's perspectives on coping. *Developmental Psychology, 24,* 247–253.

Baucom, D. H. (1987). Attributions in distressed relations. In D. Perlman & S. Duck (Eds.), *Intimate relationships: Development, dynamics, and deterioration* (pp. 177–206). Beverly Hills: Sage.

Belter, R. W., McIntosh, J. A., Finch, A. J. Jr., & Saylor, C. F. (1988). Preschoolers' ability to differentiate levels of pain: Relative efficacy of three self-report measures. *Journal of Clinical Child Psychology, 17*(4), 329–335.

Beyer, J. E., & Aradine, C. R. (1987). Patterns of pediatric pain intensity: A methodological investigation of a self-report scale. *Clinical Journal of Pain, 3*, 130–141.

Beyer, J. E., & Byers, M. L. (1985). Knowledge of pediatric pain: The state of the art. *Children's Health Care, 13*(4), 150–159.

Bibace, R., & Walsh, M. (1980). Development of children's concepts of illness. *Pediatrics, 66*, 912–917.

Bieri, D., Reeve, R. A., Champion, G. D., Addicoat, L., & Ziegler, J. B. (1990). The Faces Pain Scale for the self-assessment of pain experienced by children: Development, validation, and preliminary investigation for ratio scale properties. *Pain, 41*, 139–150.

Brown, J. M., O'Keefe, J., Sanders, S. H., & Baker, B. (1986). Developmental changes in children's cognition to stressful and painful situations. *Journal of Pediatric Psychology, 11*(3), 343–358.

Brown, R. E. Jr., & Broadman, L. M. (1987). Patient controlled analgesia for postoperative pain in adolescents. *Anesthesia and Analgesia, 66*, S22.

Burke, A. E., Solotar, L. C., Silverman, W. K., & Israel, A. C. (1987). Assessing children's and adults' expectations for child self-control. *Journal of Clinical Child Psychology, 16*(1), 37–42.

Bush, J. P. (1987). Pain in children: A review of the literature from a developmental perspective. *Psychology and Health, 1*, 215–236.

Bush, J. P. (1990). Understanding pediatric pain: A developmental perspective. In T. W. Miller (Ed.), *Chronic pain: Vol. 2* (pp. 1121–1167). Madison, CT: International Universities Press.

Bush, J. P., & Cockrell, C. S. (1987). Maternal factors predicting parenting behaviors in the pediatric clinic. *Journal of Pediatric Psychology, 12*(4), 505–518.

Bush, J. P., & Holmbeck, G. N. (1987). Children's attitudes about health care: Initial development of a questionnaire. *Journal of Pediatric Psychology, 12*(3), 429–443.

Bush, J. P., Holmbeck, G. N., & Cockrell, J. L. (1989). Patterns of PRN analgesic drug administration in children following elective surgery. *Journal of Pediatric Psychology, 14*(3), 433–448.

Bush, J. P., Melamed, B. G., Sheras, P. L., & Greenbaum, P. E. (1986). Mother-child patterns of coping with anticipatory medical stress. *Health Psychology, 5*(2), 137–157.

Compas, B. E., Malcarne, V. L., & Fondacaro, K. M. (1988). Coping with stressful events in older children and young adolescents. *Journal of Consulting and Clinical Psychology, 56*(3), 405–411.

Craig, K. D., & Best, J. A. (1977). Perceived control over pain: Individual differences and situational determinants. *Pain, 3*, 127–135.

Craig, K. D., Grunau, R. V. E., & Branson, S. M. (1987, August). *Age-related aspects of pain: Pain in children*. Fifth World Congress on Pain, Hamburg, Federal Republic of Germany.

Craig, K. D., & Prkachin, K. M. (1983). Nonverbal measures of pain. In R. Melzack (Ed.), *Pain measurement and assessment* (pp. 173–179). New York: Raven.

Curry, S. L., & Russ, S. W. (1985). Identifying coping strategies in children. *Journal of Clinical Child Psychology, 14*(1), 61–69.

Cuthbert, M. I., & Melamed, B. G. (1982). A screening device: Children at risk for dental fears and management problems. *ASDC Journal of Dentistry for Children*, *40*, 277–284.

Dixon, S., Snyder, J., Holve, R., & Bromberger, P. (1984). Behavioral effects of circumcision with and without anesthesia. *Journal of Developmental and Behavioral Pediatrics*, *5*, 246–250.

Dodd, E., Wang, J. M., & Rauck, R. L. (1988). Patient controlled analgesia for post-surgical pediatric patients ages six-sixteen years. *Anesthesiology*, *69*(3A), A372.

Dunn-Geier, B. J., McGrath, P. J., Rourke, B. P., Latter, J., & D'Astous, J. (1986). Adolescent chronic pain: The ability to cope. *Pain*, *26*, 23–32.

Dworkin, S. F. (1986). Integrating behavioral and pharmacological therapeutic modalities. *Anesthesia Progress*, *33*(1), 29–33.

Eland, J. M. (1981). Minimizing pain associated with prekindergarten intermuscular injections. *Issues in Comprehensive Pediatric Nursing*, *5*, 361–372.

Eland, J. M., & Anderson, J. E. (1977). The experience of pain in children. In A. Jacox (Ed.), *Pain: A sourcebook for nurses and other health professionals* (pp. 453–473). Boston: Little, Brown.

Elliott, C. H., & Jay, S. M. (1987). Chronic pain in children. *Behaviour Research and Therapy*, *25*(4), 263–271.

Ferrante, F. M., Orav, E. J., Rocco, A. C., & Gallo, J. (1988). A statistical model for pain in patient controlled analgesia and conventional intramuscular opioid regimens. *Anesthesia and Analgesia*, *67*, 457–461.

Fletcher, A. B. (1987). Pain in the neonate. *New England Journal of Medicine*, *317*(21), 1347–1348.

Friedman, R. (1972). Some characteristics of children with "psychogenic" pain. *Clinical Pediatrics*, *11*(6), 331–333.

Gadish, H. S., Gonzalez, J. L., & Hayes, J. S. (1988). Factors affecting nurses' decisions to administer pediatric pain medication postoperatively. *Journal of Pediatric Nursing*, *3*(6), 383–389.

Gaffney, A., & Dunne, E. A. (1986). Developmental aspects of children's definitions of pain. *Pain*, *26*, 105–117.

Gillman, J. B., & Bush, J. P. (1991). Is there a general factor in children's pain responses? A multivariate study of three types of pain in children. *The Society of Behavioral Medicine Proceedings*, 124.

Gochman, D. S., & Saucier, J-F. (1982). Perceived vulnerability in children and adolescents. *Health Education Quarterly*, *9*, 46–59.

Graves, D. A., Foster, T. S., Batenhorst, R. L., Bennett, R. L., & Baumann, T. J. (1983). Patient controlled analgesia. *Annals of Internal Medicine*, *99*, 360–366.

Grunau, R. V. E., & Craig, K. D. (1987). Pain expression in neonates: Facial action and cry. *Pain*, *28*, 395–410.

Haight, W. L., Black, J. E., & DiMatteo, M. R. (1985). Young children's understanding of the social roles of physician and patient. *Journal of Pediatric Psychology*, *10*(1), 31–43.

Harbeck, C., & Peterson, L. (in review). Children's understanding of specific pains. In J. H. Johnson & S. B. Johnson (Eds.), *Advances in child health psychology: Proceedings of the Florida Conference*. Gainesville, FL: University of Florida Press.

Harkins, S. W., Price, D. D., & Martelli, M. (1986). Effects of age on pain perception: Thermonociception. *Journal of Gerontology, 41*, 58–63.

Jay, S. M. (1985). Pain in children: An overview of psychological assessment and intervention. In A. R. Zeiner, D. Bendell, & C. E. Walker (Eds.), *Health psychology: Treatment and research issues* (pp. 167–196). New York: Plenum.

Jay, S. M., Elliott, C. H., Katz, E. R., & Siegel, S. E. (1987). Cognitive behavioral and pharmacological interventions for children's distress during painful medical procedures. *Journal of Consulting and Clinical Psychology, 55*(6), 860–865.

Jay, S. M., Elliott, C. H., & Varni, J. W. (1986). Acute and chronic pain in adults and children with cancer. *Journal of Consulting and Clinical Psychology, 54*(5), 601–607.

Jensen, B. (1981). Caudal block for postoperative pain relief in children after genital operations: A comparison of bupivicaine and morphine. *Acta Anaesthesiologica Scandinavica, 25*, 373–375.

Kane, N. E., Lehman, M. E., Dugger, R., Hansen, L., & Jackson, D. (1988). Use of patient controlled analgesia in surgical oncology patients. *Oncology Nursing Forum, 15*(1), 29–32.

Kavanaugh, C. (1983). Psychological intervention with the severely burned child: Report of an experimental comparison of two approaches and their effects on psychosocial sequelae. *Journal of Child Psychiatry, 22*, 145–156.

Kleiman, R. L., Lipman, A. G., Hare, B. D., & MacDonald, S. D. (1987). Patient controlled analgesia versus regular intramuscular injections for severe postoperative pain. *American Journal of Nursing*, 1491–1492.

Langland, J. T., & Langland, P. I. (1988). Pain in the neonate and fetus. *New England Journal of Medicine, 318*(21), 1398.

Lazarus, R. (1977). Cognitive and coping processes in emotion. In A. Monat & R. Lazarus (Eds.), *Stress and coping: An anthology* (pp. 145–158). New York: Columbia University Press.

LeBaron, S., & Zeltzer, L. (1984). Assessment of acute pain and anxiety in children and adolescents by self reports, observer reports, and a behavior checklist. *Journal of Consulting and Clinical Psychology, 52*(5), 729–738.

Lunn, J. (1979). Postoperative analgesia after circumcision. *Anesthesia, 34*, 525–555.

Maddux, J. E., Roberts, M. C., Sledden, E. A., & Wright, L. (1986). Developmental issues in child health psychology. *American Psychologist, 41*(1), 25–34.

McCaffery, M. (1977). Pain relief for the child. *Pediatric Nursing, 3*(4), 11–16.

McGrath, P. A. (1987a). The multidimensional assessment and management of recurrent pain syndromes in children. *Behaviour Research and Therapy, 25*(4), 251–262.

McGrath, P. A. (1987b). An assessment of children's pain: A review of behavioral, physiological and direct scaling techniques. *Pain, 31*, 147–176.

McGrath, P. J., Cunningham, S. J., Goodman, J. T., & Unruh, A. (1986). The clinical management of pain in children: A review. *Clinical Journal of Pain, 1*(4), 221–227.

McGuire, L., & Dizard, S. (1982). Managing pain in the young patient. *Nursing, 12*, 54–55.

McLaughlin, C. R., Hull, J. G., & Cramer, C. P. (1991). New trends in infant pain management: Potential for opiate dependence. *NIDA Research Monograph Series: Problems of drug dependence, 1990* (pp. 537–538).

Means, L. J., Allen, H. M., Lookabill, S. J., & Krishna, G. (1988). Recovery room initiation of patient controlled analgesia in pediatric patients. *Anesthesiology*, *69*(3A), A772.

Melamed, B. G., & Bush, J. P. (1985). Family factors in children with acute illness. In D. C. Turk & R. D. Kerns (Eds.), *Health, illness, and families: A life-span perspective* (pp. 183–219). New York: Wiley.

Melzack, R. (1973). *The puzzle of pain*. New York: Basic Books.

Merskey, H. (1970). On the development of pain. *Headache*, *10*, 116–123.

Morrison, R. A., & Vedro, D. A. (1989). Pain management in the child with sickle cell disease. *Pediatric Nursing*, *15*(6), 595–599.

Mulhearn, R., Horowitz, M., Ochs, J., Friedman, A., Armstrong, F. D., Copeland, D., & Kun, L. E. (1989). Assessment of quality of life among patients with cancer. *Psychological Assessment*, *1*(2), 130–138.

Osborne, R. B., Hatcher, J. W., & Richtsmeier, A. J. (1989). The role of social modeling in unexplained pediatric pain. *Journal of Pediatric Psychology*, *14*(1), 43–61.

Owens, M. E. (1984). Pain in infancy: Conceptual and methodological issues. *Pain*, *20*, 213–230.

Perlman, D., & Peplau, L. (1981). Toward a social psychology of loneliness. In S. Duck & R. Gilmour (Eds.), *Personal relationships: In disorder. Vol. 3* (pp. 31–35). London: Academic Press.

Peterson, L., & Toler, S. M. (1986). An information seeking disposition in child surgery patients. *Health Psychology*, *5*(4), 343–358.

Piaget, J. (1965). *The moral judgment of the child*. New York: Free Press.

Price, D. D. (1988). *Psychological and neural mechanisms of pain*. New York: Raven.

Price, D. D., Harkins, S. W., & Baker, C. (1987). Sensory-affective relationships among different types of clinical and experimental pain. *Pain*, *28*, 297–307.

Purcell-Jones, G., Dormon, F., & Sumner, E. (1988). Pediatric anesthesiologists' perceptions of neonatal and infant pain. *Pain*, *33*, 181–187.

Rape, R. N., Bush, J. P., & Saravia, M. (1988). Development of children's dental fears: An observational study. *Journal of Clinical Child Psychology*, *17*(4), 345–351.

Rauen, K. K., & Ho, M. (1989). Children's use of patient controlled analgesia after spine surgery. *Pediatric Nursing*, *15*(6), 589–593, 637.

Reid, V., & Bush, J. P. (1990). Ethnic factors influencing pain expression: Implications for clinical assessment. In T. W. Miller (Ed.), *Chronic pain Vol. 1* (pp. 117–145). Madison, CT: International Universities Press.

Rodgers, B. M., Webb, C. J., Stergios, D., & Newman, B. M. (1988). Patient controlled analgesia in pediatric surgery. *Journal of Pediatric Surgery*, *23*(3), 259–262.

Ross, R. S., Bush, J. P., & Crummette, B. D. (1991). Factors affecting nurses' decisions to administer PRN analgesic medication to children after surgery: An analog investigation. *Journal of Pediatric Psychology*, *16*(2), 151–167.

Ross, D. M., & Ross, S. A. (1984). Childhood pain: The school-aged child's viewpoint. *Pain*, *20*, 179–191.

Ross, D. M., & Ross, S. A. (1988). Assessment of pediatric pain: An overview. *Issues in Comprehensive Pediatric Nursing*, *11*, 73–91.

Rothbaum, F., Weisz, J. R., & Snyder, S. S. (1982). Changing the world and changing the self: A two-process model of perceived control. *Journal of Personality and Social Psychology, 42*(1), 5–37.

Saravia, M., & Bush, J. P. (1991). The needleless syringe: Efficacy of anesthesia and patient preference in child dental patients. *Journal of Pedodontics, 15*(2), 109–112.

Shearer, M. H. (1986). Surgery on the paralyzed, unanesthetized newborn. *Birth, 13*(2), 79.

Sukhani, R. (1989). Anesthetic management of the newborn. *Clinics in Perinatology, 16*(1), 43–60.

Tarnowski, K. J., Gavaghan, M. G., & Wisniewski, J. (1989). Acceptability of interventions for pediatric pain management. *Journal of Pediatric Psychology, 14*(3), 463–472.

Truog, R., & Anand, K. S. (1989). Management of pain in the postoperative neonate. *Clinics in Perinatology, 16*(1), 61–78.

Varni, J. (1984). Pediatric pain: A biobehavioral perspective. *Behavior Therapist, 7,* 23–25.

Walker, L. S., & Zeman, J. (1989, August). *Mother and father reinforcement of child illness behavior.* American Psychological Association, New Orleans.

Weinstein, P., Getz, T., Ratener, P., & Domoto, P. (1982). The effect of dentist variables on fear-related behaviors of young children. *Journal of the American Dental Association, 104,* 32–38.

Wilkie, D. J., Holzemer, W. L., Tesler, M. D., Ward, J. A., Paul, S. M., & Savedra, M. C. (1990). Measuring pain quality: Validity and reliability of children's and adolescents' pain language. *Pain, 41,* 151–159.

Wong, D. L., & Baker, C. M. (1988). Pain in children: Comparison of assessment scales. *Pediatric Nursing, 14*(1), 9–17.

Part I
Research, Clinical, and Professional Issues

2
Developmental Contributions to the Assessment of Children's Pain: Conceptual and Methodological Implications

LIZETTE PETERSON, CYNTHIA HARBECK,
JANET FARMER, AND MICHELLE ZINK

Begin by acknowledging pain as a concept, rather than an entity. Any given pain may or may not have a known physical basis, may or may not be exacerbated by anxiety or depression, may have a sudden or gradual onset, may be acute or chronic, and may possess a variety of qualities such as piercing, throbbing, burning, or aching (Johnson, 1988). Next, accept that pain is a multifaceted concept including sensory, affective, and evaluative components (Melzack & Torgerson, 1971). Pain is difficult to study even in adults, who experience few changes in sensory, affective, and perceptual functioning. Pain is subjective in nature and can be observed only through verbal descriptions of the sufferer and a limited number of nonverbal responses (Beyer, DeGood, Ashley, & Russell, 1983).

Then, place the study of pain in childhood, against an ever-changing background of cognitive and affective development, where children have limited abilities to communicate about pain. Finally, imagine the child's pain as influenced by an ever-expanding network of systems such as the family, peer, school, community, and culture. Clearly, the study of children's pain is exceptionally challenging.

This chapter describes some conceptual issues and methodological practices that may improve the study of children's coping with pain. Discussion will highlight the role of development, the importance of considering the type of painful stimulus encountered, and the need to specify whether the child is coping in anticipation of a painful stimulus or is coping with pain itself. Most of the work on children's illness or medical procedures has focused on the preparation for stressful encounters, as preparation is more lengthy and more predictable than the actual painful encounter. Research on injury-induced pain is rare indeed and, due to the nature of the event, includes only coping in response to the painful event, not preparation for such an event. Where relevant, we will integrate current research on children's responses to pain with a variety of classical developmental research methods that may prove applicable to the future study of children's pain.

This discussion also focuses on the current trend toward acknowledging the role that development plays in determining children's coping with pain.

This emphasis on development is not unique to the study of children's pain. The last decade has seen important rapprochement between the fields of classical developmental and clinical psychology (e.g., Gelfand & Peterson, 1985) and between developmental and behavioral psychology (e.g., Mash & Terdal, 1988). Pediatric psychology has historically highlighted the importance of considering the developmental level of the child (e.g., Tuma, 1975), and current descriptions of the field explicitly emphasize the contribution of developmental concepts (e.g., Peterson & Harbeck, 1988; Roberts, 1986). However, as the following research overview documents, developmental specificity is particularly important to the study of children's pain.

Finally, there is increased attention to incorporating developmental concepts into the classical literature on coping with stress. Garmezy and Rutter (1988) described a child application of the Lazarus and Launier (1978) model of stages of coping — appraisal (gathering information about a stressful stimulus), encounter (contacting the stressful stimulus), and recovery (returning to a normal state after completing contact with a stressful stimulus). This model seems especially useful in considering influences on children's coping with pain. Peterson, Harbeck, Chaney, Farmer, and Thomas (1990) recently applied that model in an empirical demonstration of differences in children's appraisal and encounter coping with invasive medical procedures. They described one dimension of appraisal coping that ranged from seeking out to avoiding information. They outlined two dimensions of encounter coping, one involving a range of withdrawing from the stressor to approaching the stimulus, and the other an internally driven versus externally driven dimension. Internally controlled withdrawal might be seen in the use of distraction, externally controlled withdrawal in tears or clinging. Internally controlled stimulus approach might involve sensory redefinition; externally controlled stimulus approach might involve aggressively failing to cooperate.

The classical coping model suggests that differing stressors will elicit differing responses from the same individual. Not only does pain as a stressor vary in terms of quality, intensity, and duration, but the source of the pain is likely to influence children's responding. Varni, Katz, and Dash (1982) suggest that there are four primary etiologies for pain: (a) pain associated with physical injury (e.g., a skinned knee or broken bone), (b) pain associated with a medical or dental procedure (e.g., a blood test or a restoration filling in a tooth), (c) pain associated with a known disease state (e.g., the ache of juvenile rheumatoid arthritis or the cramping from intestinal flu), and (d) pain not associated with a well-defined disease category or injury (e.g., chronic headache or limb pain). These different sources of pain bring a lot of "baggage" with them. The degree to which the onset is sudden, the focus of pain is visible, and the intentionality with which pain is induced by a trusted adult all are likely to influence the child's response.

The developmentally dependent resources a child has available for use when coping with pain can be artificially dichotomized into child-based qualities such as cognitive, affective, and physical abilities, which we will describe in some detail, and environmentally based influences such as caretaker attachment, familial, community, and cultural influences, which we will consider more briefly. We employ this organization to facilitate a non-comprehensive overview of potential conceptual and methodological contributions of a developmental orientation to the study of children's coping with pain. Before beginning this discussion, however, we must explicitly acknowledge the artificiality of separating these categories and emphasize the degree to which we believe that they are interactive rather than independent. For example, cognitions are clearly linked to emotion. During the appraisal of a stressful event, a child's cognitive ability (or inability) to produce a scheme or script to explain a painful medical procedure or injury may determine the extent to which the child is frightened by the event. Similarly, the degree to which a child becomes emotionally aroused is likely to influence the child's memory. Further, child-based and environmentally based aspects of the children's world are mutually interdependent. For example, secure attachment to a caregiver may moderate internal emotional responses to pain, and family models can influence the child's cognitions and beliefs about pain. Thus, although we focus on a single system at a time, we acknowledge at the outset its dynamic interaction with other systems.

Child-Based Factors That Affect Pain

Cognition

Children's Understanding of Illness and Pain

Many pediatric psychologists have commented on the importance of considering children's developmental level when evaluating their cognitive reactions to physical illness and pain. Children's ability to comprehend the causes and processes of disease have been shown to be strongly dependent on their general cognitive development. Burbach and Peterson (1986) reviewed cognitive-developmental studies of children's conceptualization of illness. Although none of these studies focused on pain per se, their general methods and conclusions are relevant to the study of pain, and in terms of specifying unique phases of development, will have to suffice. There is little published work to date documenting discrete developmental stages of children's understanding of pain analogous to the research on children's understanding of illness concepts. Like most work in the child development area, studies on illness that utilized specific stage-oriented tests of cognitive development showed a clearer relationship to stages of illness concepts than did studies that focused on age as an index of cognitive development. For the most part, gender failed to influence children's understanding of illness, although in some of the age-based studies older males showed a particular reluctance to acknowledge illness and pain, a reluctance not seen in older girls or younger children of either sex.

Within studies reviewed by Burbach and Peterson (1986), children in earlier stages of cognitive development differed from children in more mature stages in many ways. Their understanding of illness and associated pain tended to be more global and nonspecific (e.g., Natapoff, 1978), they were unlikely to consider psychological, affective, and social aspects of physical illness (e.g., Perrin & Gerrity, 1981), and they confused symptoms (e.g., sneezing, vomiting) with causes (e.g., virus; Nagy, 1951). Furthermore, children in earlier stages focused on external cues (e.g., a runny nose) more than internal cues (e.g., fatigue) to evaluate their illness (e.g., Neuhauser, Amsterdam, Hines, & Steward, 1978); they confused contagious illness with noncontagious events (e.g., Potter & Roberts, 1984); and they felt less control over illness and recovery (Bibace & Walsh, 1980) than more cognitively advanced children. Less advanced children also had more unfounded beliefs concerning relationships between their own misbehavior and illness than older children.

Very little research has examined children's cognitions about pain independent from their beliefs about illness, and all studies that have focused on children's pain have been conducted in the last decade. Research in this area has, for the most part, not been as tightly tied to developmental theory as were the studies on children's understanding of illness and has not uniformly reported age-related differences. These studies have examined not only children's understanding of the causes of pain but children's ability to describe pain.

In one of the first studies in this area, Savedra, Gibbons, Tesler, Ward, and Wegner (1982) found that younger children focused on physical causes of pain, whereas older children were more likely to consider psychological causes as well. Younger children were more likely to use terms such as "feel like crying" to describe pain, older children were more likely to use phrases such as "like an ache" or "sore." Ross and Ross (1984a) did not find clear age-related trends in the 5- to 12-year-old children they interviewed. In general, the children reported pain to be caused by external events such as "accidents," heat, surgery, or aggressive acts of others. The majority (80.9%) emphasized general discomfort when describing pain and many (nearly 70%) used phrases such as "stabbing," "burning," "squeezing," "jabbing," and "dull."

Some researchers have focused exclusively on the description of pain and have used familiar referents such as color, texture, shape, pattern, and continuous versus intermittent to assess children's descriptions of pain. Scott (1978), employing such methodology, found that elementary school–age children could describe pain in terms of sensory, evaluative, and affective components. Across age, children showed interesting agreement on some seemingly subjective aspects of pain. For example, children described the "color" of pain most often as red and the pain of a needle as "jagged" rather than "smooth." When Unruh, McGrath, Cunningham, and Humphreys

(1983) asked children 5 to 18 years of age to draw pictures of pain, they found no age-related differences in the categories generated by the types of pictures produced by children. Children most often drew pain using the colors red and black.

Gaffney and Dunne (1986) focused on children's definitions of pain in answer to the open-ended statement, "Pain is . . . ". They examined the responses of children from three age groups and argued that the responses corresponded to the Piagetian preoperational, concrete operational, and early formal operational stages of development. Specifically, younger children more often used concrete terms to describe pain (e.g., "a thing in your tummy"), whereas older children used definitions that were more abstract and suggested psychological as well as physiological origins for pain.

Harbeck and Peterson (in press) provided a more detailed description of the developmental progression of children's understanding of pain. These authors created empirically derived categories of answers from children's descriptions of pain sensations, their understanding of the reasons why pain "hurts," and their notions about the value of pain. Then, these categories were ordered into developmental steps by experts in the area. With age and increasing cognitive development, children gave more complex answers to these questions. Understanding of pain causality generally appeared to progress from the child being unable to verbalize a reason why pain hurts, to verbalizing a general, usually external cause of the pain, to finally including physiological or psychological causes. It is striking to note, however, that only 6% of the responses contained a physiological explanation and only 5% contained a psychological cause. Preschoolers, first graders, and third graders had virtually no awareness of physiological or psychological explanations; even college freshmen reported very few physiological (13%) or psychological (13%) causes. Although subjects had some difficulty identifying reasons why pain hurt, they had a much more difficult time identifying how experiencing pain might be valuable. Older subjects were better able to identify the value of pain (75% of college freshmen vs. 9% of preschoolers). However, overall, half of the subjects (54%) could not identify a value of pain. An additional 9% only identified pain values such as relief or familiarity with the pain.

Interestingly, age was a better predictor of more cognitively mature answers about pain than were measures derived from a Piagetian conservation-identity task. This may have been due to the relative insensitivity of the cognitive measure, but the authors also argued that life experiences and encounters with pain increase with age and are likely to influence cognitions about pain independent from general cognitive maturity. It appears as if both life experiences and cognitive maturity are important in the development of children's understanding about pain. Future research may be able to articulate the contribution of each.

The few studies that have been completed in this area only scratch the surface of children's cognitive-developmental understanding of pain. The researchers in this area stress the utility of an active interview process in which children are given open-ended questions (Ross & Ross, 1984b) and multiple, progressively more structured but nonleading prompts (Harbeck & Peterson, 1988). It may even be that the traditionally used interview methods would be well supplemented by other methods—for example, structured tasks such as those used by Piaget and his proponents, who used several tasks to illustrate children's inability to decenter prior to concrete operational functioning in tasks using clay, liquid in different beakers, and coins or buttons in a row (Piaget, 1970). Less mature children were unable to attend simultaneously to height and width, or to both length of and spaces between a set of items in evaluating amount of a substance. This quality of being unable to decenter combined with children's poor ability to evaluate temporal parameters, may contribute to young children's exceptionally negative response to injections and venipunctures, which many children report to be more fear provoking than anesthesia or postoperative recovery (Eland & Anderson, 1977; Poster, 1983). These are procedures with high intensity and short duration. If a child is unable to evaluate two aspects of the stimulus at the same time, then the short duration (e.g., "it will only hurt for a minute") would not meaningfully detract from the evaluation of anticipated intense pain. These and similar concepts might be profitably assessed using tasks that elicit the simultaneous use of different stimulus attributes.

The Role of Memory

Application of developmental principles of cognition to pediatric psychology has typically involved the use of Piagetian-like stage theories (e.g., Bibace & Walsh, 1980). However, some of the classic work on information processing and on memory also has great potential for elucidating children's responses to pain. To give one very simple example, it is clear that young children's recognition memory is quite a bit better than their recall abilities. Thus, the prior work on memory for toys or pictures (e.g., Myers & Perlmutter, 1978), and more recent work on real-world memory in medical settings (Ornstein, Gordon, & Larus, in press), would suggest that when a parent asks the child to spontaneously recall the last injection experienced, only a minority of young children (2 to 5 years of age) will be able to do so. However, because their recognition memory is more effective in the stimulus setting, where the appropriate physical equipment, smells, personnel, and so forth are available, the memory may come flooding back to the majority of young children when they arrive at the clinic or hospital, leaving the children little time following the appraisal to organize their resources to cope with encountering a painful stimulus like an injection. Laboratory studies and limited work on real-world memory would predict that older children, in contrast to younger children, will have substantial recall from their prior encounter with injections before being exposed to that stimulus situation and so can prepare for the next experience at their leisure. Future research may profit from methodologies that assess recognition as well as recall by using both open-ended questions and props such as syringes and venipuncture equipment when querying children about medical events.

Another, slightly more complex extrapolation is drawn from the hypothesis that semantic memory (that is, organized general knowledge) grows out of episodic memory (that is, the child's own memory of personally experienced events). Some believe this transition is the quintessential description of the development of memory in children (Nelson & Brown, 1978). One way such specific personal experiences become incorporated as a general understanding of the world is through the development of scripts, or organized representations of common sequences of events (e.g., Nelson, 1986). The degree to which a given sequence has been repeatedly experienced should determine the existence of a script. Thus, fairly young children may be familiar with the script "I climb up, I slip, I fall, I hurt." In contrast, a script in which a trusted adult dresses the child nicely, takes him or her to visit another adult, holds the child down, and allows another adult to stick a needle into the child is likely to be a very unfamiliar event for the young child who lacks experience with the health care system. A child who has previously been exposed to health care procedures will have a doctor-dentist-nurse script that may incorporate such painful events and thus cue effective coping behavior.

Most of the research on memory seems more relevant to children's ability to appraise pain as a stressor before the event occurs, rather than dealing with it only during stimulus encounter. However, some of the literature on children's active encounters with pain suggests that memory plays an important role. As the child's ability to think about pain develops, the child may respond to encountering a new pain by remembering a coping method that was effective with a past pain experience. This demonstrates that the different sensations are being regarded under the common rubric of "pain." So we see children reporting that they would blow on a cut, possibly because of the success of this maneuver with a burn, and later describing quite sophisticated strategies such as imagery or stimulus redefinition for use across very dissimilar types of pain (Harbeck & Peterson, 1988). To date, few studies have probed children's actual memory for their own painful events or have attempted to explore how past coping attempts may influence what is remembered. These seem exceptionally important questions when structuring interventions to enhance encounter coping.

We have selected only a few from many potential applications of current basic research on children's memory to illustrate their potential contributions to the problem of pediatric pain. It remains for future research to utilize these conceptualizations and methodologies to investigate the influence of memory on children's cognitive appraisal of a painful stressor.

Language

As was noted earlier, pain is a subjective experience and the most common method of evaluating another's pain is to solicit verbal descriptions. When attempting to assist a child in the appraisal of a potentially painful stressor, the child's ability to understand and correctly interpret linguistic descriptions of the pain is thus critical. Such ability is at least partially determined by developmental level. Most pain descriptions employed by adults are likely to be adjectives (e.g., intense) or metaphors (e.g., it felt like an elephant dancing in my head), two of the last speech forms to be learned by children. Further, such descriptors often employ a fairly concrete action term (e.g., burning or stabbing) in an abstract fashion that can be very confusing to a young child. Finally, the words used to describe the parameters of pain ("for a minute") are not terms readily understood by young children. To a small child, his or her tummy is almost the entire thorax and words like "thigh" or "shin" are unknown. Thus, it is essential for both practitioners and researchers to obtain information on children's understanding of appraisal information.

There is also some degree of circularity in linguistic references to pain, in that a person is unlikely to be able to interpret another's description of pain during appraisal unless that person has experienced very similar pain. Certainly, lay descriptors for different pains are confusing and inadequate. For example, the "ache" we get in our muscles following a day of exercise bears little resemblance to a "headache" and that, in turn, is nothing like a "stomachache" which can mean anything from nausea and vomiting to cramping diarrhea to ulcer-induced pain to a ruptured appendix.

Parmelee (1986) raised a fascinating issue in his presidential address to the Society for Research in Child Development when he argued that children could learn a great deal about perspective taking and empathy by observing family members catching, enduring, and recovering from the same day to day colds and flu experienced by the child. If this is the case, it would argue for clear verbalizations of subjective states to be produced by the ill adults to allow the child to acquire labels for differing types of pain. In this fashion, children could be exposed to a richer linguistic basis for communicating about pain at the same time they are exposed to the virus! (However, we will consider adult pain models later in this chapter, and that discussion will suggest some prudent limits for such communications.)

Not only are linguistically and experientially immature children less able to profit from verbal descriptions of pain, but some research would suggest that their ability to *think* about pain and form a general concept of pain is at least partially dependent on having words to describe differing types of pain (e.g., Kay & Kempton, 1984). This ties the present discussion back to the earlier described studies on children's spontaneous cognitions about pain. However, it also suggests the value of examining how well children interpret what is said *to* them about pain (a very different question than how they themselves describe pain) and how they go about assigning meaning to pain descriptors given to them by others.

The flip side of studying how children interpret linguistic cues they receive about pain during their appraisal phase is the investigation of how children themselves produce linguistic cues during real encounters with pain. Although most children are skillful at an early age in registering discomfort, specifics such as where, how much, and how long cannot be described well nonverbally. Although some effort has been made to develop nonverbal methods of assessing pain in children (e.g., Eland, 1986), such measures typically deal only with intensity and are not successful in very young children. The quality or nature of a sensation may be even more critical to know than intensity or other parameters. Yet quality of pain is even less likely to be linguistically produced by a small child because of its specificity and level of abstraction. Although the average vocabulary of a 3½-year-old is around 1,222 words and a 6-year-old around 2,526 words (Carey, 1978; Smith, 1926), most of these words are concrete nouns and verbs. The use of abstract adjectives such as those describing the quality of pain develop much later.

At first, children may use a word to describe pain only in the precise situation in which it was learned, showing a rigidity likely born of imitating a word that is not yet understood. Later in toddlerhood, it becomes more common for the child to use a more general term like "hurts" or even an inaccurate term like "sting" to describe what might be a very different discomfort such as nausea. (We know one toddler who used the word "headache" for any unpleasant intrabody sensation. After rubbing his abdomen during an intestinal flu attack, he exclaimed, "I have a bad headache right here.") The overextension of a term from one meaning to another is described by the semantic feature hypothesis (Clark, 1973). This and similar theories about children's early language use could make important contributions to research on children's pain by clarifying methods of interpreting and evaluating developmental differences in children's ability to express experienced pain.

Although most pediatric psychologists have considered developmental contributions to the study of children's medical and psychological difficulties, they have traditionally considered only the influence of cognition, and thus our discussion places most emphasis there. However, the child's emotional and physical spheres also have been the focus of contributions by developmentalists and, as will be seen in the next section, these literatures may also be useful in directing future research on children's pain.

Emotion

The study of children's emotional development has gained much needed attention in recent years (Cicchetti & Hesse, 1982; Lewis & Michalson, 1983; Strayer, 1985). Although definitions and terminology related to the study of emotion vary considerably, "emotion" often refers to a biologically prewired phenomenon involving both physiological responses and subjective experience (Lewis & Michalson, 1983). At birth, emotion and pain seem to be relatively undifferentiated, with physical comfort equivalent to psychological well-being (Piers & Curry, 1985). However, over the course of development, more distinct basic emotions appear including joy, anger, disgust, surprise, fear, sadness, sexual ardor, and affection (Campos, Barrett, Lamb, Goldsmith, & Stenberg, 1983).

Developmental Aspects of Emotion and Pain

Not surprisingly, given the typically cognitive orientation of developmentalists described earlier, much of the basic research on children's emotions has actually focused on children's cognitions about and labels for emotions. Although such research programs fail to access children's emotions directly, insight into children's reactions to emotions at different developmental levels may have implications for the study of children's pain. For example, Graham and Weiner (1986) have found that young children tend to label their emotional experience on the basis of the positive or negative outcomes of events, with a relatively undifferentiated reaction of "happy" or "sad." With development, children come to identify their emotions in a more differentiated fashion due to the attributions they make about the causes of events. For instance, if the basic outcome of an event is negative and the attribution is that the event was caused by oneself, the emotion experienced is guilt. However, if a negative event has occurred and the attribution is that the fault belongs to another, anger is experienced. Graham and Weiner's (1986) formulation would suggest that understanding children's cognitions about blameworthiness for an injury or illness would allow prediction of the emotion experienced, which in turn may have the potential to predict the pain response, at least in children sufficiently mature to have acquired the relevant attribution-emotion links.

Nannis and Cowan (1987) offer another explanation, drawing from Piaget's developmental theory. They describe four levels of a child's understanding of emotion. In the first level, feelings are a concrete entity based on a facial expression, like a smile, or on an event, like receiving a gift or playing an exciting game. In level two, feelings are still concrete but now they are tied to an internal entity like an organ ("My heart is sad"). In the third level, feelings are more abstract and active; people have control over their feelings and feelings are internally generated. Finally, in the fourth and highest level, both physiological and psychological explanations of the feelings and thoughts plus one's perceptions of events, are thought to influence feelings. This conceptualization suggests that enjoining small children to control their emotions during a painful event may not seem possible to those children who still view emotion as an automatic outcome of an event.

The study of children's knowledge about situations that provoke emotions (Harris, 1985) complements Nannis and Cowan's (1987) stage theory of emotional development. Younger children (6 years old) tend to think that there is a direct link between the nature of a situation and the emotional response that one makes. That is, young children associate a situation such as two friends quarreling with anger in the form of overt angry facial expressions, stamping of feet, and fighting. Older children (11 years old) are much more likely to make a distinction between the situation, inner feelings, and their behavioral reaction to the situation. Thus, young children believe that it is necessary to change the situation in order to modify one's feelings. In contrast, older children are more aware that redirecting one's thoughts can be effective in modifying emotional reactions. The close situation-emotional response link found in young children underscores the need to study children's reactions to specific types of painful situations (i.e., related to illness, injury, or medical procedures) as suggested by Harbeck and Peterson (1988).

Because their emotional reaction is mediated by inner cognitive processes, older children can conceive of discrepancies between one's inner emotional state and one's facial expression and behavior (Harris, 1985), and they exhibit more knowledge about display rules for emotional expression (Saarni, 1979). Although cognitive-developmental changes undoubtedly play a role in expression of internal states, developmentalists are also currently examining the impact of socialization on emotions, including factors such as parent-child attachment (Field & Fogel, 1982), emotional contagion and social referencing (Strayer, 1985), and familial and cultural rules for expressing emotions (Lewis & Saarni, 1985). Both the experience and expression of pain may be closely linked to the socialization of emotion. These topics will be further explored in the section on external factors that influence children's pain.

Emotion is linked to memory development as well. For example, there is a growing literature suggesting that children retrieve memories more efficiently when experiencing the same mood as was experienced during encoding (Bartlett & Santrock, 1982). That is, children who are sad are likely to recall memories stored when they were unhappy, and events that, at the time, provoked positive feelings, are more readily recalled when they are happy. This may have important implications for children's preparation for medical events. For instance, it may be necessary to maintain the same mood through appraisal of and encounter with a medical stressor, if appraisal cognitions are to be recalled accurately. In addition, the memory of an emotionally charged pain situation may have an important carryover effect on repeat contact with a painful stimulus.

What kinds of emotions are provoked by the experience of pain? How is pain likely to influence and be influenced by emotion? We consider these questions in the next section.

Emotional Reactions to Pain

For most children, fear and anxiety are the immediate emotional responses associated with painful stimuli. In fact, Johnson (1988) points out that it is almost impossible to behaviorally distinguish between children's perceived pain and anxiety, they are so intimately related. Siegel (1988) argues that this relationship between anxiety and pain is reciprocal. There is clear evidence that fear exacerbates pain, and pain in turn appears to promote fear and anxiety, thus creating a spiraling increase in experienced pain. Both medical and psychological treatments for pain frequently involve reducing arousal and altering the child's focus on fear-provoking aspects of an injury, illness, or medical procedure.

Many factors such as the child's temperament, the perceived intensity of the pain, and the way in which the child appraises the painful stimulus may influence the extent of the child's emotional reaction. For example, Williams, Murray, Lund, Harkiss, and DeFranco (1985) found that children with a history of refusing dental treatment were rated by their parents as being anxious at the thought of pain or discomfort. On a measure of temperament, these children were also rated as having more difficulty approaching new situations, being more resistant to change, and experiencing more negative moods relative to a control group of nonrefusing children. Interestingly, although the group of previous dental refusers was rated much higher in anticipatory anxiety, their self-reported distress during the actual dental procedure did not differ from controls.

As suggested by the Williams et al. (1985) study, anticipatory fear that is generated during appraisal of the stressor can cause more physical and emotional discomfort than the stressful stimulus itself. One adult subject reported that the stomachaches she experienced whenever she knew she must have an injection were undoubtedly worse than the injection pain ultimately experienced. In such cases, appropriate preparation to limit anxiety, or if this is not possible, to limit the extent of appraisal would seem important.

Most of the literature on preparation for surgery (e.g., Melamed, Dearborn, & Hermecz, 1983; Melamed & Siegel, 1975; Peterson & Shigetomi, 1981) describes factors in preparation that influence level of fear. For example, if the child understands the description of the stressor (i.e., the preparation is at an appropriate developmental level and is sensitively administered), this is likely to cause less fear than if the child has an unclear or exaggerated expectation of the stimulus. If sensations are described in a familiar, nonthreatening, yet accurate manner ("Your mouth will be heavy and tingly and have little feeling, like when your foot is asleep"), this seems to be less fear provoking (Siegel & Peterson, 1980).

When severe discomfort such as postsurgical pain is anticipated, Janis (1958) has suggested that some degree of fear may be necessary to promote "the work of worrying" needed to plan successful coping. This concept is difficult to investigate, particularly in children. It is quite clear that adults and children who are very anxious prior to surgery continue to be more anxious following the experience (Auerbach, 1973; Melamed, 1982). However, children who actively seek out information and plan their responses tend to cope more adaptively than children who deny or ignore their anticipation of a medical procedure (Peterson, 1989). Further, young children who may have fewer coping resources tend to be more fearful than older children (Peterson & Mori, 1987).

How do other emotions such as anger or sadness influence the experience of pain? An important area almost devoid of empirical study in children is the impact of moods like depression on pain perception. Anecdotal reports of children's reactions to injuries such as burns (Kelley, Jarvie, Middlebrook, McNeer, & Drabman, 1984) and to chronic pain such as that experienced by hemophiliacs (Varni, 1983) suggest that anxiety, sadness, and negative mood all may exacerbate the experience of pain. Interventions that focus on reducing negative affect and increasing positive affect need increasingly to be a part of pain treatment.

It is important not to overlook the potential power of positive emotions. Children spontaneously report using positive imagery as a method of dealing with pain (Peterson et al., 1990). Further, training in positive mental imagery has been used successfully as a preventive treatment for child surgery patients (e.g., Peterson & Shigetomi, 1981). In a study by Kuttner, Bowman, and Teasdale (1988), pleasant imagery was shown to be more effective in reducing pain and anxiety in young children undergoing bone marrow aspirations than attempts to draw their attention away from the painful sensations and onto other interesting persons and objects in the treatment room. Imagery involvement was differentially more helpful for children aged 3 to 6 years compared to 7- to 10-year-old children, whose observed anxiety and pain decreased under both distraction and positive imagery conditions. Research is needed that continues to explore the actual changes in mood accompanying such interventions at different developmental levels in order to clarify the role of positive affect in blocking the experience of pain.

The explicit consideration of the influence of cognitions and emotions on children's pain perception is typical of a pediatric psychological approach. In our last section on child factors, we will describe the small amount of data on developmental differences in the physical bases of pain, and consider how these differences should influence clinical research and practice.

Physiological Factors

A review of several major neurology texts (Adams & Victor, 1985; Kandel & Schwartz, 1985; Rowland, 1984) shows little or no attention to the physical basis of pediatric pain. These texts contain scant information on pain and no information on the development of pain perception. Similarly, Wall and Melzack's initial edition (1984) of the *Textbook of Pain* contained over 800 pages, with only three pages on pain in children listed in the index. The second edition (Wall & Melzack, 1989) devotes one chapter to pain in children, with the rest of the book describing pain in adults.

There is growing concern about misinformation on the physical basis of pain in infants and children. Early studies on responses of neonates to pain suggested limited perception or localization of pain (e.g., McGraw, 1943), and it has been traditionally accepted in the medical community that neonates are incapable of experiencing "real" pain (Wallerstein, 1985). The anatomical basis for this belief has been the absence of myelination in the neonatal nervous system (Shearer, 1986).

However, in the adult nervous system, pain perception occurs in fibers that are unmyelinated (C-polymodal fibers) and very thinly myelinated (A-delta fibers) (Schulte, 1975). It is clear that myelination is not essential for signal transmission but that its presence does increase the velocity of the signal. In infants, it is likely that the decrease in velocity due to lack of myelination is offset by shorter interneuronal distances (Linneweh, 1968). Further, a variety of forms of evidence ranging from facial expression, body movement, and crying to cardiac activity and plasma cortisol levels suggest that infants have the physical basis for experiencing pain, and that they react to painful stimuli in a variety of ways indicating nociception (Owens, 1984).

Anand, Phil, and Hickey (1987) provide an excellent overview of the development of the physical basis for pain in neonates, describing neuro-transmission, development of intracortical connections, incorporation of the thalamus, cortical involvement, and development of the endogenous opioid system. They conclude that the pathways, and the subcortical and cortical centers necessary for pain perception, are well developed before birth and that neurochemical systems necessary for pain transmission are functional at birth. Despite such data, surgeries continue to be performed on unanesthetized infants (Shearer, 1986), and as noted in other chapters of this text, infants and children remain demonstrably undermedicated for pain.

It should not come as a surprise that little is known about developmental changes in the child's nervous system that may result in changes in pain perception. In our literature search, only two studies were located that addressed the issue of children's developing pain thresholds. McGraw (1963) used a pinprick to evaluate the responses of 75 infants. A few hours after birth, infants showed little response to the pinprick. By 1 week they responded to the pinprick with diffuse body movements and local withdrawal reflex, and at 1 month they showed increasing response specificity and organization. In a study by Haslam (1969), children aged 5 to 18 were asked to report when pressure applied to the tibia began to "hurt." A low but significant correlation between age and pain threshold suggested that the threshold for pain may be higher for older children. Clinical evidence also supports this finding (Lollar, Smits, & Patterson, 1982).

It is noteworthy that the two empirical studies that we were able to locate that examined physical development of pain thresholds were conducted over two decades ago. It seems likely that ethical concerns prevent many researchers from studying physiological factors in the development of pain perception, if such study requires inducing pain in infants and children. However, study of developmental differences in perception of the same sensations would seem to necessitate control over the aversive stimuli. Such control is not possible in regularly occurring medical events that are most often the source of our knowledge of infants' and children's responses to pain (Owens, 1984).

Environmentally Based Systems Factors

In the previous sections we have considered at some length child-based factors that affect pain; in the next sections we will consider more briefly the environmentally based factors that affect pain such as parent-child attachment, pain modeling, and other events occurring in the child's life, learning, and culture.

Parent-Child Attachment

Infants' relationships with their caregivers may impact their early experiences with pain. For example, infants' first contacts with noxious sensations involve events such as becoming hungry, being wet, feeling too warm or cold, and encountering a painful stimulus like a diaper pin or a phenylketonuria (PKU) blood test stick. Typically such stimuli provoke crying, which promotes a caregiver to intervene (Ainsworth, Blehar, Waters, & Walls, 1978). Indeed, initially, successful coping in the infant demands only the ability to cue the caregiver.

What happens when the caregiver does not respond appropriately to the cue? Consider the young child who experiences sensitive caregiving to most basic needs but who experiences regular and painful stimuli that are not removed by the caregiver. Some classical developmental theory (e.g., Erikson, 1959) posits that the young infant develops trust that the caregiver will successfully eliminate noxious stimuli. If the caregiver fails to effectively do so, does such trust fail to develop? Are attachment bonds weakened? For mothers who are depressed or otherwise incapacitated, this may be the case (Gaensbauer, Harmon, Cytryn, & McKnew, 1984; Radke-Yarrow, Cummings, Kucynski, & Chapman, 1985; Zahn-Waxler, Cummings, McKnew, & Radke-Yarrow, 1984). However, it seems noteworthy that most infants with repeated pain from colic, for example, far from rejecting their caregiver, are soothed and assisted in dealing with the discomfort by contact with the caregiver. Early experiences with colic or other painful events such as surgery may influence the child's later response to painful events as well. Using attachment paradigms to study infants who are experiencing pain may yield more information about this process.

Similarly, later in life, presence of a caregiver may affect a child's pain in either a positive or negative direction. Shaw and Routh (1982) and Gross, Stern, Levin, Dale, and Wojnilower (1983) found that children were more likely to cry and complain when parents were present during an injection and a blood test, respectively, than when parents were absent. However, these authors suggested that the children may have been less anxious even though they fussed more when parents were present. Alternatively, the complaints may have resembled an extinction burst as the child increasingly demanded that the parent intervene to halt the procedure. Future research might use some of the microscopic (moment to moment) observational methodologies used by developmentalists who study mother-infant bonding to assess the source of these effects.

Some authors have begun to use such methods. Bush, Melamed, Sheras, and Greenbaum (1986), for example, observed children and their parents during the waiting periods in an outpatient clinic using a sensitive observational system that analyzed small units of interaction. They found that children's crying and fear-related verbalizations were positively related to observable parental agitation and anxious reassurance of the child. Children's crying and complaining of fear were also related to parents' self-reported anxiety and fear. Parental distraction of the child, in contrast, was correlated with less crying and fewer verbalizations of fear. Future investigations that not only consider anxiety but that also address pain directly may be essential to understanding how parents influence children's pain. Because fear and pain are often closely connected, one might hypothesize that similar parental factors would affect a child's fear and pain experiences.

Family Factors

Modeling

Adults not only affect a child's current pain experience in a medical setting, but they may also affect the way in which the child typically responds to pain and may even influence the acquisition and maintenance of chronic pain. Several studies have reported a relationship between parental and offspring pain symptomatology; however, most of these studies have been conducted with adults. Violon and Giurgea (1984), for example, reported that of their adult chronic pain patients, 78% reported a history of pain in other members of their families; in contrast, only 44% of pain-free patients had a family history of pain. Similarly, Turkat, Kuczmierczyk, and Adams (1984) reported that a high percentage of adult headache sufferers versus nonsufferers could be identified by using the presence or absence of a headache model in the family history as the predictor variable.

Edwards, Zeichner, Kuczmierczyk, and Boczkowski (1985) studied familial pain models in 168 college students. They asked the subjects to complete the Parameters of Pain Questionnaire, which assesses the frequency, duration, and intensity of 10 common pain symptoms. Similar to the previously reported studies, more pain models were present in the families of students who reported a higher level of current pain complaints.

A more recent study (Harbeck & Peterson, 1988) used a wide age range (3 to 18) to examine the relationship between child and parental pains. In this study, children were asked to identify all pains that they and their parents had experienced. A correlation of .68 was found between subjects' pains and their reports of their parents' pains. Similarly, Routh and Ernst (1984) reported a higher incidence rate of somatization disorder in relatives of children with "functional" rather than "organic" pain.

Family Health and Stress

Perhaps the high correlation between parental and offspring pains is related to the way the family thinks about health issues. Mechanic (1964) suggested that definitions of symptoms and patterns of use of medical resources are acquired within the family, and that the child's ability to define his or her symptoms is learned from family members who initially define the illnesses and teach him or her to attend selectively to various symptoms. Hughes and Zimin (1978) found that families of children with recurrent abdominal pain frequently used bodily sensations, physical explanations, and medical or surgical procedures to deal with psychic distress. In addition, family histories of these pediatric chronic pain patients were replete with illnesses and somatic complaints of various family members as well as deaths of close relatives. Parents were preoccupied with health concerns. Mothers appeared overly concerned about their child's illness, but were usually poorly informed about children's basic needs and stresses such as friends, school activities, and plans.

Hodges, Kline, Barbero, and Flanery (1984) also found a high degree of health-related stressors in families of children with recurrent abdominal pain (see also chapter 10, this volume). They compared children with recurrent abdominal pain (RAP) and their families to families of behavior disordered (BD) and healthy children. They found that both BD and RAP children experienced significantly more life events and reported more stress associated with those events than did the healthy children. In comparison to the healthy control children, RAP children reported more serious illness/hospitalization and deaths of significant others, decreased arguments with and between parents, and change in acceptance by peers. In addition, differences were found between the BD and RAP children, suggesting that the RAP children had experienced more negative life events related to health than the BD children.

Familial Rewards for Pain

Other researchers (Fordyce, Roberts, & Sternbach, 1985; Fordyce & Steger, 1979) propose that families may help maintain a child's pain through socially reinforcing the pain. The reinforcer may not be the initial cause of the pain, but may be the maintaining factor. For example, a child may get a severe headache and find that pain complaints elicit expressions of comfort as well as privileges from his or her parents. The child may then learn to use complaints of pain in order to obtain certain reinforcers. The pain may even be shaped by such reinforcers, even though the child might consciously prefer to be healthy.

Adults are aware of secondhand gain in children's pain but often avoid considering a psychological cause for the children's pain (Peterson & Harbeck, 1988). In addition, many children are aware of the reinforcing consequences of pain. For example, Ross and Ross (1984b) questioned a sample of almost 1,000 5- to 12-year-olds about maladaptive pain usage. They found that 19.7% reported that they had used pain for secondary gain on one occasion and 15.7% reported more than one case of using pain for such gain. These children most often used pain to obtain increased parental and peer attention, and to avoid school and athletic activities. According to the authors, this maladaptive pain usage could be the antecedent for later instances of chronic pain.

Family Systems Influence

Family dynamics may also affect a child's pain. According to Minuchin, the initiation or maintenance of pain may be influenced by four family characteristics: enmeshment, overprotectiveness, rigidity, and low conflict threshold (Minuchin, Rosman, & Baker, 1978). These characteristics combine to form a family with a very low tolerance for conflict. As a result, problems are not negotiated or resolved; the child with pain plays a role in the family's avoidance of conflict by presenting a focus for concern. The system then reinforces his or her behavior in order to preserve its pattern of conflict avoidance.

Using similar family features, Olson and his colleagues developed the Circumplex Model of Marital and Family Systems (Olson, Sprenkle, & Russell, 1979). According to this model, well-functioning families have moderate levels of cohesion and adaptability. Cohesion is defined as the emotional bonding family members have with one another and the degree of individual autonomy a member experiences within the family system. Adaptability concerns the ability of the family system to change its power structure and role relationships in response to situational and developmental stress. Although little research has explored this model in relation to children's pain, researchers have begun to apply the circumplex model to other aspects of pediatric chronic illness such as disease process and medication compliance (Chaney & Peterson, 1989; Hanson, Henggeler, Harris, Burghen, & Moore, 1989; Holden, Friend, Gault, Kager, Foltz, & White, 1991). Future research could profitably explore the relationship between family cohesion and adaptability and children's pain initiation and maintenance.

Culture

Not only do family systems affect children's perceptions of, and coping with, pain, but other interacting systems such as peers, schools, and communities may also influence children's reactions to pain. In particular, it seems as if the culture in which children live may also affect their pain experience. Although this is an appealing idea, little research is available that examines cultural influences on pain. In one rare exception, Moore, Miller, Weinstein, Dworkin, and Liou (1987) had Chinese, Anglo-American, and Scandinavian subjects describe pain and pain coping perceptions. Data from interviews and a card-sorting task revealed universal dimensions of pain. However, culture-specific dimensions were seen as well. For example, Chinese subjects described *suantong* or "sour pain" as a multivariate pain of bone, joints, teeth, and gingiva. Similarly, Western subjects, but not Chinese subjects, described "real" versus "imagined" pains. Abu-Saad (1984) also reported that children from various cultures describe pain differently. He reported that Arab-American and Latin-American children were more likely to use sensory words to describe pain, whereas the Asian-American children tended to use relatively more words in the affective and evaluative domains. It seems likely that cultural values affect not only pain descriptions, but also pain expression and pain perception. In a culture where children are bombarded with exhortations to take Anacin, Tylenol, Bufferin, Nuprin, etc., when one has a headache, muscle aches, menstrual pain, flu, colds, arthritis, or any discomfort, tolerance for pain might be anticipated to be minimal, and locus of control for pain management external.

Methodological Issues for the Future

Throughout this discussion of both applied and basic research relevant to children's pain, we have repeatedly noted how future research can profit from and even improve on methods used in the past. In this final section, we offer a brief, explicit consideration of these methodological issues raised earlier. First, we will explore some stumbling blocks typical to past research in this area and then examine some extensions of current research methods that might be valuable for future study.

Methodological Inadequacies

Many of the studies reviewed here are limited by problems in subject selection and description, subject number, measurement and analysis problems, and an absence of control over extraneous variables.

We are often not told how the particular subjects who served and not others came to be included as participants. Because most of the work in this area is descriptive, it seems particularly important to establish the representativeness of subjects. Are these subjects randomly drawn from a population or are they children whose parents are particularly interested in pain as a topic? If a clinical population is used, are these children more or less ill, more dependent on the medical system, or more cooperative than other children with the same diagnosis?

If children's cognitive level is an issue, is that explicitly measured or is age used as an inaccurate proxy? Are the influences of gender and interactions between gender and developmental level explicitly considered? Are other variables such as prior medical experience, socioeconomic status, parental presence, etc., controlled?

If a control group is present, is it clear what is being controlled? An ill, chronic pain group might be better contrasted with an ill-but-without-pain group than a healthy community control. Optimally, both controls would be used.

Are measures standardized or are appropriate psychometrics given for measures? (Given the small amount of literature in this area, this is almost never the case.) If an interview is used, is there a balance between open-ended and structured questions to allow both recall and recognition of information? Is the interview too leading? Is it developmentally appropriate, especially in regard to length and potential fatigue? Is the interviewer well trained to deal with children and yet uninformed as to child status (e.g., ill or healthy) or experimental hypotheses?

Are there sufficient children to afford appropriate statistical power? (Small n may be one of the biggest problems in this area.) Are analyses appropriately conservative, with at least 10 to 20 children per variable in multiple regression solutions, at least 10 per cell in analysis of variance solutions, and some kind of alpha control used for multiple tests? This area can benefit from multimodal measurement, but only if the measures are handled correctly in data analysis.

Extensions from Past Research

There is a tradition in this area for field research, and on-site testing of children actually experiencing pain is a vitally important part of understanding pediatric pain. On the other hand, this review has described a variety of laboratory studies with methods relevant to the study of children's pain. A combination of these approaches may be valuable for future research.

The past emphasis both in classical developmental psychology and in the study of children's pain has been on child-based factors, primarily on cognitive factors. These can continue to be explored profitably, as this subarea is still in its infancy. However, it is important to extend the focus to affective and physical components as well, for a more holistic approach to understanding pain in children.

Similarly, there are few studies examining the role of the caregiver and the entire family in influencing children's responses to pain and the area will be much enriched if these themes are explored in further research. In addition, it may be useful in the future to consider peer models, community and school influence, and even to study the impact of United States cultures on children's perception of pain. Each level of analysis would seem to have its own unique contribution.

Conclusions

This presentation has merely sampled from the content and methodological contributions that developmental psychology can make to the study of children's pain. Because this is such a new area, with the parameters still undefined, it is particularly important to continue to examine the applicability of existing findings and research methods to understanding pain in children. There are many difficulties with investigating this subjective, internal phenomenon, particularly on a developing cognitive, affective, and social background. However, many potent tools are available and many important questions have already been posed. As the remainder of this book will demonstrate, some significant answers are already flowing in. In addition, we believe the coming decade can produce a flood of knowledge on pediatric pain, where so little understanding currently exists.

References

Abu-Saad, H. (1984). Cultural group indicators of pain in children. *Maternal-Child Nursing Journal, 13*, 181–196.

Adams, R. D., & Victor, M. (1985). *Principles of neurology* (3rd ed.). New York: McGraw-Hill.

Ainsworth, M., Blehar, M., Waters, E., & Walls, S. (1978). *Patterns of attachment.* Hillsdale, NJ: Erlbaum.

Anand, K. J. S., Phil, D., & Hickey, P. R. (1987). Pain and its effects in the human neonate and fetus. *New England Journal of Medicine, 317*, 1321–1329.

Auerbach, S. M. (1973). Trait-state anxiety and adjustment to surgery. *Journal of Consulting and Clinical Psychology, 40*, 264–271.

Bartlett, J. C., & Santrock, J. (1982). Emotional mood and memory in young children. *Journal of Experimental Child Psychology, 34*, 59–76.

Beyer, J. E., DeGood, D. E., Ashley, L. C., & Russell, G. (1983). Patterns of postoperative analgesic use with adults and children following cardiac surgery. *Pain, 17*, 71–81.

Bibace, R., & Walsh, M. E. (1980). Development of children's concepts of illness. *Pediatrics, 66*, 912–917.

Burbach, D., & Peterson, L. (1986). Children's concepts of physical illness: A review and critique of the cognitive developmental literature. *Health Psychology, 15*, 307–325.

Bush, J. P., Melamed, B. G., Sheras, P. L., & Greenbaum, P. E. (1986). Mother-child patterns of coping with anticipatory medical stress. *Health Psychology, 5*, 137–157.

Campos, J. J., Barrett, K. C., Lamb, M. E., Goldsmith, H. H., & Stenberg, C. (1983). Socioemotional development. In M. M. Haith & J. J. Campos (Eds.), *Handbook of child psychology. Vol. 2: Infancy and developmental psychobiology* (4th ed., pp. 783–915). New York: Wiley.

Carey, S. S. (1978). The child as word learner. In M. Halle, J. Bresnan, & G. A. Miller (Eds.), *Linguistic theory and psychological reality* (pp. 264–293). Cambridge, MA: MIT Press.

Chaney, J. M., & Peterson, L. (1989). Family variables and disease management in juvenile rheumatoid arthritis. *Journal of Pediatric Psychology, 14*, 389–403.

Cicchetti, D., & Hesse, P. (1982). *Emotional development*. San Francisco, CA: Jossey-Bass.

Clark, E. V. (1973). What is in a word? On the child's acquisition of semantics in his first language. In T. E. Moore (Ed.), *Cognitive development and the acquisition of language* (pp. 27–62). New York: Academic Press.

Edwards, P. W., Zeichner, A., Kuczmierczyk, A. R., & Boczkowski, J. (1985). Familial pain models: The relationship between family history of pain and current pain experience. *Pain, 21*, 379–384.

Eland, J. (1986). Management of pain. In M. J. Hockenberry & D. K. Coody (Eds.), *Pediatric oncology and hematology: Perspectives on care* (pp. 394–406). St. Louis, MO: C. V. Mosby.

Eland, J. M., & Anderson, J. E. (1977). The experience of pain in children. In A. K. Jacox (Ed.), *Pain: A source book for nurses and other health professionals* (pp. 453–473). Boston: Little, Brown.

Erikson, E. (1959). *Identity and the life cycle*. New York: Norton.

Field, T., & Fogel, A. (Eds.). (1982). *Emotion and early interaction*. Hillsdale, NJ: Erlbaum.

Fordyce, W. E., Roberts, A. H., & Sternbach, R. A. (1985). The behavioral management of chronic pain: A response to critics. *Pain, 22*, 113–125.

Fordyce, W. E., & Steger, J. C. (1979). Chronic pain. In O. Pomerleau & J. Brady (Eds.), *Behavioral medicine: Theory and practice* (pp. 125–153). Baltimore: Williams & Wilkins.

Gaensbauer, T. J., Harmon, R. J., Cytryn, L., & McKnew, D. H. (1984). Social and affective development in children with manic-depressive parents. *American Journal of Psychiatry, 141*, 223–229.

Gaffney, A., & Dunne, E. A. (1986). Developmental aspects of children's definitions of pain. *Pain, 26*, 105–117.

Garmezy, N., & Rutter, M. (Eds.). (1988). *Stress, coping and development in children*. Baltimore: Johns Hopkins University Press.

Gelfand, D. M., & Peterson, L. (1985). *Child development and psychopathology*. Beverly Hills, CA: Sage.

Graham, S., & Weiner, B. (1986). From attributional theory of emotion to developmental psychology: A round trip ticket? *Social Cognition, 4*, 152–179.

Gross, A. M., Stern, R. M., Levin, R. B., Dale, J., & Wojnilower, D. A. (1983). The effect of mother-child separation on the behavior of children experiencing a diagnostic medical procedure. *Journal of Consulting and Clinical Psychology, 51*, 783–785.

Hanson, C. L., Henggeler, S. W., Harris, M. A., Burghen, G. A., & Moore, M. (1989). Family systems variables and the health status of adolescents with insulin dependent diabetes mellitus. *Health Psychology, 8*, 239–253.

Harbeck, C., & Peterson, L. (1988, April). Children's understanding of specific pains. Presented at the Florida Conference on Child Health Psychology, Gainesville, FL.

Harbeck, C., & Peterson, L. (in press). "Elephants dancing in my head": Children's perceptions of specific pains. *Child Development*.

Harris, P. (1985). What children know about the situations that provoke emotion. In

M. Lewis & C. Saarni (Eds.), *The socialization of emotions* (pp. 161–185). New York: Plenum.

Haslam, D. (1969). Age and the perception of pain. *Psychonomic Science, 15,* 86–87.

Hodges, K., Kline, J. J., Barbero, G., & Flanery, R. (1984). Life events occurring in families of children with recurrent abdominal pain. *Journal of Psychonomic Research, 28,* 185–188.

Holden, E. W., Friend, M., Gault, C., Kager, V., Foltz, L., & White, L. (1991). Family functioning and parental coping with chronic childhood illness: Relationships with self-competence, illness adjustment and regimen adherence behaviors in children attending diabetes summer camp. In J. H. Johnson & S. B. Johnson (Eds.), *Advances in child health psychology: Proceedings of the Florida conference* (pp. 265–276). Gainesville, FL: University of Florida Press.

Hughes, M. C., & Zimin, R. (1978). Children with psychogenic abdominal pain and their families: Management during hospitalization. *Clinical Pediatrics, 17,* 569–573.

Janis, I. L. (1958). *Psychological stress.* New York: Wiley.

Johnson, S. B. (1988). Chronic illness and pain. In E. J. Mash & L. G. Terdal (Eds.), *Behavioral assessment of childhood disorders* (pp. 491–527). New York: Guilford.

Kandel, E. R., & Schwartz, J. H. (1985). *Principles of neural science* (2nd ed.). New York: Elsevier.

Kay, P., & Kempton, W. (1984). What is the Sapir-Whorf hypothesis? *American Anthropologist, 86,* 65–79.

Kelley, M. L., Jarvie, G. J., Middlebrook, J. L., McNeer, M. F., & Drabman, R. S. (1984). Decreasing burned children's pain behavior: Impacting the trauma of hydrotherapy. *Journal of Applied Behavior Analysis, 17,* 147–158.

Kuttner, L., Bowman, M., & Teasdale, M. (1988). Psychological treatment of distress, pain and anxiety for young children with cancer. *Journal of Developmental and Behavioral Pediatrics, 9,* 374–381.

Lazarus, R. S., & Launier, R. (1978). Stress-related transactions between person and environment. In L. A. Pervin & M. Lewis (Eds.), *Perspectives in interactional psychology* (pp. 287–326). New York: Plenum.

Lewis, M., & Michalson, L. (1983). *Children's emotions and moods: Developmental theory and measurement.* New York: Plenum.

Lewis, M., & Saarni, C. (1985). Culture and emotions. In M. Lewis & C. Saarni (Eds.), *The socialization of emotions* (pp. 1–17). New York: Plenum.

Linneweh, F. (1968). *Fortschrifte der paedologie* (Vol. 2). Berlin: Springer-Verlag.

Lollar, D. J., Smits, S. J., & Patterson, D. L. (1982). Assessment of pediatric pain: An empirical perspective. *Journal of Pediatric Psychology, 7,* 267–277.

Mash, E. J., & Terdal, L. G. (Eds.). (1988). *Behavioral assessment of childhood disorders.* New York: Guilford.

McGraw, M. (1943). *The neuromuscular maturation of the human infant.* New York: Columbia University Press.

McGraw, M. (1963). *The neuromuscular maturation of the human infant.* New York: Harper.

Mechanic, D. (1964). The influence of mothers on their children's health attitudes and behavior. *Pediatrics, 33,* 444–453.

Melamed, B. G. (1982). Reduction of medical fears: An information processing analysis. In J. Boulougouris (Ed.), *Learning theory approaches to psychiatry* (pp. 205–218). New York: Wiley.

Melamed, B. G., Dearborn, M., & Hermecz, D. A. (1983). Necessary considerations for surgery preparation: Age and previous experience. *Psychosomatic Medicine, 45*, 517–525.

Melamed, B. G., & Siegel, L. J. (1975). Reduction of anxiety in children facing hospitalization and surgery by use of filmed modeling. *Journal of Consulting and Clinical Psychology, 43*, 511–521.

Melzack, R., & Torgerson, W. S. (1971). On the language of pain. *Anesthesiology, 34*, 50–59.

Minuchin, S., Rosman, B., & Baker, L. (1978). *Psychosomatic families*. Cambridge, MA: Harvard University Press.

Moore, K. A., Miller, M. L., Weinstein, D., Dworkin, S. F., & Liou, H. H. (1987). Cultural pain perceptions and pain coping preferences among patients and dentists. *Proceedings of the Fifth World Congress on Pain of the International Association for the Study of Pain, 4*, 5351.

Myers, N., & Perlmutter, M. (1978). Memory in the years from 2 to 5. In P. Ornstein (Ed.), *Memory development in children*. Hillsdale, NJ: Erlbaum.

Nagy, M. H. (1951). Children's idea of the origin of illness. *Health Education Journal, 9*, 6–12.

Nannis, E. D., & Cowan, P. A. (1987). Emotional understanding: A matter of age, dimension, and point of view. *Journal of Applied Developmental Psychology, 8*, 289–304.

Natapoff, J. (1978). Children's view of health: A developmental study. *American Journal of Public Health, 68*, 995–1000.

Nelson, K. (1986). *Event knowledge*. Hillsdale, NJ: Erlbaum.

Nelson, K., & Brown, A. L. (1978). The semantic-episodic distinction in memory development. In P. A. Ornstein (Ed.), *Memory development in children* (pp. 233–241). Hillsdale, NJ: Erlbaum.

Neuhauser, C., Amsterdam, B., Hines, P., & Steward, M. (1978). Children's concepts of healing: Cognitive development and locus of control factors. *American Journal of Orthopsychiatry, 48*, 335–341.

Olson, D., Sprenkle, D., & Russell, C. (1979). Circumplex model of marital and family systems: I. Cohesion and adaptability dimensions, family types, and clinical applications. *Family Process, 18*, 3–28.

Ornstein, P. A., Gordon, B. N., & Larus, D. M. D. (in press). Children's memory for a personally experienced event: Implications for testimony. *Applied Cognitive Psychology*.

Owens, M. E. (1984). Pain in infancy: Conceptual and methodological issues. *Pain, 20*, 213–230.

Parmelee, A. H., Jr. (1986). Children's illnesses: Their beneficial effects on behavioral development. *Child Development, 57*, 1–10.

Perrin, E., & Gerrity, P. S. (1981). There's a demon in your belly: Children's understanding of illness. *Pediatrics, 67*, 841–849.

Peterson, L. (1989). Coping by children undergoing stressful medical procedures: Some conceptual, methodological, and therapeutic issues. *Journal of Consulting and Clinical Psychology, 57*, 380–387.

Peterson, L., & Harbeck, C. (1988). *The pediatric psychologist: Issues in professional development and practice*. Champaign, IL: Research Press.

Peterson, L., Harbeck, C., Chaney, J., Farmer, J., & Thomas, A. (1990). Children's coping with medical procedures: A conceptual overview and integration. *Behavioral Assessment, 12*, 197–212.

Peterson, L., & Mori, L. (1987). Multimodal behavioral assessment of children in stressful medical settings. In R. Prinz (Ed.), *Advances in behavioral assessment of children and families* (pp. 35–36). Greenwich, CT: JAI.

Peterson, L., & Shigetomi, C. (1981). The use of coping techniques to minimize anxiety in hospitalized children. *Behavior Therapy, 12*, 1–14.

Piaget, J. (1970). Piaget's theory. In P. E. Mussen (Ed.), *Carmichael's manual of child psychology* (Vol. 1, 3rd ed., pp. 703–732). New York: Wiley.

Piers, M. W., & Curry, N. E. (1985). A developmental perspective on children's affects. *Journal of Children in Contemporary Society, 17*, 23–35.

Poster, E. C. (1983). Stress immunization: Techniques to help children cope with hospitalization. *Maternal-Child Nursing Journal, 12*, 119–134.

Potter, P. C., & Roberts, M. C. (1984). Children's perceptions of chronic illness: The roles of disease symptoms, cognitive development and information. *Journal of Pediatric Psychology, 6*, 275–292.

Radke-Yarrow, M., Cummings, E. M., Kucynski, L., & Chapman, M. (1985). Patterns of attachment in two- and three-year-olds in normal families with parental depression. *Child Development, 56*, 884–893.

Roberts, M. C. (1986). *Pediatric psychology: Psychological interventions and strategies for pediatric problems*. New York: Pergamon.

Ross, D. M., & Ross, S. A. (1984a). Childhood pain: The school-aged child's viewpoint. *Pain, 20*, 179–191.

Ross, D. M., & Ross, S. A. (1984b). The importance of type of question, psychological climate, and subject set in interviewing children about pain. *Pain, 19*, 71–79.

Routh, D. K., & Ernst, A. R. (1984). Somatization disorder in relatives of children and adolescents with functional abdominal pain. *Journal of Pediatric Psychology, 9*, 427–437.

Rowland, L. P. (1984). *Merritt's textbook of neurology* (7th ed.). Philadelphia: Lea and Febinger.

Saarni, C. (1979). Children's understanding of display rules for expressive behavior. *Developmental Psychology, 15*, 424–429.

Savedra, M., Gibbons, P., Tesler, M., Ward, J., & Wegner, D. (1982). How do children describe pain? A tentative assessment. *Pain, 14*, 95–104.

Schulte, F. J. (1975). Neurophysiological aspects of brain development. *Mead Johnson Symposium on Perinatal and Developmental Medicine, 6*, 38–47.

Scott, R. (1978). "It hurts red." A preliminary study of children's perception of pain. *Perceptual and Motor Skills, 47*, 787–791.

Shaw, E. G., & Routh, D. K. (1982). Effect of mother presence on children's reaction to adverse procedures. *Journal of Pediatric Psychology, 7*, 33–42.

Shearer, M. H. (1986). Surgery on the paralyzed, unanesthetized newborn. *Birth, 13*, 79.

Siegel, L. J. (1988). Dental treatment. In D. K. Routh (Ed.), *Handbook of pediatric psychology* (pp. 448–459). New York: Guilford.

Siegel, L. J., & Peterson, L. (1980). Stress reduction in young dental patients through coping skills and sensory information. *Journal of Consulting and Clinical Psychology, 48*, 785–787.

Smith, M. E. (1926). An investigation of the development of the sentence and the extent of vocabulary in young children. *University of Iowa Studies in Child Welfare*, *3*, No. 5.

Strayer, J. (1985). Current research in affective development. *Journal of Children in Contemporary Society*, *17*, 37–55.

Tuma, J. M. (1975). Pediatric psychology? . . . Do you mean clincial child psychology? *Journal of Clinical Child Psychology*, *4*, 9–12.

Turkat, I. D., Kuczmierczyk, A. R., & Adams, H. E. (1984). An investigation of the etiology of chronic headache: The role of headache models. *British Journal of Psychiatry*, *145*, 665–666.

Unruh, A., McGrath, P. J., Cunningham, S. J., & Humphreys, P. (1983). Children's drawings of their pain. *Pain*, *17*, 385–392.

Varni, J. W. (1983). *Clinical behavioral pediatrics: An interdisciplinary biobehavioral approach*. New York: Pergamon.

Varni, J. W., Katz, E. R., & Dash, J. (1982). Behavioral and neurochemical aspects of pediatric pain. In D. C. Russo & J. W. Varni (Eds.), *Behavioral pediatrics: Research and practice* (pp. 117–224). New York: Plenum.

Violon, A., & Giurgea, D. (1984). Familial models for chronic pain. *Pain*, *18*, 199–203.

Wall, P., & Melzack, R. (Eds.). (1984). *Textbook of pain* (1st ed.). London: Churchill Livingstone.

Wall, P., & Melzack, R. (Eds.). (1989). *Textbook of pain* (2nd ed.). London: Churchill Livingstone.

Wallerstein, E. (1985). Circumcision: The uniquely American medical enigma. *Urology Clinics of North America*, *12*, 123–132.

Williams, J. M. G., Murray, J. J., Lund, C. A., Harkiss, B., & DeFranco, A. (1985). Anxiety in the child dental clinic. *Journal of Child Psychology and Psychiatry*, *26*, 305–310.

Zahn-Waxler, C., Cummings, E. M., McKnew, D. H., & Radke-Yarrow, M. (1984). Affective arousal and social interactions in young children of manic-depressive parents. *Child Development*, *55*, 112–122.

3
Assessment of Pediatric Pain

PAUL KAROLY

The assessment of pediatric pain is, paradoxically, one of the most complex and one of the simplest acts a health professional can perform. The physician suturing a wound, for example, can readily observe the physical damage, can hear the child's cries as the procedure ensues (even after an anesthetic has been administered), or can feel the tension in the child's limbs should the hurt youngster elect to remain silent. "It'll be over soon," is a familiar utterance by the doctor, nurse, or parent who unerringly senses that he or she is in the presence of suffering. Therefore, asking the child how much she hurts appears to be as unnecessary as it is unkind.

On the other hand, there are those who endeavor to understand the nature and meaning of children's nociceptive experiences, who monitor/evaluate the effects of surgical or pharmacological pain treatments, or whose job involves predicting the degree of psychopathology likely to attend chronic illness or children's exposure to invasive therapies. These health professionals are extremely interested in and dependent upon metrically sound, reliable, and clinically sensitive methods for accessing and quantifying children's pain. This chapter, written for this second group of investigators, seeks to offer some small comfort in the face of a sobering reality: that as data rapidly accumulate in the field of pediatric algology, the task of relating new information to existing conceptual formulations (of pain) and to pressing clinical responsibilities seems to grow increasingly difficult.

Conceptual Underpinnings

Methods of pain assessment are derived, explicitly or implicitly, from models or conceptualizations of the fundamental nature of the pain experience. By far the most common organizing framework is *biomedical*, within which pain is defined as an unpleasant sensory reaction: to bodily events, usually trauma or tissue damage, to relatively stable pathophysiological conditions such as cancer, or to invasive medical or dental (diagnostic or treatment) procedures. Even this seemingly clean and uncluttered definition contains some perplexing elements — for example, the conjunction of pain as a sensation and as a by-product of that sensation, as an objectively definable occurrence and as a subjective judgment, and as an emotional response as well as a natural mode of adaptation (cf. Beyer & Knapp, 1986; Karoly, 1988; Melzack & Wall, 1983). Despite some inherent limitations, the biomedical definition has well served the hurt, injured, and diseased, guiding physicians and allied health professionals in their assessment and interventive efforts.

Nonetheless, children and adults may be better served by a more comprehensive model, one that *contextualizes* and *individualizes* the pain experience, that highlights *motivational* elements and their *developmental* origins, and that fully addresses the *social* as well as the *cognitive* nature of pain. A number of behavioral scientists have offered alternatives to the biomedical viewpoint (e.g., Keefe & Gil, 1986; Leventhal & Everhart, 1979; Melzack & Wall, 1983; Turk & Flor, 1987), adding individual facets to a one-dimensional framework, such that, today, the scientific study of pain — algology — is beginning to assume dynamic and multidimensional proportions. To illustrate the overall shape of the "new look" in pain analysis, I shall briefly describe the psychosocial elaboration model (PEM), a heuristic for systematically conceptualizing pain across a variety of relevant levels. Although not a consensus viewpoint, the PEM brings together a number of perspectives and fits within what Chapman (1989) calls the classical theory tradition of measurement. That is, from a classical viewpoint, measurement is always (a) context dependent, (b) based on latent and/or manifest variables, and (c) an ongoing process of modeling reality, rather than an effort to capture the "truth" and express it as a single score.

Psychosocial Elaboration Model (PEM)

Any symptom, including pain, is considered the product of interacting forces both within the person and in the external world. Any suprathreshold symptom capable of affecting adjustment is likely to produce one or more of six basic reactions: autonomic arousal, an emotional response (or responses), a communicative or expressive reaction, motor activity, efforts at understanding or justification ("Why is this happening to me?"), and efforts at symptom management. The individual need not be consciously aware of processing any of these six potential symptom sequelae. Further, the potency of any of these kinds of response will be a complex function of many variables, including aspects of the setting in which the symptom occurs and the individual's physiologically based (constitutionally determined) style of reactivity/sensitivity. In the setting, the presence (or absence) of other people, rules of conduct, models (exemplars) of how to act, and physical constraints upon action serve to set boundaries on how much emotion is displayed and whether symptoms are enacted or suppressed. Temperament likewise sets boundaries on symptom experience (e.g., someone with a low arousability threshold is more apt to become excited at the sensory level than is a high-threshold person). If a symptom is recurring, the repeated activation of one or more of the six reaction types will lead, over time, to the creation of a symptom "set point," categorical structure, or reference standard. The individual becomes selectively attuned to this standard (it becomes focal in the person's conscious experience when activated by contextual cues) and may develop a strong expectation that, all things being equal, this is the way he or she is usually going to feel. Finally, at an even higher level of processing, the individual develops an implicit theory relating the symptom, its precipitating conditions, and their adjustmental implications — a theory or mental model capable of flexibly influencing lower order reactions, including attention, perception, and problem solving (see Figure 3.1).

In contrast, the typical biomedical view of symptom experience takes into account the so-called precipitants and the sensory-perceptual response. Research emanating from this model has sought to identify the conditions under which specific precipitants evoke specific sensations and the interventions (surgical or pharmacologic) that might alter these connections. As obviously useful as this perspective has been (and continues to be), it essentially ignores the right side of the elaboration model (postperceptual processing) and offers little guidance to the clinician who has exhausted all tissue-centered modes of diagnosis and remains uninformed about a particular patient's habits of symptom presentation (a frequent occurrence).

Why might a child's symptoms worsen as she gets older and the physical condition is presumably improving? Why might a child in a family with somatizing parents display more severe symptoms than one with a similar disorder reared in a "healthy" family environment? Why do chronic pain problems improve in the summer and flare up again as the new school year approaches? It is toward the resolution of such questions as these that the PEM is directed. It is in these areas that the traditional sensory view of pain reaches the limits of its analytic power.

Among the most desirable features of an elaborated view of pain-related symptoms are the following:

1. Developmental Relevance. Neonates, toddlers, children, and adolescents experience pain, although their ability to invest the experience with personal meaning varies (cf. Schechter, 1985). Accepting the basic premise of the gate-control and other modern theories of pain, that central modulation of nociceptive experience is possible, investigators must begin to systematically assess age- and experience-based differences in symptom processing. Although not a theory of development, the PEM nonetheless serves to delineate areas of potential importance, such as children's evolving capacities to store and retrieve information, to conceptualize bodily functions (their causes and consequences), to formulate plans and goals, and to self-regulate affect, attention, and instrumental behavior.

62

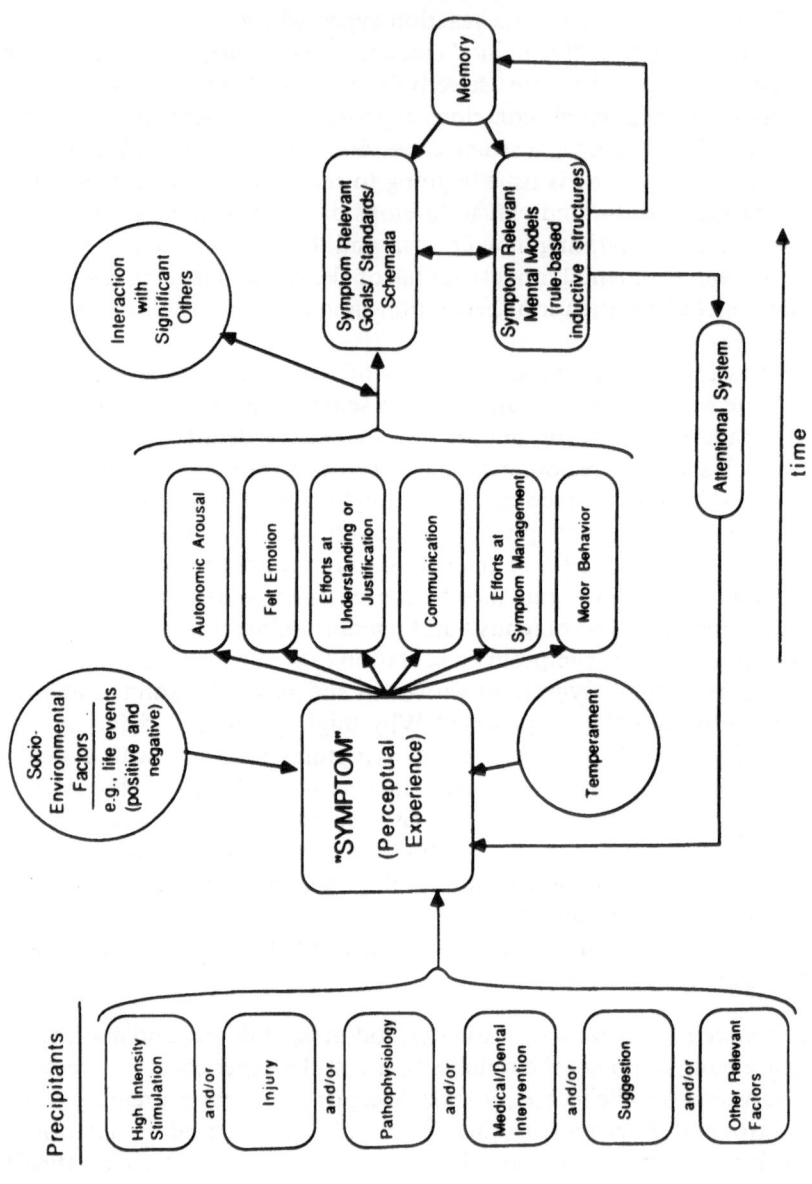

FIGURE 3.1. The psychosocial elaboration model (PEM) of symptom experience.

2. Ecological Relevance. Although biology and disease parameters provide an important context for pain and symptom experience, so too does the family environment (Turk, Flor, & Rudy, 1987), the health care system (McGrath & deVeber, 1986), the school (Isaacs & McElroy, 1980), and the peer group (Sigelman & Begley, 1987). The PEM acknowledges socioenvironmental forces and the link between persons and their contexts that extends over time (Bolger, Caspi, Downey, & Moorehouse, 1988).

3. Motivational Relevance. The traditional definition of acute or chronic pain as unpleasant feeling states establishes escape or avoidance as principal motivational constructs. Indeed, prolonged pain in combination with failed attempts at escape or avoidance can be expected to lay the groundwork for eventual interpersonal and intrapsychic disruption (psychopathology). The PEM enlarges the scope of clinical analysis by noting the cognitive, "sensemaking" activities of the pain patient and the relation between pain cognitions and broader aspects of self-knowledge and personal goals. The juvenile arthritic, for example, may not only work hard to minimize her physical discomfort but also to prove to significant others that she can achieve academically, socially, and physically. Thus, the PEM would extend motivational assessment questions from an exclusive focus on modes of avoidance to an equal concern with *approach tendencies* (goal-directed) in children and the relation of these tendencies to long-term patterns of adjustment (cf. also Karoly & Jensen, 1987). However, it is important to note that *cognitive avoidance* strategies (such as distraction, use of fantasy, reinterpretation of sensations, and the like) may operate in the service of long- or short-term adjustment or symptom management, and thus may be labeled *coping* mechanisms (cf. Siegel, 1988).

The Assessment Model

Having argued that a symptom such as pain is not simply a sensory event, but a *psychosocial construction*,[1] it is necessary that a coherent framework be offered that can serve as a guide to specifying *why* certain aspects of the pain experience should be targeted for measurement and *how* that measurement can best be accomplished. Although, from a logical point of view, knowing what and why to assess should precede the selection of measurement devices, in actual practice the clinician is often restrictively guided by

---

[1]Other more precise ways exist for describing a recurrent symptom. However, the terminology soon becomes cumbersome. For example, a symptom is a cognitive representation that is influenced by current interpersonal events as well as by the individual's accumulated experiences. Therefore, although it would be more accurate to describe chronic pain as an "historically embedded, socially negotiated cognitive representation", the term *psychosocial construction* is a bit more maneuverable.

his or her training experiences, special interests, and/or by the ready availability of certain measurement instruments. Despite its widespread occurrence, this tail-wagging-the-dog phenomenon should be strenuously avoided.

Because pain may be assessed at different levels and in varying contexts, it is incumbent upon the assessor to be aware of the doors that are being simultaneously opened and closed when a particular avenue of assessment is pursued. For example, consider the clinician who conducts relaxation training with children to help them prepare for bone marrow aspiration procedures. Do the relaxation treatments affect perceived pain? To address this question, the clinician plans to ask children to complete visual analogue scales of pain intensity prior to the formal introduction of therapy and at the end of training. If significant reductions in rated intensity are recorded pre- and postintervention, the assessor will conclude that a useful therapeutic regimen had been employed.

Why was pain assessed only twice? Couldn't repeated measures have been taken during the bone marrow aspiration procedure? Why was intensity of pain the sole index of the child's nociceptive experience? Couldn't relaxation have affected the discomfort threshold or pain duration as well as or instead of intensity? Why were self-reports employed rather than direct behavioral observations? Questions such as these should be thought through prior to the mounting of any assessment program. What follows is a scheme for explicitly considering what are, too often, implicit decisions in pain assessment. The multidimensional assessment frame (MAF), as I call it, like Cattell's (1988) "Data Box," should serve as a check on whether an investigator's procedures match his conceptual intent.

Multidimensional Assessment Frame (MAF)

The clinician is advised to consider the following seven dimensions when planning an assessment program:

1. The Contexts of Measurement. Whenever pain is displayed (in whatever form) it is best considered a "message" with a recipient who is primed to interpret it in accordance with some preexisting theoretical or pretheoretical framework. An interpretative context can be associated with a fundamental organizing question. For example, within what has been dubbed context I, the "biomedical context," the basic question is, Why does this patient hurt? (cf. Karoly & Jensen, 1987). It leads to the conduct of a health history and physical examination, along with laboratory tests designed to assist in the formulation of a medical diagnosis. If, on the other hand, one wishes to understand better how the patient is currently acting and feeling, the interpretative context is distinct from, although related to, the biomedical. This second investigative stance is called the "focal/experiential context," and is associated with a different set of information-collection strategies directed at clarifying the sensory-perceptual, emotional, motoric, social, expressive, and cognitive attributes that jointly comprise the child's experience of hurt and suffering (Melzack & Wall, 1983; Schechter, 1985). This stance (context II) is the traditional province of social and behavioral science. Finally, a third mode of approach to pain is termed the "meaning/relational context," and addresses, along several key dimensions, the question, What difference does the pain make? The assessor working out of context III doesn't only view a child's pain as cancer-caused or as extremely intense with an overlay of anger and depression (although these are useful avenues of description), but rather as a set of reaction tendencies that can influence and be influenced by motivation (to go to school or to perform physical therapy exercises), psychological adjustment, family dynamics, self-perception, problem-solving, and the like. Clearly, a systematic pain assessment program requires that all three interpretative frameworks be adopted (cf. Karoly & Jensen, 1987, for a more complete discussion of the multiple assessment contexts).

2. Assessment Foci. Having assumed an interpretative mindset, the clinician must still decide which attribute(s) to examine. Within context II, for example, one can elect to study psychophysiologic correlates of arousal, instrumental pain behaviors, or subjective self-appraisals. In a context III analysis of pain's effect upon school performance, the focus could be upon grades, teachers' reports, or peer opinions of a target child's popularity. The selection of foci of assessment is dictated usually by the constraints of the setting, the expense of the assessment or its logistic complexity, issues relating to informed consent and ethical standards, professional expertise, and one's theoretical leanings. Although I offer no rules of thumb about how to focus within a particular assessment context, I caution assessors against a "standard battery" of tests to be used in all situations. Unless such a battery is comprehensive, touching all possible analytic bases, it is bound to omit some dimensions whose inclusion is dictated by the assessor's organizing question(s).

3. Time Frame. Measures of pain can be taken on a relatively frequent basis over the course of diagnosis, treatment, and/or follow-up or they can be intermittent. Even when obtained over multiple testing occasions, measures can either be aggregated or their temporal patterns can be preserved in a time series fashion. Summary approaches are generally best if the purpose is descriptive, whereas a "process analysis" usually calls for the tracking of pain reactions in real time and over extended periods of observation. If a process question is raised (e.g., How do youngsters cope with pain?), a pre-post change score type of analysis cannot provide a very useful answer.

4. Situational Frame. Pain is often assessed where it happens and often it is measured at times and in places "convenient" for the patient or clinician. One's situational frame should not be left to chance, however. Chronic pain in particular may not be as "portable" as acute pain; and the selection of an assessment site can substantively influence the generalizability of one's conclusions. For example, if a clinician needs an index of pain intensity to help determine analgesic dosage level, then the intensity measure should be simple and short enough to be administered in the setting where pain is occurring, e.g., in bed, on the ward, in the playroom, etc. Complex projective measures of intensity are often administered at times and places far removed from the actual pain experience, and, thus, are unlikely to assist physicians or nurses in drug level determinations.

5. Data Collection Strategy. Assuming the appropriate time, place, and pain attributes are decided upon, the assessor still has a wide choice of information sources from which to draw. These include the "medical" strategies of physical examination and physiochemical analysis as well as broader, social science methods such as standardized psychometric tests, self-reports of illness and health patterns, key informant reports, direct observations of behavior, physiologic and telemetric monitoring, structured interviews, projective tests, the analysis of archival records, and epidemiologic surveys (Karoly, 1985a). A richer portrait of the child's pain experience generally emerges when more than one strategy is employed; yet multimethod assessment is also costly, time-consuming, and subject to internal inconsistencies (Karoly & Jensen, 1987). As shall be demonstrated later in this chapter, assessment operations usually possess a strong degree of domain specificity, each one especially useful in addressing a particular class of diagnostic questions. Again, the assessor is advised to select methods on a case by case basis rather than relying upon habit or mere convenience.

6. Psychometric Model. Because the assessment process always involves implicit assumptions about the *what* and *why* of measurement that undergird the selection of specific strategies, the clinician is committed to a psychometric model whether he or she is cognizant of it or not. For example, viewing pain as a sensory event pledges one to some variant of a *signal detection* approach to scaling. Pain intensity becomes a magnitude estimate or discriminative response that can be more or less accurate depending upon the strength of the sensory signal, an individual's sensitivity to stimulation, and a subjective judgment rule (cf. Dember & Warm, 1979; Karoly, 1985b). A cognitive-behavioral pain model, such as reflected in the PEM, on the other hand, implies that pain is a theoretical construct or *latent variable* to be inferred on the basis of relationships among manifest indicators (cf. Hayduk, 1987). To date, most empirical investigations of pain as a latent construct have relied upon factor analytic or regression analyses. However, as Rudy (1989) has pointed out, structural equation modeling holds considerable promise as a means of testing the goodness-of-fit between pain data and complex descriptive approaches (such as the PEM). So-called bias free and sample-independent methods associated with latent trait theory (item response theory) may also prove to be useful psychometric paradigms for the pain assessor (Rudy, 1989).

7. Corollary (Relational) Assessment. The reader will recall that the first MAF dimension highlighted three interpretative "contexts," the last of which involved indexing various pain attributes to outcomes such as mental health, social relationships, scholastic goals, and the like. The assessor is here reminded that careful attention should be paid to determining the nature of these corollary targets. Developmental factors such as the level of cognitive skills, family constellation, and physical maturity are relevant to the selection of these so-called meaning dimensions.

Review of Measurement Strategies in Pediatric Pain

Having addressed the *what, where,* and *why* of pain assessment, it is now time to turn to pragmatic considerations — the *how*(s). Despite differences in the systems by which pain measures are classified, most authors agree that methods for assessing pain in children should include direct and indirect; body-centered, intrapsychic, and social; and objective and subjective — all having to demonstrate adequate reliability, validity, and versatility to insure their inclusion in the arsenal of the pediatric pain specialist (McGrath, 1987a; Owens, 1984; Turk & Flor, 1987).

I shall selectively review assessment strategies under eight general headings, illustrating in particular how the modalities of measurement relate to the key organizing questions of contexts I, II, and III (see above).

1. Interview Methods. Since clinical judgment is a commodity with fluctuating market value, the clinical interview seems to move in and out of favor, at least in the empirical literature. Also, because pain patients, young and old, tend to be demanding, impatient, and sometimes disrespectful of authority, the appeal of paper-and-pencil approaches is often magnified. However, notwithstanding their disadvantages, interviews with children in pain provide a flexible diagnostic method, uniquely suited for clarifying information obtained from other sources, for probing beyond children's concrete responses, and for alleviating children's situational discomfort so as to encourage honest and uncensored answers. Further, *feedback interviews* serve to provide didactic and therapeutic information to children and their parents. Hence, there is no substitute for face-to-face data collection/ dissemination.

Interviews can be conducted on an unstructured, semistructured, or structured basis, with the latter two types preferred for psychometric reasons. To date, structured (all questions fixed) and semistructured (some questions fixed) interviews have been developed to gauge children's sensory and emotional experiences, their interpretations of the causes and consequences of pain, their use of coping maneuvers, and their characteristic ways of expressing pain verbally and motorically (e.g., Abu-Saad, 1984a; McGrath, 1987b; Perrin & Gerrity, 1981; Ross & Ross, 1984).

As suggested by the PEM, interviews with children in pain should not be confined to the collection of pain-specific information. Family history data, information on current situational influences on adjustment and on the presence of nonpain symptoms, should be obtained as well, in order to contextualize the child's complaint. Structured interviews (of children and/ or their parents) have been employed, for example, to explore the role of social modeling on unexplained pain (Osborne, Hatcher, & Richtsmeier, 1989) and to determine the relation between "functional" abdominal pain and patterns of somatization in first- and second-degree relatives (Routh & Ernst, 1984).

When youngsters and their parents are both interviewed, the data often fail to converge, leading to the wholly unjustified practice of restricting the data collection to parents or other caretakers. Certain types of context II information (concerning experiential attributes of pain) simply cannot logically be obtained from informants, no matter how close they are to the child in pain. Furthermore, beliefs about the excessive unreliability of children as reporters of their bodily states are not well grounded, and may reflect a reluctance on the part of clinicians to deal with the admittedly difficult task of interviewing children. As far as the discordance between adult and child reports is concerned, it is best seen as a function of differential epistemic vantage points (Achenbach, McConaughy, & Howell, 1987).

Unfortunately, some of the mechanisms relevant to pain adaptation that are inaccessible to key informants may be just as inaccessible to children, at least through direct questioning. As I have previously noted:

. . . many of the most salient aspects of pain processing may be automatic, implicit, or beyond the child's normal self-monitoring capabilities. Thus, whether a child doesn't know, doesn't notice, or knows differently (compared to other sources of information) is never easy to discern. (Karoly, 1988, p. 374)

I shall review (below) some techniques that are better equipped to obtain information on higher order forms of information processing than are structured and semistructured interviews.

2. Self-Report Methods. For the sake of convenience (speed and ease of administration), children's perceptions of their nociceptive experience — its immediate cues and consequences, its presumed mediators, and its impact on their lives in general — can be obtained via self-report scales and questionnaires. When such instruments are standardized and empirically validated, they provide an important source of clinical and research insight into the pain experience. Paper-and-pencil devices focus on single or multiple aspects of the sensory-perceptual facet of pain or upon elaborational (reactive) components, such as depression, anger, or coping style.

By a wide margin, self-reports have been concerned with reliably gauging *intensity*, as if this were the cardinal feature and the most clinically accessible aspect of pediatric pain (cf. Karoly, 1985a, 1988; McGrath, 1987b; Varni, Jay, Masek, & Thompson, 1986). Probably because making pain "hurt less" has been the prime objective of pharmacologic and surgical interventions, the intensity dimension has garnered the lion's share of psychometric attention. I shall, therefore, discuss pain intensity ratings first, even though (a) modern behavioral and cognitive intervention programs teach *living with* intense or frequent pain rather than pain intensity reduction, and (b) intensity may be only weakly related to indices of clinical pain adjustment (Jensen & Karoly, 1989).

Indices that are designed to be minimally reliant upon language are among the most popular rating scales for pediatric pain intensity.[2] Graded lines that quantify the amount of pain experienced, picture scales (e.g., with faces representing varying degrees of upset), or thermometers marked off by degrees of hurt are *discrete* numerical measures, whereas ungraded lines anchored by descriptions of *no pain* on one end to *severe pain* on the other can be seen as *continuous*.

An example of the former is a measure called the Oucher, designed to assess intensity of pain among children from 3 to 12 years of age (Beyer, 1984; Beyer & Aradine, 1986, 1987). Arguing that there is little evidence for the validity and reliability of other intensity measures, the developers of the Oucher mounted a two-dimensional assault on the problem: their instrument contains a 0 to 100 numerical scale (marked off in increments of 10) and a series of six photographs of a Caucasian preschooler ordered to display increasing levels of discomfort and indexed to the 0, 20, 40, 60, 80, and 100 points on the numerical scale. Children can select either the numerical scale (if they are able to count to 100) or the pictures to assist them in expressing their pain intensity. Children generally agree with the sequencing of the photographs, and the numerical and pictorial scales tend to correlate with each other when both are used.

Among the other popular indices of intensity are the visual analogue scale (a 10-cm line arranged horizontally or vertically, with verbal anchors on either end) and the Poker Chip Tool (Hester, 1979) in which different colored poker chips are used to express degree of hurt (e.g., one white chip equals "no hurt" and four red chips equals "the biggest hurt you could ever have"). Although the clinician benefits from the availability of alternate methods, with some more appealing to children than others, the empirical yield is less obvious. Are intensity measures reliable, particularly when employed by children under seven? Are these measures sensitive to interventions designed to alter pain intensity? And are the instruments cost-effective in terms of professional effort?

---

[2]So-called nonverbal tests for children three and younger do not, in fact, possess special qualities that allow them to be readily understood. The child must have a concept of number to employ numerical rating scales and a spatial awareness to use visual analogue scales. In addition, all tests make use of instructions by the examiner, even "nonverbal" devices. Thus, some language skills and a degree of social sensitivity are required on the part of the child. When youngsters are cognitively impaired, immature, unfriendly, or noncooperative, the assessor tends to rely upon *behavioral* indicators of pain.

Generally, the data seem to support the use of visual analogue or numerical rating scales for youngsters over five (Abu-Saad & Holzmer, 1981; McGrath, 1987a, 1987b). More complex and time-consuming methods for assessing intensity (such as projectives) do not appear warranted. And what of the two-dimensional Oucher? To their credit, the developers of the Oucher have sought to compare it to other measures in order to establish its "convergent and discriminant validity" (Beyer & Aradine, in press). As expected, the Oucher scales did not correlate with measures of fear (lending divergent validity) and did correlate strongly with the visual analogue and poker chip scales. But because so few subjects chose the picture scale, the Oucher's numerical rating scale appears the device of choice. However, given the ease of constructing a 0 to 100 rating scale, investigators need not use the Beyer-Aradine device at all. It is unfortunate that the Oucher's faces scale, designed to be used with children under five, has yet to be proven reliable, valid, or cost-effective. Indeed, its inclusion now confuses the assessment process, as it is not clear how much influence it has over the child's numerical ratings. Further, the pictures are of a Caucasian child. The development of black, Hispanic, Oriental, and other versions may take several years to complete. It is not clear to this reviewer that the continued search for a quantified pictorial index of intensity is justified, especially in view of the neglect of other experiential dimensions. Similarly, research on the use of *verbal* rating scales with children (9 and older) has not yet clearly established the incremental utility of this approach over simple and economical numerical rating and visual analogue scales (cf. Karoly, 1988; Savedra, Gibbons, Tesler, Ward, & Wegner, 1982).

Among the important, if relatively overlooked, aspects of the pain experience that require systematic assessment for purposes of treatment planning and evaluation are (a) coping activities, (b) nonpain symptoms, (c) temperament, and (d) the child's perception of stressful life events. Self-report methods can also be useful in tapping what I have called "corollary" pain-related outcomes, including mental health, self-esteem, scholastic performance, body awareness, social skills, and the like.

Multidimensional assessment devices have been expressly designed to contextualize a child's pain, and have included many, but by no means all of the experiential dimensions (in addition to intensity and frequency) and relational factors herein discussed. Among the multiple indicator and multiple dimension devices are: the Pediatric Pain Questionnaire (PPQ) (Tesler, Ward, Savedra, Wegner, & Gibbons, 1983), the Varni-Thompson Pediatric Pain Questionnaire (VT-PPQ: Thompson & Varni, 1986; Varni, Thompson, & Hanson, 1987; Walco & Varni in chapter 12), and the Children's Comprehensive Pain Questionnaire (CCPQ) (McGrath, 1987a, 1987b). The VT-PPQ and the CCPQ are being actively evaluated and refined, and are extremely promising instruments. The former, modeled after the well-known McGill Pain Questionnaire (Melzack, 1975), has available not only a child self-report form, but parent and adolescent forms as well. The child form addresses pain intensity and location as well as evaluative and affective components. The parent form asks about similar dimensions and includes a family health history and questions about socioenvironmental factors that may be influencing the child's pain. The VT-PPQ makes use of a variety of reporting formats — open and closed-ended questions, verbal, numerical, and pictorial ratings, color codings, and the like. A visual analogue scale for use by physicians or other health professionals is also included. The CCPQ is similarly extensive and multidimensional, including measures of coping, expectations of future pain relief, parents' ideas on pain causation, and parent and sibling reactions during the child's pain episodes.

3. Pain Diaries and Self-Monitoring Systems. Notwithstanding their descriptive and predictive value, retrospective reports by children and their caretakers are experiential summaries of the child's encounters with pain. Questionnaires and interviews can only indirectly tap pain's temporal flow and contextual embeddedness (the dynamics of the pain experience in real time). However, self-observation records attempt (albeit imperfectly) to capture the feelings, thoughts, and actions of the pediatric pain patient as they occur (or soon after they occur) as well as the environmental conditions within which pain/coping episodes are enacted. To be effective, self-monitoring needs to be carried out systematically and consistently; it is, clearly, *not* the assessment of choice for very young, preverbal children or for youngsters requiring extensive supervision.

Visual analogue scales, numerical and verbal rating scales, symptom checklists, and the like become self-monitoring instruments when utilized in vivo in accordance with predetermined schedules. Thus, it isn't the content of the devices that necessarily requires attention, but the manner in which they are used by children when direct, adult supervision is unavailable. The essential point to be made here is that this category of measurement often involves *extensive training of children* prior to and during the assessment period. Parental involvement in the training and subsequent utilization of self-monitoring by children is a helpful adjunct.

Another format for self-recording is the *pain diary*. Such an instrument usually contains familiar rating scales for pain intensity and related sensory features, for emotional reactions, for environmental events (pain triggers or pain inhibiting stimuli) as well as open-ended questions designed to assess unexpected or complex occurrences.

Although used more extensively with adults (see Karoly & Jensen, 1987), pain diaries have proven to be useful for children in third grade or higher. For example, Richardson, McGrath, Cunningham, and Humphreys (1983) asked children, aged 9 to 17, with migraine headaches to record headache intensity four times per day for a period of 4 weeks. Instructions, role playing, and feedback were used to teach diary-keeping to the children and a parent. In addition to intensity ratings, diary keepers noted symptoms (e.g., nausea, vomiting, dizziness, etc.), medication taken, and possible causes of the headache episode. Using the weighted kappa to determine parent-child concordance, the investigators found fair to high levels of agreement. In this instance, the type of pain being monitored (migraine) was associated with observable sequelae (such as vomiting and dizziness), permitting a reasonable degree of overlap between parent and child report. Such a finding would be less likely in the case of pain that is not so clearly linked to overt correlates, such as abdominal pain.

The self-assessment approach to pain measurement possesses great potential for illuminating the mechanisms involved in context III–type processes. However, much more work is needed in the design, refinement, and psychometric verification of self-monitoring devices before their clinical potential is realized.

4. Direct Observation Methods. The subjective distress of acute and chronic pain often finds avenues of expression in facial, verbal, and motor responses. Further, adaptive and maladaptive ways of coping with pain are readily indexed behaviorally, as in medication-taking, sleeping, exercising, academic/vocational activities, etc. Infants and young children in particular "show the world" their pain in a host of directly perceptible ways (Keefe & Gil, 1986). Of the various methods available for indexing overt pain expression (including global ratings by health professionals and archival data, such as school days missed) the use of trained observers who code and log ongoing activity for specified periods is among the most well researched, reliable, and popular.

Observational methods have generally been used to gather data on specific, treatment-related sorts of pain-distress reactions in infants (e.g., circumcision) or children (e.g., bone marrow aspiration, burn debridement, postoperative reactions, lumbar punctures, etc.). Coding systems typically focus upon children's pain and anxiety and related dysfunctional reaction tendencies rather than seeking to capture the full range of contextually relevant action and reaction.

Pediatric oncology has been the site of several well-known scale development programs. For example, the Procedure Behavioral Rating Scale (PBRS) was developed by Katz and his colleagues (Katz, Kellerman, & Siegel, 1980) to assess various categories of pain response to procedures such as the lumbar puncture and bone marrow aspiration. Observers noted the occurrence of 11 behaviors during three periods over the course of the procedure. The PBRS and its revised version have revealed important aspects of children's reactivity to procedural pain, such as age and sex differences.

Based in part on the PBRS, Jay and her associates (Jay, Ozolins, Elliott, & Caldwell, 1983) developed the Observational Scale of Behavioral Distress (OSBD). The OSBD permits continuous sampling throughout the painful medical procedure, with 15-second recording intervals. Eleven operationally defined behaviors are the subject of this instrument (including crying, screaming, muscular rigidity), with a weighting system based upon severity (e.g., screaming = 4.0, muscular rigidity = 2.5, and information seeking = 1.5). In a recent intervention study, Jay and her colleagues reported a between-observer reliability of .98 and interobserver agreements for each of the eleven behaviors ranging from 67 to 100%, with a mean of 84% (Jay, Elliott, Katz, & Siegel, 1987).

The Pain Behavior Checklist (PBCL) of LeBaron and Zeltzer (1984) utilizes an 8-category observation system, and allows the observer to code intensity levels for each action recorded (from 1, very mild to 5, extremely intense). Like the other two indices, the PBCL can be reliably applied and is correlated with children's self-ratings and with global pain ratings.

Postoperative pain is the target of the Children's Hospital of Eastern Ontario Pain Scale (CHEOPS) developed by P. J. McGrath and his colleagues (McGrath et al., 1985). Six behaviors are rated at 30-second intervals, with values assigned in accordance with judged pain severity. Preliminary data are encouraging, but more psychometric work is needed on this observational instrument.

Recently, the assessment focus has begun to widen in the behavior analysis realm, with investigators concerning themselves with positive or coping responses in addition to pain-distress reactions, and with the cuing and reinforcing role of adults (e.g., medical staff during acute pain episodes or parents in hospital-based or naturalistic exchanges with their chronically ill children). Blount and his colleagues (Blount, Corbin, Powers, Sturges, & Maieron, 1988; Blount et al., 1989; Blount, Corbin, & Wolfe, 1987) have sought to develop a measure that includes codes for children's distress, neutral and coping behaviors as well as for adult neutral, coping, and distress reactions. The careful measurement of coping is needed, they point out, not only because it supplies information about the neglected positive side of children's pain repertoires, but because it can assist clinicians in distinguishing between the absence of effective responding versus children's failure to emit coping behaviors at the proper time, place, rate, or manner (cf. Blount et al., 1988). Similarly, the role of adult responding prior to and during medical procedures and the reciprocal effect of children's distress upon adults' performance represents a long overdue context III perspective on pain, one capable of rendering our assessment programs truly "dynamic" in nature.

To accomplish their objectives, Blount and his colleagues constructed the Child-Adult Medical Procedure Interaction Scale (CAMPIS), containing 35 verbal content codes (19 for adults, 16 for the child), 16 child behavior codes (corresponding to their verbal codes) that include both distress-related actions (crying, screaming) and coping behaviors (humor, therapeutic breathing), a set of affect codes (e.g., neutral, positive, sad, whiny), and a set of codes for staff/parent behavior during the bone marrow aspiration or lumbar puncture procedures (e.g., reassuring comments, apologies, praise, commands to employ a coping strategy, etc.). Consistent with a perspective that views pain as an "emergent" rather than a fixed response to a specific level of neural stimulation, the recommended handling of CAMPIS data is via lag sequential analysis (Sackett, 1979).

Notwithstanding the considerable precision and theory-testing power associated with observational procedures, limitations need also to be considered. These methods have been largely restricted to assessments of procedural pain in the hospital setting. The behavior of children with acute pain when outside the hospital may differ dramatically from their responses when "under the knife." Further, their behavior while being operated upon might itself change as a function of time, personnel, and distal environmental forces. Certainly the behavior of youngsters with *chronic* pain conditions while at home, at play, and at school merits careful observational assessment as well. Finally, the limitations of the "pain as motor/verbal behavior" construct should be recognized. As noted by Turk and Flor (1987), cognitive appraisal processes can be overlooked, whereas immediate environmental events are often presumed to function as reinforcers or punishers without sufficient validation. Moreover, the PEM calls for attention to covert processes removed in time from pain episodes and possibly inaccessible to the direct introspection of the patients. I shall turn momentarily to a consideration of methods for accomplishing the assessment of intrapsychic and distal influences on pain.

5. Physiochemical Methods. In the biomedical context, assessment of the physiologic and neurochemical aspects of pain is fundamental. Specialized knowledge of anatomy, chemistry, and electronic monitoring are necessary to obtain valid and reliable data on sensory transmission and the impact of injury, disease, and psychosocial events on pain, anesthesia, and normal transduction. Among the commonly targeted "indicators" of pain and/or distress are heart rate, respiration rate, blood pressure, skin conductance (electrodermal response), blood plasma cortisol levels, endorphin concentrations in the blood, and various indices of the brain's electrical activity as well as the electrical activity associated with particular muscle groups (Karoly & Jensen, 1987; McGrath, 1987b). As with overt behaviors and self-reports, physiological and neurochemical measures represent a useful "level of analysis" of pediatric pain/distress, yielding data that sometimes converge with (yet sometimes diverge from) data obtained through other means. Note that *both* pain and distress (anxiety, depression, fear) are referred to as the assessment target; no biochemical or electrophysiological index can yet be taken as a "pure" or specific measure of one or the other.

Although relatively rare, assessments of infants or children that employ physiochemical analyses in concert with other measurement modalities can reveal the conditions under which bodily systems co-vary with subjective states and can facilitate the testing of "psychosomatic" or "somatopsychological" hypotheses. Too often, however, measures are combined atheoretically.

Abu-Saad (1984b) obtained eight sets of measurements on each of 10 children who had undergone surgery (the children were tested on their first and second postoperative days). A checklist was used to note behavioral pain indicators (grunting, screaming, groaning, sobbing, etc.), the child completed a visual analogue scale, provided verbal descriptors, and was assessed for pulse rate, respiration, and blood pressure. Abu-Saad found that all of the so-called behavioral indicators were displayed, including vocalizations, facial expressions, and body movements, and that these overt responses were related to the pain scale responses. However, there was no relationship between pain scale responses and the physiological measures taken. The author offered no speculation concerning the absence of a relationship between the psychological and autonomic indicators, but suggested that, in the future, all of the modalities (including the physiologic) be employed to assess children's pain, combined into what she called a "multidimensional tool."

This report illustrates the weaknesses of ad hoc multielement assessment. First, when a variety of measures are included in a protocol, shortcuts are often involved: no single modality is given the care and attention it deserves. Further, a box score approach is taken. Since the physiologic measures didn't pan out, they are barely mentioned. If the facial expressions had not co-varied with the other behavioral indicators, they no doubt would have likewise been discounted. Finally, the physiologic measures were not justified conceptually. They were included (I surmise) because they are normally part of the charting that nurses perform on the postoperative service. Although it is fashionable to conduct multiaxial diagnoses, care is still required in the selection and operationalization of one's axes.

An example of a careful, hypothesis-testing approach to assessment, employing physiologic measures, is the study of Feuerstein, Barr, Francoeur, Houle, and Rafman (1982). These investigators sought to examine the hypothesis that children with recurrent abdominal pain (RAP) might be especially susceptible to stressful events or unable to recover quickly after stressful encounters. This hypothesis seemed reasonable in view of the frequent finding that youngsters with RAP are physiologically and biochemically unremarkable. To test their predictions, the authors compared RAP children to normal and hospital controls on measures of heart rate (cardiovascular system functioning), forearm muscle activity (somatic system functioning), facial expression, and subjective intensity perception (using a visual analogue scale), among others. To simulate stress, the children were exposed to a cold pressor (ice-water immersion of the hand) task. Findings failed to support the differential susceptibility notion, as no differences emerged among the groups across the baseline, cold pressor, and recovery periods of the experiment.

6. Projective and Drawing Methods. Because pain is a complex, multi-tiered, subjective experience and may be perceived with heightened arousal and palpable confusion by youngsters (especially preverbal children), the inference that many pediatric pain assessors have drawn is that the experience might best be approached indirectly (because the "unconscious knows"). Thus, children have been asked to draw their pain, associate it to a specific color, and/or to identify with various animals depicted in distressing or dangerous situations or poses. Contemporary cognitive science perspectives and the PEM similarly propose that nonconscious processes may influence emotions, memories, attentional strategies, mood states, preferences, decisions, and the social exchanges that comprise our day-to-day efforts at adjustment, whether or not we are symptomatic. However, the difference between cognitive-behavioral research touching upon nonconscious or automatic processing and much of the work based on some version of the "projective hypothesis" is that those in the former camp seek to index the inferred phenomena reliably and then demonstrate their relationship to measurable outcomes. Projectivists, on the other hand, are often content with describing or categorizing the putative effects of primitive forces (e.g., calculating the percentage of children who describe their pain intensity with the color red vs. other colors) while failing to show "how qualitative differences in children's responses constitute quantitative differences in their pain attitude, experience, or expression" (McGrath, 1987b, p. 163). Furthermore, many of the projective tools, some quite elaborate (requiring time both to administer and score), have been directed at assessing perceived pain intensity, a practice that (a) perpetuates the field's narrow experiential focus and (b) is patently cost-ineffective in view of the simpler methods of intensity measurement that are already available.

As projective approaches have not been tested rigorously, it would be inappropriate to conclude that they *cannot* be of use to the pediatric pain assessor. The question of their value is, of course, empirical, and it awaits further exploration.[3]

7. Informant Judgment/Rating Procedures. Global judgments by parents, physicians, nurses, teachers, and other adults about the *quality* of pediatric pain experiences are, in many ways, like children's projective responses — that is, you can obtain them, but it isn't clear exactly what they predict or how they might be used in treatment planning. However, informant judgments or ratings need not be relegated to the questionable status of a mind-reading exercise if they are directed at the many tangible effects that a child's pain experience has on those around him/her. Even peer and sibling judgments can have a place in context III-inspired measurement operations.

The VT-PPQ and the CCPQ, reviewed above, are good examples of contemporary pain inventories that ask parents to provide data about their target child *and about themselves* that may have great practical significance. Indeed, it has only recently become clear, with the advent of systems models, why a clinician would want to inquire about the thoughts, feelings, or

---

[3]With adults, pain drawings are often used in a more straightforward manner to depict where on the body pain is felt. Amount of body area colored in by patients is sometimes linked to questionnaire measures of psychopathology (e.g., hypochondriasis). However, even here, the evidence is weak (Ginzburg, Merskey, & Lau, 1988).

actions of significant others when the task is to assess a child's pain problem. Presently, in accordance with current and emerging models of illness adaptation, assessors may wish to incorporate existing measurement devices into their pediatric pain armamentarium — tests such as the Family Environment Scale (Moos, 1974), the Family Adaptability and Cohesion Evaluation Scales (FACES) and its revisions, FACES II and III (cf. McCubbin & Thompson, 1987), and other recent family-systems–based instruments (McCubbin & McCubbin, 1988). For further discussion of how families can be included in the pain assessment process, see Flor, Turk, and Rudy (1987). As these authors point out, there are as yet no psychometrically sound *pain-specific* family assessment devices; thus, this should constitute a high priority for future test development.

Another area in need of attention is the application of observational coding systems in the natural environment. Key informants such as parents and teachers can be trained to monitor the activities of youngsters with chronic pain conditions in order to gather precise and contextually sensitive information on precipitating and reinforcing stimuli, on children's naturally occurring coping behaviors, and on the transactional patterns that undergird the maintenance of adaptive and/or maladaptive adjustment.

8. Cognitive Process Analyses. No assessment of childhood pain, taking its inspiration from cognitive-behavioral models, can afford to overlook intrapsychic processes, whether accessible to conscious awareness or inaccessible (under normal circumstances). However, as I earlier noted (Karoly, 1988):

Because of the traditional algesimetric interest in molecular spheres of analysis (pain intensity perceptions, pain tolerance times, etc.) and because of the avoidance of higher order (complex) tasks in the study of child pain, the two-way link between cognition and sensory encoding has not been widely explored. (pp. 380–381)

Certainly contributing to the relative neglect of children's pain/symptom cognition is the absence of consensus on a vocabulary of cognitive processing terms and on a methodology — beyond the interview or questionnaire — for obtaining the relevant data, uncontaminated by age-related language skill differences and situational demand characteristics.

The higher order capacities with which I am concerned (based on information processing, control theory–oriented models such as the PEM) center on sense-making, metacognitive, representational mechanisms that are perhaps most clearly if indirectly evident in the regularities of young children's play, communicative speech, and goal-directed behavior patterns. Understanding oneself, understanding the world, and getting one's needs/wants met by coordinating self–world transactions are the important (if unfinished) tasks of childhood and adolescence that can be studied empirically and should be examined in the context of chronic or acute pain. Because the rules, images, "if-then" action structures, goals, autobiographic memories, etc., that guide child behavior are implicit, the investigator must devise reliable procedures for accessing them. The imperative in the preceding sentence derives from my conviction that these unstudied cognitive processes can serve to mediate the effects of life stressors and pain-inducing events on children's social adjustment. They no doubt serve also to influence children's scalable perceptions of pain and suffering.

Several other potential avenues of assessment unlike those previously discussed also merit brief consideration. First, I suggest that clinicians can readily create diagnostic procedures from those used by child development researchers to address aspects of cognitive maturation.

To study toddlers and young children, developmentalists code natural language use patterns. Such patterns can reveal the child's "rudimentary theory" of self and others. Of particular interest is the child's ability to show that he or she can distinguish mental and physical events inside his or her own body from events outside. Children as young as four can apparently make such discriminations and even understand how situational factors can influence their internal worlds and the internal worlds of other people. According to Bretherton and Beeghly (1982), the child's ability to speak about internal states occurs in the latter part of the 2nd year and develops in year 3. By observing 28-month-olds at play or interacting with an adult, a catalogue of "internal state language" was obtained by Bretherton and Beeghly as well as a collection of "causal utterances" in which internal states were involved (e.g., "I scared of shark. Close my eyes," and "I'm hot. Coat off."). Using the Bretherton-Beeghly codes to analyze the state and state-change language of children with chronic and acute pain may reveal errors or distortions in causal reasoning about bodily events (especially pain) and/ or about the relations between somatic events and perceived antecedents and consequences. Data obtained in this manner could be integrated with information about the frequency of crying or whining obtained via more familiar observational procedures.

Developmentalists also ask young children to make simple judgments, choices, or comparisons among prearranged stimuli, necessitating only that they give yes/no responses or merely point. By analyzing the underlying patterns, investigators can draw inferences about how the stimuli (in our case, descriptions or pictures of children in distress) are represented or how the child solves problems relevant to adaptive success.

The analysis of older children's propositional knowledge structures, inferences, problem-solving heuristics, scripts, plans, or goals can be accomplished by asking them to write or tell stories in response to viewing a videotape of a child dealing with physical discomfort or pain. Models for coding such productions are available (e.g., Graesser & Clark, 1985).

Because the ideas in this section have not yet been systematically applied to the assessment of children's pain, I will not belabor the need to move in the directions noted. Certainly, different is not always better. However, given the gaps in our knowledge of children's pain, the limited success we have achieved by applying the previously noted seven procedural approaches, and the growing interest in cognitive models, the sorts of analytic methods I have suggested seem to me neither radical nor premature.

Summary

In this chapter, I have considered both the conceptual and practical concerns of the pediatric algologist. To help chart the territory, I offered the psychosocial elaboration model, which described in very broad strokes how any recurrent physical symptom, including pain, can be more than the mere physiological consequence of disease, injury, or medical intervention. I have simply assumed that we humans are basically sense-making, social, and emotion-laden creatures who, over time, incorporate these fundamental constituents into a *construction* called pain. Secondly, I presented the multi-dimensional assessment frame as an organizing framework for the assessor, one that renders the implicit questions of *what* to assess, *why*, and *when* more fully explicit. Finally, I categorized the *how* of pediatric pain assessment into eight procedural formats and reviewed the specifics of each.

Strengths, weaknesses, and speculative solutions to difficult problems in the various domains of pain assessment were noted. The field is anything but cut-and-dried. It is also far from dull. I trust that readers of this volume will perceive that the "glass is half full" and work toward raising the water level in the years ahead.

References

Abu-Saad, H. (1984a). Cultural components of pain: The Arab-American child. *Issues in Comprehensive Pediatric Nursing, 7,* 91–99.

Abu-Saad, H. (1984b). Assessing children's responses to pain. *Pain, 19,* 163–171.

Abu-Saad, H., & Holzmer, W. L. (1981). Measuring children's self-assessment of pain. *Issues in Comprehensive Pediatric Nursing, 5,* 337–349.

Achenbach, T. M., McConaughy, S. H., & Howell, C. T. (1987). Child/adolescent behavioral and emotional problems: Implications of cross informant correlations for situational specificity. *Psychological Bulletin, 101,* 213–232.

Beyer, J. E. (1984). *The Oucher: A user's manual and technical report.* Evanston, IL: Judson Press.

Beyer, J. E., & Aradine, C. R. (1986). Content validity of an instrument to measure young children's perceptions of the intensity of their pain. *Journal of Pediatric Nursing, 1,* 386–395.

Beyer, J. E., & Aradine, C. R. (1987). Patterns of pediatric pain intensity: A methodological investigation of a self-report scale. *Clinical Journal of Pain, 3,* 130–141.

Beyer, J. E., & Aradine, C. R. (in press). The convergent and discriminant validity of a self-report measure of pain intensity for children. *Children's Health Care.*

Beyer, J. E., & Knapp, T. R. (1986). Methodological issues in the measurement of children's pain. *Children's Health Care, 14,* 233–240.

Blount, R. L., Corbin, S. M., Powers, S. W., Sturges, J. W., & Maieron, M. J. (1988). Toward a more comprehensive conceptualization of pediatric pain and distress. *Newsletter of the Society of Pediatric Psychology, 12,* 14–20.

Blount, R. L., Corbin, S. M., Sturges, J. W., Wolfe, V. V., Prater, J. M., & James, L. D. (1989). The relationship between adults' behavior and child coping and distress during BMA/LP procedures: A sequential analysis. *Behavior Therapy, 20,* 585–601.

Blount, R. L., Corbin, S. M., & Wolfe, V. V. (1987, March). *The child-adult medical procedure interaction scale (CAMPIS).* Paper presented at the Southeastern Psychological Association Meetings, Atlanta, GA.

Bolger, N., Caspi, A., Downey, G., & Moorehouse, M. (1988). Development in context: Research perspectives. In N. Bolger, A. Caspi, G. Downey, & M. Moorehouse (Eds.), *Persons in context: Developmental processes* (pp. 1–24). Cambridge, England: Cambridge University Press.

Bretherton, I., & Beeghly, M. (1982). Talking about internal states: The acquisition of an explicit theory of mind. *Developmental Psychology, 18,* 906–921.

Cattell, R. B. (1988). The data box: Its ordering of total resources in terms of possible relational systems. In J. R. Nesselroade & R. B. Cattell (Eds.), *Handbook of multivariate experimental psychology* (2nd ed., pp. 69–130). New York: Plenum.

Chapman, C. R. (1989). The concept of measurement: Coexisting theoretical perspectives. In C. R. Chapman & J. D. Loeser (Eds.), *Issues in pain measurement* (pp. 1–16). New York: Raven.

Dember, W. N., & Warm, J. S. (1979). *Psychology of perception* (2nd ed.). New York: Holt, Rinehart & Winston.

Feuerstein, M., Barr, R. G., Francoeur, T. E., Houle, M., & Rafman, S. (1982). Potential biobehavioral mechanisms of recurrent abdominal pain in children. *Pain, 13,* 287–298.

Flor, H., Turk, D. C., & Rudy, T. E. (1987). Pain and families. II. Assessment and treatment. *Pain, 30,* 29–45.

Ginzburg, B. M., Merskey, H., & Lau, C. L. (1988). The relationship between pain drawings and the psychological state. *Pain, 35,* 141–146.

Graesser, A. C., & Clark, L. F. (1985). *Structures and procedures of implicit knowledge.* Norwood, NJ: Ablex.

Hayduk, L. A. (1987). *Structural equation modeling with LISREL: Essentials and advances.* Baltimore: Johns Hopkins University Press.

Hester, N. (1979). The preoperational child's reaction to immunizations. *Nursing Research, 28,* 250–254.

Isaacs, J., & McElroy, M. R. (1980). Psychosocial aspects of chronic illness on children. *Journal of School Health, 50,* 318–321.

Jay, S. M., Elliott, C. H., Katz, E. R., & Siegel, S. E. (1987). Cognitive-behavioral and pharmacologic interventions for children's distress during painful medical procedures. *Journal of Consulting and Clinical Psychology, 55,* 860–865.

Jay, S. M., Ozolins, M., Elliott, C. H., & Caldwell, S. (1983). Assessment of children's distress during painful medical procedures. *Health Psychology, 2,* 133–147.

Jensen, M. P., & Karoly, P. (1989). *Psychosocial dimensions of adjustment to chronic pain: A factor analytic investigation.* Unpublished manuscript, Department of Psychology, Arizona State University, Tempe, AZ.

Karoly, P. (1985a). The logic and character of assessment in health psychology: Perspectives and possibilities. In P. Karoly (Ed.), *Measurement strategies in health psychology* (pp. 3–45). New York: Wiley.

Karoly, P. (1985b). The assessment of pain: Concepts and procedures. In P. Karoly (Ed.), *Measurement strategies in health psychology* (pp. 461–515). New York: Wiley.

Karoly, P. (1988). Pain assessment in children. I: Concepts and measurement strategies. In P. Karoly (Ed.), *Handbook of child health assessment* (pp. 357-386). New York: Wiley.

Karoly, P., & Jensen, M. P. (1987). *Multimethod assessment of chronic pain*. Oxford: Pergamon Press.

Katz, E. R., Kellerman, J., & Siegel, S. E. (1980). Behavioral distress in children with cancer undergoing medical procedures: Developmental considerations. *Journal of Consulting and Clinical Psychology*, *48*, 356-365.

Keefe, F. J., & Gil, K. M. (1986). Behavioral concepts in the analysis of chronic pain. *Journal of Consulting and Clinical Psychology*, *54*, 776-783.

LeBaron, S., & Zeltzer, L. (1984). Assessment of acute pain and anxiety in children and adolescents by self-reports, observer reports, and a behavior checklist. *Journal of Consulting and Clinical Psychology*, *52*, 729-738.

Leventhal, H., & Everhart, D. (1979). Emotion, pain, and physical illness. In C. Izard (Ed.), *Emotions in personality and psychopathology* (pp. 263-299). New York: Plenum.

McCubbin, M. A., & McCubbin, H. I. (1988). Family systems assessment. In P. Karoly (Ed.), *Handbook of child health assessment* (pp. 227-261). New York: Wiley.

McCubbin, H. I., & Thompson, A. I. (Eds.). (1987). *Family assessment inventories for research and practice*. Madison, WI: University of Wisconsin.

McGrath, P. A. (1987a). The multidimensional assessment and management of recurrent pain syndromes in children. *Behaviour Research and Therapy*, *25*, 251-262.

McGrath, P. A. (1987b). Assessment of children's pain: A review of behavioral, physiological, and direct scaling techniques. *Pain*, *31*, 147-176.

McGrath, P. A., & deVeber, L. L. (1986). The management of acute pain evoked by medical procedures in children with cancer. *Journal of Pain and Symptom Management*, *1*, 145-150.

McGrath, P. J., Johnson, G., Goodman, J. T., Schillinger, J., Dunn, J., & Chapman, J. (1985). CHEOPS: A behavioral scale for rating post-operative pain in children. In H. L. Fields, R. Dubner, & F. Cervero (Eds.), *Advances in pain research and therapy* (Vol. 9, pp. 395-402). New York: Raven Press.

Melzack, R. (1975). The McGill Pain Questionnaire: Major properties and scoring methods. *Pain*, *1*, 277-299.

Melzack, R., & Wall, P. D. (1983). *The challenge of pain*. New York: Basic Books.

Moos, R. (1974). *Family Environment Scales*. Palo Alto, CA: Consulting Psychologists Press.

Osborne, R. B., Hatcher, J. W., & Richtsmeier, A. J. (1989). The role of social modeling in unexplained pediatric pain. *Journal of Pediatric Psychology*, *14*, 43-61.

Owens, M. E. (1984). Pain in infancy: Conceptual and methodological issues. *Pain*, *20*, 213-230.

Perrin, E. C., & Gerrity, S. (1981). There's a demon in your belly: Children's understanding of illness. *Pediatrics*, *67*, 841-849.

Richardson, G. M., McGrath, P. J., Cunningham, S. J., & Humphreys, P. (1983). Validity of the headache diary for children. *Headache*, *23*, 184-187.

Ross, D. M., & Ross, S. A. (1984). Childhood pain: The school-aged child's viewpoint. *Pain*, *20*, 179-191.

Routh, D. K., & Ernst, A. R. (1984). Somatization disorder in relatives of children and adolescents with functional abdominal pain. *Journal of Pediatric Psychology*, *9*, 427-437.

Rudy, T. E. (1989). Innovations in pain psychometrics. In C. R. Chapman & J. D. Loeser (Eds.), *The measurement of pain* (pp. 51-61). New York: Raven Press.

Sackett, G. P. (1979). The lag sequential analysis of contingency and cyclicity in behavioral interaction research. In J. D. Osofsky (Ed.), *Handbook of infant development* (pp. 623-649). New York: Wiley.

Savedra, M., Gibbons, P., Tesler, M., Ward, J., & Wegner, C. (1982). How do children describe pain? A tentative assessment. *Pain, 14,* 95-104.

Schechter, N. L. (1985). Pain and pain control in children. *Current Problems in Pediatrics, 15,* 1-67.

Siegel, L. J. (1988). Measuring children's adjustment to hospitalization and to medical procedures. In P. Karoly (Ed.), *Handbook of child health assessment* (pp. 265-302). New York: Wiley.

Sigelman, C. K., & Begley, N. L. (1987). The early development of reactions to peers with controllable and uncontrollable problems. *Journal of Pediatric Psychology, 12,* 99-115.

Tesler, M., Ward, J., Savedra, M., Wegner, C., & Gibbons, P. (1983). Developing an instrument for eliciting children's description of pain. *Perceptual and Motor Skills, 56,* 315-321.

Thompson, K. L., & Varni, J. W. (1986). A developmental cognitive-biobehavioral approach to pediatric pain assessment. *Pain, 25,* 283-296.

Turk, D. C., & Flor, H. (1987). Pain > pain behaviors: The utility and limitations of the pain behavior construct. *Pain, 31,* 277-295.

Turk, D. C., Flor, H., & Rudy, T. E. (1987). Pain and families. I. Etiology, maintenance, and psychosocial impact. *Pain, 30,* 3-27.

Varni, J. W., Jay, S. M., Masek, B. J., & Thompson, K. L. (1986). Cognitive-behavioral assessment and management of pediatric pain. In A. D. Holzman & D. C. Turk (Eds.), *Pain management* (pp. 168-192). New York: Pergamon Press.

Varni, J. W., Thompson, K. L., & Hanson, V. (1987). The Varni-Thompson Pediatric Pain Questionnaire: I. Chronic musculo-skeletal pain in juvenile rheumatoid arthritis. *Pain, 28,* 27-38.

4
Intervention and Management

Patricia A. McGrath

Interest in the alleviation of children's pain has increased at an unprecedent-ed rate during the past 5 years (for review, see Barr, 1989; McGrath, 1990; McGrath & Unruh, 1987; Ross & Ross, 1988; Schechter, 1989; Tyler & Krane, 1990). Special attention has been focused on the management of acute pain in infants, recurrent pain in otherwise healthy and pain-free children, and pain caused by repeated medical procedures for children with chronic disease. Both clinical practice and research investigations have shared a dual emphasis: to develop valid, reliable, and practical techniques for evaluating a child's pain complaint, and then to select the most effective intervention for alleviating his/her pain.

Our understanding of how pain is experienced has changed dramatically since Melzack and Wall proposed the gate control theory of pain modula-tion (Melzack & Wall, 1965). The traditional concept, that there was a fixed and direct pathway from a noxious stimulus to the brain, implied that human pain perception was determined only by the quality and extent of tissue damage. However, we now know that the sensory system for pain is complex with many sites in the nociceptive system, where the signals initi-ated by a noxious stimulus can be modified to alter pain perception. The nociceptive system is now regarded as plastic and complex because pain may be altered by many factors. The knowledge that a child's pain is plastic and complex has led to the gradual realization that many nonpharmacological interventions may be ideally suited for children. Consequently, this chapter reviews the primary interventions for controlling children's pains, with a focus first on the principles of analgesic administration for children, and subsequently on the guidelines for integrating physical, cognitive, and be-havioral interventions into routine clinical practice.

Pain management begins with a thorough assessment of a child's pain complaint. Because the pain produced by a relatively constant noxious stim-ulus can be different for each child, depending on his or her expectations, perceived control, and the significance attached to the source of pain, it is essential to assess many factors when evaluating a child's pain experience. The model shown in Figure 4.1 depicts the factors that influence a child's

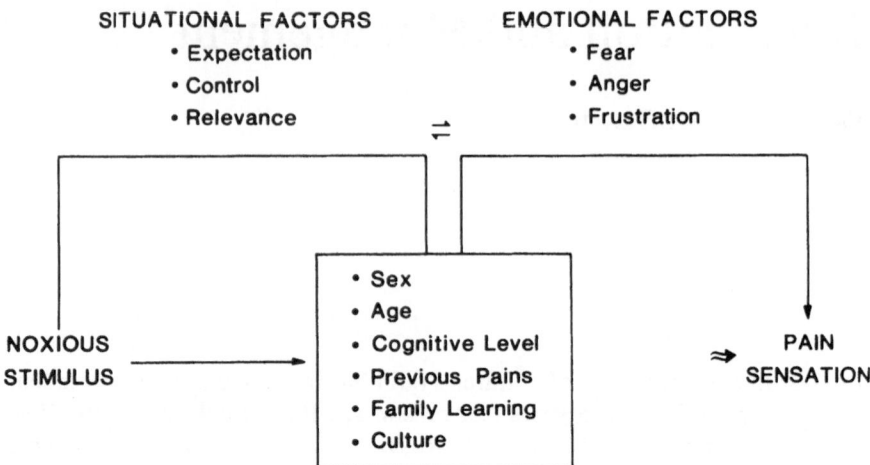

FIGURE 4.1. A model depicting the factors that influence a child's experience of pain. (From *Pain in children: Nature, assessment & treatment* [p. 22] by P. A. McGrath, 1990, New York: Guilford. Copyright 1990 by Guilford Publications, Inc. Reprinted by permission.)

pain. The pain produced by a noxious stimulus depends on the developmental, familial, situational, and emotional factors illustrated. In designing effective programs for managing pain in infants and children, then, it is essential to recognize the role of these factors in determining which interventions are required for which children.

Optimal pain management is not based solely on an identification of the noxious stimulus. Pain assessments must be conducted to identify not only the source of noxious stimulation, but also the relevant situational, emotional, and familial factors that modify neuronal processing to augment or reduce a child's pain. In this manner, the most effective pharmacological and nonpharmacological treatments can be selected (for review of specific measures used for different types of childhood pain, see McGrath, 1990).

Pharmacological Interventions

A surplus of over-the-counter and prescription drugs is available for alleviating pain and suffering. Yet, despite the availability of many pain control drugs, the prescription and administration of analgesics to infants, children, and adolescents represents a controversial issue. Much attention has been focused recently on the special problem of undermedication. Investigators have reported major discrepancies in the prescription or subsequent administration of analgesics between adults and children (Beyer, DeGood, Ashley, & Russell, 1983; Eland, 1974; Schechter, Allen, & Hanson, 1986; Swafford & Allan, 1968). Retrospective chart reviews, in which the prescription and administration of drugs (type of drug, dosage, administration route, and efficacy, as assessed by voiced pain complaints) are recorded, were compared for adults and children who had similar medical problems and presumably similar pain experiences. Swafford and Allan (1968), in a survey of children admitted to an intensive care unit during a 4-month period, reported that only 14% of the children (26 of 180) received any narcotics for pain relief. In a later study, Eland (1974) compared differences in the type and administration of analgesics between 18 adults and 25 children. Although the children had medical conditions similar to the adults, the adults received 372 opioid and 299 nonopioid analgesic doses during their hospitalization, whereas the children received only 24 analgesic doses. In fact, 13 children received no analgesics, despite diagnoses that included traumatic amputation of the foot, excision of neck mass, and heminephrectomy. This trend to undermedicate children remains evident in more recent studies (Beyer et al., 1983; Schechter et al., 1986).

Mather and Mackie (1983) surveyed the incidence of pain in 170 children (69 girls, 101 boys) recovering from surgery. This study is unique in that it consists of a prospective interview with children and a pain assessment during their surgical recovery rather than only a retrospective chart review. Although approximately 90% of the patients were premedicated prior to surgery, primarily with a commercially available mixture of papaverine and hyoscine, postoperative medications were ordered for 84% of the patients. Meperidine and acetaminophen were the most frequently ordered opioid and nonopioid medications. The primary drugs (the more potent analgesic drugs, including opioids) that were ordered were not administered to approximately 40% of the children (when opioids were the primary drugs prescribed, they were not delivered in 29% of the cases). Although nonopioid analgesics, principally acetaminophen, were generally substituted for opioid analgesics, no analgesics were administered to 16% of the children. Overall, only 25% of patients were pain free on the operative day regardless of the medication that they received and approximately 40% of the patients experienced moderate or severe pain. There was no apparent relationship between type of surgery and prescription of analgesic medication. The incidence of moderate or severe pain reported by children during the postoperative period was high, regardless of their analgesic treatment. In addition, the prescribing patterns of medical staff who managed these patients were not consistent. The interpretation of the analgesic medication orders by nursing staff, which often led to substitutions of nonopioid for more potent opioid analgesics, also contributed to poor pain control for children.

Beyer et al. (1983) compared the postoperative prescriptions and administrations of analgesics after cardiac surgery for 50 children and 50 adults. Children were prescribed significantly fewer opioids. They received only 30% of all the analgesics that were prescribed, whereas adults received 70%. Schechter et al. (1986) conducted a chart review to investigate analgesic usage in which they examined the records of 90 children and 90 adults who were selected randomly from hospital charts. They then matched children with adults according to their sex and four diagnostic categories: hernias, appendectomies, burns, and fractured femurs. Adults received an average of 2.2 doses of opioids per day, whereas children received only 1.1 doses. Significant differences in dosing practices were also noted among diagnostic categories. For example, adults received more opioids than children for medical diagnoses that required a longer hospital stay. There were also significant differences in dosing among different hospitals, an urban hospital administering more doses per day than a rural hospital. Opioids were ordered less often for infants and young children than for older children; but, when ordered, the frequency of administration was similar for all children.

Several issues critical to the management of children's pain are evident in these studies. In many cases, medications were not adequately ordered. Since the majority of orders were written for opioid primary and nonopioid secondary medication, the attending nurse decided which medication was actually administered, based on the child's needs. In addition, most orders were written p.r.n. (pro re nata, as necessary or according to circumstances), which requires further judgment as to the time intervals between drug administration. Although in theory p.r.n. should provide the optimum treatment since medication administration is scheduled by patient need, there are difficulties with this administration route. Patients are usually required to experience and report pain before medication is administered. There is a large variability in dosage regimens, both in the size of doses and in the minimal time interval specified between doses. As an example, some high-clearance drugs with typical plasma lives of 3 to 4 hours require dosing intervals of 3 to 4 hours for effective pain relief. For some children the intervals between doses were too long to provide sufficient analgesia. Also, individual variability should be recognized and doses adjusted accordingly.

The extent to which infants and children are undermedicated, whether due to a failure to recognize their pain or to a general reluctance to assume responsibility for the selection and administration of appropriate analgesics, is not known, but evidence suggests that it is quite substantial.

Analgesics

The term *analgesic* describes a category of drugs that act to reduce pain selectively without producing a general loss of consciousness. Ninety-nine percent of all analgesic prescriptions derive from only two families of compounds—the aspirin type and the opium type. (For review, see Beers & Bassett, 1979; Dundee & Loan, 1983; Gladtke, 1983; Huskisson, 1984; Jaffe & Martin, 1980; McCaffery & Beebe, 1989.) In general, drugs reduce pain either centrally by inhibiting transmission of nociceptive signals to the brain, or peripherally by inhibiting the metabolism of pain-producing substances in body tissues. Opioid analgesics relieve pain by acting on the central nervous system, whereas aspirin-type drugs relieve pain by acting on the peripheral nervous system. Analgesics vary in their pain reducing potency, in the extent to which they cause undesirable side effects, and in their probable mode of action. Selection of an appropriate analgesic for children requires consideration of the nature of the pain and the potency, side effects, and physiological properties of the available analgesics.

The nonopioid analgesics include antipyretic drugs to lower body temperature and anti-inflammatory drugs to reduce swelling. These are the drugs of choice for controlling low-intensity pain, fever, and inflammation. The most commonly prescribed antipyretic analgesics for children are aspirin compounds and acetaminophen. Antipyretic drugs have a long history of therapeutic use, with a high level of effectiveness, low level of toxicity, and limited abuse potential.

Antipyretic Drugs

Aspirin

In 1763, the Reverend Edward Stone wrote to the Royal Society in London to describe that the extract of willow bark reduced fever and alleviated suffering from rheumatism. Leroux identified the active ingredient in the willow extract in 1827 and named it "salicin" for the scientific name of the tree from which it was isolated, Salix Alba. The subsequent synthesis of acetylsalicylic acid replaced the analgesic use of salicylates derived from naturally occurring sources. Dreser introduced acetylsalicylic acid into the medical formulary in 1899 and it was later marketed by Bayer as aspirin. Aspirin, the drug of choice for the relief of mild to moderate pain, is most effective for controlling pain associated with inflammation. Aspirin is contraindicated for children with liver disease, hemophilia, vitamin K deficiency, or platelet coagulation deficiencies because it interferes with platelet aggregation. Caution is also recommended in the administration of aspirin to children with influenza because of a possible role in the development of Reye's syndrome (American Academy of Pediatrics, Committee on Infectious Diseases, 1982).

Aspirin has been mixed with many compounds to buffer its gastrointestinal effects, but generally these compounds are less effective buffers than when children swallow aspirin with food, milk, or antacids. Acetylsalicylic acid preparations are available for children in tablets, gums, and suppositories. The specific doses required for optimal analgesia vary with the form of the drug due to differences in absorption.

Acetaminophen

Acetaminophen, also known as paracetamol, (e.g., Tylenol, Panadol, and other brands), was introduced by Von Mering as an analgesic and antipyretic in 1893. It is the major metabolite of phenacetin and acetanilid. Phenacetin was introduced into medicine as an analgesic in 1887. However, it was removed from the market because it had serious toxicity. Acetaminophen has antipyretic and analgesic properties equivalent to aspirin, but lacks aspirin's anti-inflammatory properties. It also does not have aspirin's gastrointestinal and hematologic side effects or the possible connection with Reye's syndrome. Acetaminophen is probably the most commonly administered analgesic for mild to moderate pains in children. Its antipyretic properties make it a popular choice for the treatment of colds and influenza. However, since acetaminophen does not have anti-inflammatory properties, it is not as effective as aspirin for pain of an inflammatory origin. Acetaminophen is available in elixirs, tablets, drops, and suppositories.

Combination Drugs

A variety of combination analgesics have been developed to combine the analgesic effects of aspirin or acetaminophen with compounds to reduce possible side effects or to elevate mood. These include primarily buffers against gastrointestinal irritation and caffeine. Combination drugs may also include antihistamines or antispasmodics with aspirin or acetaminophen. As yet, though, no over-the-counter combination drugs have been demonstrated as more effective for the reduction of mild to moderate pain in children than aspirin or acetaminophen.

Non-Steroidal Anti-Inflammatory Drugs

Non-steroidal anti-inflammatory drugs (NSAIDs) are similar in potency to aspirin and are used primarily to treat inflammatory disorders and acute pain of mild to moderate intensity. The most commonly used drugs include ibuprofen (Motrin), naproxen (Naprosyn), tolmetin (Tolectin), and indomethacin (Indocin). The NSAIDs inhibit prostoglandin synthesis. And, like aspirin, their anti-inflammatory and analgesic effects occur peripherally, while the antipyretic effects occur centrally. The actions of NSAIDs on platelet function are reversible and are clinically milder than those of aspirin. Recently, NSAIDs such as ibuprofen have become available in elixir form for children. More research must be conducted to evaluate which NSAIDs offer more analgesia than aspirin. Since most NSAIDs have not yet been approved as analgesics for children, it is probable that many multicenter efficacy studies will be conducted soon on NSAIDs for children.

Opioid Analgesics

Morphine

Opioid analgesics refer to a class of drugs with similar pain-reducing properties, traditionally described as narcotics. The term *narcotic* is derived from the Greek word for stupor, *narcosis*, because these analgesics produce a drowsy stupor along with pain relief. The term *opioid* is now used to describe this class of drugs as analgesics, to avoid the negative connotation associated with the undesirable side effects and abuse potential if self-administered without medical supervision for only its mood-altering effects. Opium, a drug extracted from the dried juice of the unripe capsule of the opium poppy, has been used as an analgesic, antitussive, and antidiarrheal for many centuries. The first medical document, the Ebers Papyrus of 1550 B.C., recommends opium for crying children, presumably for its sedative and analgesic properties. The Greeks dedicated opium to the gods of night, death, sleep (Hypnos), and dreams (Morpheus). Hippocrates prescribed it as a hypnotic. However, in the Roman era, Galen used opium specifically to reduce pain. Morphine was isolated from opium in 1803 by Serturner and named after Morpheus. Morphine, the standard analgesic drug for the relief of severe acute and chronic pain, represents the current standard against which the analgesic properties of all opioid drugs are compared.

Although morphine produces selective analgesia in that it does not alter other sensory systems, morphine has several adverse effects such as lightheadedness, dizziness, sedation, nausea, vomiting, and sweating. Dose-related respiratory depression accompanies acute morphine administration due to a decrease in responsiveness in the brain stem respiratory center. Morphine stimulates the chemoreceptor trigger zone that leads to nausea and vomiting. There may be a vestibular component to this phenomenon because more ambulatory than recumbent patients become nauseated. Morphine has the potential for drug abuse because it can produce mental and physical dependency.

Codeine

Codeine, a naturally occurring opium alkaloid, is structurally related to morphine. Codeine is the primary weak opioid analgesic used to control moderate pain. Codeine is approximately $1/12$ as potent as morphine parenterally (administered nonorally), but between $1/3$ and $1/4$ as potent orally. Codeine is also used as an antitussive to relieve exhausting nonproductive coughs that do not respond to nonopioid antitussives. Its most common side effects are nausea, constipation, dizziness, and sedation. Codeine has a fairly low addictive potential, and codeine tolerance develops very slowly.

Codeine is available as pure preparations or as combination drugs with aspirin or acetaminophen. Although the comparative efficacy of these drugs has not been described precisely for children, the combination drugs may provide more analgesia than codeine, aspirin, or acetaminophen alone. Codeine is not as effective as aspirin for reducing pain due to inflammation since opioids do not have anti-inflammatory properties.

Synthetic and Semisynthetic Opioids

Several synthetic and semisynthetic derivatives of codeine and morphine have been used clinically since the early 1900s. These drugs are obtained by a relatively simple structural modification of the morphine or codeine molecule (semisynthetic) or by production of a compound with a structural resemblance to the molecule (synthetic). The drugs are classified according to their structural similarity to morphine or codeine, their analgesic potency relative to morphine or codeine, their agonist (facilitating) or antagonist (blocking) relationship to morphine, their abuse potential, and their adverse side effects. Meperidine (Demerol), hydromorphone (Dilaudid), fentanyl citrate (Sublimaze), oxycodone (Percocet, Percodan) and pentazocine (Talwin) are among the most commonly prescribed synthetic and semisynthetic opiate drugs. These drugs were developed to yield the quality of analgesia produced by morphine without the problems of loss of consciousness, tolerance, and addiction. Although an ideal opioid analgesic drug, with maximal pain-reducing potency and no side effects, has not yet been developed, these derivatives provide valuable alternative analgesics that vary in potency, duration of action, and side effects. Drugs may be selected according to the specific needs of the patient and according to the nature of the pain. As an example, fentanyl (Sublimaze), produces profound analgesia for a much shorter period (15 to 30 min) than morphine. Consequently, this drug is useful for relatively short-duration invasive medical investigations in children, such as cardiac catheterizations.

Diamorphine hydrochloride (heroin), a semisynthetic derivative of morphine, produces analgesia more quickly, but for a shorter time period. Heroin produces more respiratory depression than morphine. Other side effects include vomiting, constipation, and sedation. Heroin is strictly controlled in Great Britain for use with adult patients who have severe pain due to malignant disease, but is not approved for use in the United States and Canada. Although there are few controlled studies comparing the analgesic efficacy of heroin to that of morphine, these studies suggest that morphine and heroin produce similar analgesia and have similar adverse effects (Levine, Sackett, & Bush, 1986). Many individuals have advocated the use of heroin for terminal patients with severe pain. The use of heroin represents an emotionally charged issue because of the common fear that patients' pain cannot be controlled adequately with only morphine. However, there has been insufficient research to substantiate this fear. The mechanisms of heroin-induced analgesia are similar to those of morphine; heroin is converted within the body into morphine and presumably affects comparable supraspinal sites. Although more research should be conducted to unequivocally resolve the question of whether heroin can provide better analgesia for adults with chronic pain than morphine, the issue is not yet relevant to pediatrics. Sufficient data are not available about the prevalence and control of chronic pain associated with malignant disease in children and the possible need for other opioid analgesics. Until data are available to show that the proper prescription and administration of the available opioid analgesics is not adequate for children, it is premature to consider the use of heroin for pediatric pain control.

Methadone (Dolophine) is not closely related to morphine but produces similar analgesic and respiratory effects. Methadone analgesia has a longer duration than morphine analgesia. Unlike morphine, methadone has good oral absorption with a parenteral to oral ratio of 1:2, so that it is the most effective orally administered potent opioid. Orally administered methadone is recommended for the control of moderate to severe pain. Methadone produces less nausea and vomiting than morphine. Although physical dependence can occur, methadone is used to treat opioid addiction. It enables individuals to function without euphoric and sedative side effects and prevents physiological withdrawal.

Oral Opioids

Oral opioids have been mixed with other drugs to provide medication that enhances analgesia while minimizing aversive side effects. The Brompton Cocktail, probably the best known mixture, was developed at Brompton Hospital in England. The cocktail initially contained morphine, cocaine, gin, and honey to provide an effective opioid-stimulant combination. The name is now used to describe several different analgesic mixtures that usually combine morphine, cocaine, and alcohol. The particular ingredients in the various cocktails are often selected according to the specific needs of the patient. Some mixtures include phenothiazines to potentiate the analgesic effects of morphine and to relieve anxiety. Although several cocktails are used for children, children may find the taste of some of the inactive ingredients, particularly alcohol, aversive (Twycross, 1979). It should be possible to adjust the ingredients so that the aversiveness of the solution is not a major problem. Methadone, with better oral absorption than morphine, should provide a better oral opioid mixture.

Since children tend to prefer to swallow pain medications, oral opioid mixtures can provide a practical administration route for a combination of drugs selected according to the needs of the children. These mixtures have been quite useful for relieving pain and anxiety in children scheduled for invasive medical procedures in ambulatory clinics.

Adjunctive and Combination Drugs

Adjunctive drugs, such as tranquilizers and antidepressants, do not have specific analgesic properties, but may help relieve children's pain by elevating their moods, reducing anxiety, minimizing the adverse side effects of the primary analgesic ingredients, or potentiating analgesia. Other combination analgesics, consisting of aspirin or acetaminophen with an opioid such as codeine, are often used to obtain maximal pain relief by activating both central and peripheral mechanisms to increase analgesia.

Physical Drug Dependency

The fear of drug dependency represents one of the common explanations for why children may receive inadequate doses of opioid analgesics for the control of severe pain. Yet, there is little evidence that fear of addiction is a valid concern for pediatrics. Although drug dependency is possible, there are no published reports describing physical or psychological dependency to opioid analgesics in children. Drug dependence occurs when children become accustomed to the effects (physiological or psychological) of a drug so that they require the drug on a continuous or periodic basis. Children may develop tolerance to a drug, so that they require progressively higher doses to achieve the same physiological effect. Children with prolonged pain may require progressively higher doses of opioids to achieve adequate analgesia. Yet drug tolerance should not be equated with drug addiction. Physical dependence develops when an individual's body requires the drug to function; there is a physical disturbance if the drug is withdrawn. Drugs that produce physical dependence include morphine, morphine-like substances, some tranquilizers, barbiturates, and alcohol.

Physical dependence is a common phenomenon and mild withdrawal symptoms are evident in most patients who have taken opioid analgesics for over 2 weeks and then stop taking them. Mild symptoms such as restlessness, rhinorrhea, or sleeplessness, may develop approximately 8 to 12 hours after the last dose of an opioid. Major withdrawal symptoms, such as irritability, tremor, nausea, diarrhea, or muscle pains, will develop 48 to 72 hours after the last dose. Although dependency can be easily controlled by gradually tapering medication and usually does not constitute a major problem for the clinician or patient, the term *dependency* is often used somewhat synonymously with the term *addiction*, resulting in exaggerated fears associated with opioid use with children. Unlike dependence, which is common, addiction is extremely rare in patients entering the hospital for control of pain. Addiction represents a pattern of drug use in which an individual is wholly absorbed in the compulsive use and procurement of a drug, and has a tendency to relapse after withdrawal (Yaffe, 1980). Twycross (1978) described a low incidence of addiction even in adult patients with terminal malignancies who received opioids for prolonged periods of time. Although the majority of patients with severe chronic pain due to malignant disease are adults, not children, and the majority of studies on the potential of dependency to opioid analgesics are conducted with adults, there is little empirical evidence to indicate that children should be denied opioid analgesics for fear of dependency or addiction.

Guidelines for Analgesic Administration

A variety of analgesics are available to control pain in infants and children. The primary concern in pediatric pain control is how to select and administer the most appropriate analgesic to reduce a child's pain. Several guidelines for analgesia administration in children are listed in Table 4.1. It is first necessary to evaluate the severity and etiology of the pain, that is, the peripheral or central origins of the pain and the probable role of inflamma-

TABLE 4.1. Guidelines for analgesic administration.

Determine children's pain level
    Mild   —   Aspirin and acetaminophen

    Moderate   —   Codeine

    Strong   —   Morphine, methadone
Evaluate physical source
    Peripheral or central
    Inflammatory processes
Consider situational and emotional factors
Select appropriate administration route, dosage, and dosing interval
Consider need for adjunctive drugs
    Tranquilizers
    Antidepressants

From *Pain in children: Nature, assessment & treatment* (p. 126) by P. A. McGrath, 1990, New York: Guilford. Copyright 1990 by Guilford Publications, Inc. Reprinted by permission.

tory mechanisms. The drug's pharmacologic properties, indications, side effect liability, adverse reactions, and dosage routes must then be considered. The rational prescription of analgesics for children requires matching the analgesic efficacy of a drug or combination of drugs with pain level, after careful consideration of the drug's side effects and the onset and duration of analgesic action. Specific dosing regimens, analgesic potencies, side effects, and contraindications are listed in hospital formularies and in the Pediatric Drug Handbook (Benitz & Tatro, 1981; Goodman & Gilman, 1985; Shannon & Berde, 1989).

The mode of administration of an analgesic drug is a more important consideration for children than for adults. Children's typical fear of injections may lead them either to not request pain medication or to deny pain when checked by medical staff. Optimal analgesic administration for children thus requires flexibility in selecting routes of administration. Analgesics may be administered: orally in tablets, elixirs, or gums; by intravenous, intramuscular, or subcutaneous injections; and by suppositories. The use of portacatheters has increased in pediatrics, particularly for children who require administration of multiple drugs at weekly intervals. Catheters are surgically implanted within a vein with a small tube extending to the outside of the skin. Drugs are injected directly into the external tube. Intermittent subcutaneous and intramuscular injections are problematic for children with bleeding diathesis. Continuous intravenous or subcutaneous infusions with constant infusion pumps can provide excellent pain relief for these children. Continuous infusion techniques are indicated for children with severe pain for whom oral and intermittent parenteral opioids provide insufficient pain relief or for whom intractable vomiting prevents the use of oral analgesics.

Since continuous infusion techniques can provide uninterrupted and safe pain control, they are now used more frequently for children with postoperative pain. Spinal administration of opioid drugs and local anesthetics has been developed as an alternative method of pain control for adults with cancer pain (for review, Bromage, 1984; Cousins & Mather, 1984; Moulin & Coyle, 1986; Yaksh, 1981). During the past few years, the injection of analgesics and anesthetics into the subarachnoid (intrathecal administration) and epidural spaces has been initiated with children (Attia, Ecoffey, Sandouk, Gross, & Samii, 1986; Finholt, Stirt, & DiFazio, 1985; Glenski, Warner, Dawson, & Kaufman, 1984; Krane, Tyler, & Jacobson, 1989; McIlvaine, 1990; Shapiro, Jedeikin, Shalev, & Hoffman, 1984).

Since the analgesic potency of drugs varies according to the administration route, the route for a desired analgesic must be selected primarily on the basis of which route will provide maximal analgesia within the necessary time frame. Although children prefer to swallow pain medications rather than receive injections, their choices are not based solely on a common fear of more painful injection routes. Usually children have not received any consistent instructions about their need to receive pain medication or about how to cope with injections, such as specific suggestions about how to reduce the painfulness. Children often perceive the injections as more threatening because they do not understand many aspects of their hospitalization and treatment. Most events, including the times and methods for receiving treatments, seem beyond their control. There may be less consistency among personnel in conducting procedures, particularly invasive procedures that will hurt children. The preparation of a body site, the position in which a child is placed, and the manner in which a child may be distracted or encouraged to participate should be consistent to enable children to understand and comply with treatments. Behavioral management programs, in which even toddlers receive painful treatments in a structured consistent manner to allow them some control and to provide them with accurate expectations about what will happen, will facilitate an easier and less painful procedure.

The literature on pain control clearly recommends that pain medication be prescribed in anticipation of pain and to prevent its recurrence, rather than to eliminate a strong pain after it has developed. This is particularly important for children who may not understand that they can be pain free despite a major injury. They may associate pain with their condition and with their general anxiety about hospitals or medical personnel so that they do not realize that they can be comfortable even while their injury heals and while they are in the hospital. The constant experience of even mild pain may lead to behavioral and emotional problems that can intensify existing pain. When pain is immediately and effectively managed, children's anxiety is reduced because they realize that their suffering can be controlled.

Medication should be administered prophylactically in a time-contingent manner, rather than prescribed on a p.r.n. basis. Otherwise, children must experience pain before they are able to obtain relief. Furthermore, since higher doses of opioids are necessary to relieve existing pain than to prevent the recurrence of pain, p.r.n. dosing schedules do not provide optimal analgesia. A pain problem may develop when children are hospitalized for a long period and receive analgesic medication according to a p.r.n. schedule. There may be variable or lengthy delays between the time children request pain relief and the time they receive it, particularly if there is a shift change in nursing staff or if drugs are ordered during a busy period in the hospital pharmacy. Children may begin to request their medication at progressively shorter time intervals or may develop exaggerated pain behaviors in an effort to convince medical staff that they truly need their medication. These problems generally do not occur when children receive analgesics on a time-contingent basis when the dosing interval has been determined according to the drug's duration of action and the child's need for pain relief.

Patient-controlled analgesia (PCA), in which patients press a button to administer incremental analgesic doses delivered through an intravenous catheter connected to a portable infusion system, has been used successfully by adults to control their pain, particularly postoperative pain. More recently, PCA has been used by children and adolescents (Brown & Broadman, 1987; Dodd, Wang, & Rauck, 1988; Means, Allen, Lookabill, & Krishna, 1988; Rodgers, Webb, Stergios, & Newman, 1988; Tyler, 1987). Children from 6 to 18 have used PCA and received excellent pain relief with minimal side effects and adverse complications. Children can easily understand how to use the PCA button to titrate their analgesic requirements. In fact, studies indicated that children use less analgesia postoperatively on the PCA system than when drugs were administered in more conventional routes and schedules. Children also preferred PCA.

In addition to the proper drug choice, administration route, and dosing interval, it is necessary to remember that the children are the patients and that pain and pain control should be evaluated from children's perspectives. Parents may make decisions about how children should receive medication or how children should cope during treatments from their adult and personal perspectives. As an example, some parents believe that children should not be informed in advance about a painful injection. Also, they can inadvertently teach children to fear injections because they protect, soothe, and reassure children during treatments, without allowing them to also learn to cope on their own and to make choices. Although some parents may prefer to "not look" during injections, their children may prefer to watch what happens. Their intent concentration during the procedure may lessen their pain. There are many simple tools that children can use to reduce pain during analgesic administrations (for review, McGrath, 1990). They need to evaluate and choose which tool is best for them.

When children's pain is evaluated by considering the source of noxious stimulation in relation to their unique characteristics, children feel they have more control over their hospitalization, treatments, and pain so that the aversiveness associated with their illness and treatment is diminished. They are more able to cope positively with their illness, pain, and painful analgesic administrations. Although young children may not be able to make valid decisions about their needs for analgesic medication, it is wrong to assume that all children are incapable of making any decisions about how to receive their medications and how to cope with their pain. Children should participate in various aspects of their medical treatment. When possible, they should be encouraged to choose an injection site, to learn some simple pain-coping strategies that can be transferred to all situations in which they receive invasive medical procedures, and to evaluate the efficacy of a sedative or analgesic. Children who are 3 to 5 years old have been able to make decisions about whether they prefer sedation, nonpharmacological methods such as relaxation or hypnosis, or a combination of drug and nondrug interventions prior to and during lumbar punctures or bone marrow aspirations (McGrath, 1990). Although it requires more time to teach children in a concrete, age-appropriate manner about their treatment choices, the benefits are enormous. Children are generally less anxious and apprehensive about treatments and they are even more responsive to the effects of sedative drugs (McGrath, 1990). Not all children, even older children, will want to share decisions about their medical treatments or medications. However, most children are curious, interested, and motivated to participate actively in decisions with their parents and medical staff.

It is essential to remember that environmental, behavioral, cognitive, and pharmacological interventions for pain control are not mutually exclusive. In fact, pain management is a special discipline with direct relevance to Pediatrics. Education programs must be provided to teach all health professionals that pain management in infants and children is not simply a corollary of disease management. It is the author's experience that most pediatric departments and children's hospitals do not subscribe to any of the three journals that are exclusively devoted to publications about pain and pain control. Many medical schools still promote the concept of a rigid nociceptive system that dictates a relatively inflexible approach to pain control. More education is needed to dispel myths about children's nociceptive processing, their endogenous pain inhibitory systems and the factors that can activate them, their abilities to use valid and reliable pain measures, and the efficacy of pharmacological interventions for controlling their pain. Much more research is necessary to evaluate the analgesic efficacy of the over-the-counter and prescription medications available for controlling pain in children, in accordance with the guidelines for the ethical conduct of drug studies in infants and children (American Academy of Pediatrics, Committee on Drugs, 1977; Cohen, 1980).

Nonpharmacological Interventions

Nonpharmacological interventions include a wide variety of techniques that are categorized as physical, behavioral, or cognitive, according to whether the intervention is focused primarily on modifying an individual's sensory systems, behaviors, or thoughts and coping abilities. Table 4.2 lists some of the nonpharmacological methods of pain control that have been used for children. Although interventions are listed within a principal category, the three categories are not mutually exclusive. Instead, most nonpharmacological methods vary in the particular combination of physical, behavioral, and cognitive modulation that is involved. As an example, although hypnosis may be considered primarily a cognitive intervention because patients learn to reduce pain by intense mental concentration, an hypnotic induction process usually includes a physical component, progressive muscle relaxation, and often includes a behavioral component, such as suggesting that a patient alter his or her behaviors at home to increase general activity level.

Some of the current interventions listed in Table 4.2 are similar to those originally cited by Avicenna when he wrote the Canon of Medicine in 900 A.D. (Gruner, 1930). Avicenna described several physical methods, such as stimulation by the application of heat and cold, various poultices, massage, and relaxing exercise, specifically "walking about gently for a considerable time" to soften the tissues and relieve pain (Gruner, 1930, p. 529). In addition, he cited cognitive methods such as listening to agreeable music and "being occupied with something very engrossing." Although these interventions are quite similar to the physical, behavioral, and cognitive techniques in wide use many centuries later, much more is now known about how they modify pain and why they should be included in most pain management programs with children.

Since space precludes a review of all nonpharmacological methods, only the behavioral and cognitive methods that have been used to alleviate children's pain are described in this section. (Please refer to McGrath, 1990, for a review of physical interventions and their probable modes of action.)

Behavioral Methods

Since the perception of pain depends on many physical, familial, emotional, situational, and behavioral factors, it should be possible to alter children's pain by modifying each of these factors. Behavioral techniques for reducing

TABLE 4.2. Nonpharmacological pain interventions.

Physical	Behavioral	Cognitive
Surgical techniques	Exercise	Distraction
Anesthetic blocks	Operant conditioning	Attention
Pressure, massage	Relaxation	Imagery
Hot and cold stimulation	Biofeedback	Thought stopping
Electrical nerve stimulation	Modeling	Hypnosis
Acupuncture	Desensitization	Music therapy
	Art and play therapy	Psychotherapy

From *Pain in children: Nature, assessment and treatment* (p. 133) by P. A. McGrath, 1990, New York: Guilford. Copyright 1990 by Guilford Publications, Inc. Reprinted by permission.

pain typically consist of methods that target either the children themselves or the adults who respond to them when they experience pain. The primary objectives are to modify behaviors that may initiate, maintain, or exacerbate children's pain by assessing the children's behaviors prior to and during painful experiences as well as the behaviors of the adults that care for them (McGrath, 1990).

Children who tense specific muscles or restrict their general behaviors because they fear that they will increase their pain, may actually cause or exacerbate pain as a consequence of the physical changes associated with their altered behaviors. It is essential to recognize that pain intensity is not determined solely by activity in nociceptive pathways, but is also determined by activity in nonnociceptive pathways with the result that abnormal sensory input due to a child's abnormal physical restrictions can exacerbate pain. Parents, teachers, physicians, or nurses may inadvertently respond to children so that their anxiety, fear, distress, and pain are increased. Children may be rewarded for their pain complaints when they receive special attention, reduced expectations for achievement, and permission to stay home from school, so that their pain complaints are maintained. Recognition of the manner in which the behaviors of children and adults may influence children's pain is essential for the optimal management of any acute, recurrent or chronic childhood pain (Gross & Gardner, 1980; McGrath, 1990; Thompson & Varni, 1986; Varni, 1984). Several methods may be used to modify behaviors to reduce pain problems for children such as physical exercise, operant conditioning, biofeedback, modeling, art therapy, and play therapy.

Operant and Classical Conditioning

Operant or instrumental conditioning is a type of learning in which an individual learns by the direct consequences of his or her actions on other people in the environment. General actions and specific behaviors that lead to positive outcomes will continue to occur, and those that lead to negative outcomes will decrease. A child's behaviors when he or she experiences pain are inevitably shaped by the reactions of significant others. Behaviors such as crying, seeking reassurance, grimacing, or withdrawing from other family members may be inadvertantly rewarded by increased attention, empathy, comfort, or reduction of work and performance expectations. These positive outcomes, whether implicitly or explicitly communicated, will encourage the child to repeat the behaviors that elicited the favorable responses of others.

Thus, some pain behaviors represent learned or conditioned behaviors rather than spontaneous responses to pain. Conditioned maladaptive behaviors are those that lead not only to exaggerated pain symptomatology but also possibly to increased pain for children. When parents respond to children's pain complaints by increased attention, and by encouraging children to cope solely by relying on them or on medication, this leads to children's increased passiveness, decreased control over the situation or disease, and reduced ability to learn independent methods for reducing pain. Also, the aversiveness of the procedure or disorder increases. These situational factors increase children's anxiety, distress, and pain (McGrath, 1990).

Children with recurrent pain are at risk for developing exaggerated pain symptomatology because they experience frequent episodes of strong pain in the absence of well-defined organic etiology that necessitates medical treatment. The usual reassurance that "nothing is wrong" despite recurrent pain may lead to the development of more symptoms or increased pain complaints, as children attempt to convince their parents that the pain is real and requires attention. Children whose parents do not respond consistently to their pain complaints often may develop conditioned pain behaviors that are directly related to the intermittent responses of their parents. These parents generally vary in their responses, either providing excessive emotional and physical support or indicating that they do not have time to assist the child. The implicit message that many children receive from these inconsistent responses is that their pain or pain complaints need to be stronger to convince their parents that they now need the same level of support they have sometimes received.

Children with recurrent pain syndromes are also prone to the development of classically conditioned pain triggers, environmental stimuli or situations that can initiate a painful episode. Classical conditioning is a type of learning in which an individual learns indirectly by an association between events. As an example, a child who develops headaches during math class learns to relate the two events in a causal manner. The longer otherwise healthy children experience frequent headaches, abdominal pains, or limb pains in the absence of a well-defined cause, the more likely they are to develop beliefs that the environmental stimuli that were associated in time or place with the pain episode actually caused the pain. Although clearly some foods, weather conditions, and social situations may lead to a headache, the usual cause is not the environmental factor but rather the parents' and child's anxiety about that factor (McGrath, 1990).

Special attention has been focused on the role of conditioning for maintaining pain behaviors and invalidism for adults with persistent pain and the benefits of changing the responses of health staff to encourage more natural behaviors. Although the pain was initially caused by injury, the subsequent therapy of rest, medication, and individual care may facilitate the pain persisting beyond the usual time period required for healing. Fordyce (1976, 1978) provides a comprehensive and practical description of how the principles of operant conditioning are relevant for adults with chronic pain. More recently, Masek, Russo, and Varni (1984) reviewed how these principles are relevant for children with chronic pain. Essentially, the use of operant conditioning to reduce pain and pain behaviors is similar for adults and children. It is necessary first to identify all pain behaviors (verbal and nonverbal) and to evaluate the responses of significant persons (family, medical, school, work, peer) to the patient's pain. Then, a plan is designed to modify the responses of these significant persons to minimize maladaptive pain behaviors and maximize adaptive behaviors that reduce pain. Children's pain behaviors are often inadvertently reinforced by concerned parents and medical staff, when children perceive that the special concern they receive is contingent on their needs for pain relief and comfort. Behaviors that lead to immediate, increased child-staff or child-parent interactions will generally increase, even if the behaviors themselves prolong disability and reliance on parents or medication.

The application of operant conditioning for pain management in children requires a comprehensive program to monitor and modify both parents' and children's behaviors. First, a thorough assessment of the child's pain, pain behaviors, and the relevant emotional, situational, and familial factors is conducted. Then, the most disruptive or pain-increasing behaviors are targeted for modification. Positive coping behaviors are selected according to the child's age, sex, and pain problem. A reward system is designed that will effectively motivate the child such as stickers, points toward a treat, special time with parents, or increased social activities with peers.

Both parents and medical staff (if appropriate) must agree to consistently follow the program, with rewards contingent on the child fulfilling well-defined behavioral criteria. Appropriate selection of behaviors and rewards is critical to the success of the program. The child must be able to achieve the positive behavioral criteria. Only one maladaptive behavior at a time should be targeted for reduction, with other behaviors added after children have consistently modified previous behaviors. It is essential that parents and children understand the objectives of the program, so that parents do not reward the targeted behavior and therefore reduce the efficacy of the intervention. Similarly, the program should not be used indiscriminately with all children with similar types of pain, since not only should the behaviors and rewards be selected for each child but, more importantly, the same overt pain behaviors (stalling, withdrawing, and screaming during an injection) may represent very different levels of fear, anxiety, emotional distress, and learning for different children. These differences necessarily indicate that individual combinations of cognitive and behavioral programs, designed to meet the needs of each child and family, are required for optimal pain control. Although specific program goals will differ, the general principles and goals are consistent.

Although operant conditioning is usually one of the components of an integrated cognitive and behavioral approach to pain control, it may be the only approach required for children whose pain complaints are related solely to familial or environmental reinforcers. Operant conditioning has been successfully incorporated into several multistrategy pain management programs to reduce children's acute, recurrent, and chronic pain (McGrath, 1990).

Relaxation

Pain usually causes tension and irritability, so many behavioral interventions are designed to relax patients (physically and mentally) to minimize pain associated with the physiological changes of muscle tension and anxiety. Progressive muscle relaxation, yoga, meditation, and biofeedback are now widely used to alleviate anxiety, distress, and pain for both adults and children. The physiological changes that are associated with the "relaxation response" are consistent with a general decrease in sympathetic nervous system activity (for review see Benson, Pomeranz, & Kutz, 1984). There is decreased oxygen consumption and respiratory rate, increased skin resistance, and production of cerebral alpha waves. However, the precise mechanisms by which the relaxation response reduces pain is not yet known.

Various relaxation techniques have been incorporated into treatments to alleviate children's burn pain (Wakeman & Kaplan, 1978), acute pain from necessary cancer treatments (Jay, Elliott, Ozolins, Olson, & Pruitt, 1985; McGrath & deVeber, 1986), sickle cell anemia (Zeltzer, Dash, & Holland, 1979), headaches (Diamond, 1979; McGrath, 1983), and arthritic pain in hemophilia (Varni, 1981; Varni, Gilbert, & Dietrich, 1981). The most common techniques for assisting children to relax are deep breathing exercises, progressive muscle relaxation, and biofeedback. Children learn to breathe calmly, deeply and rhythmically to relax their bodies when they are tense during painful procedures or when they experience recurrent or chronic pain. The slower and deeper their breathing, the more their bodies seem to relax. The specific suggestions used to teach children about the pain-reducing effects of relaxation depend on the child's age, cognitive level, and pain source. In general, children younger than 7 require concrete examples and coaching assistance when they use relaxation to reduce pain. They benefit from listening to music, listening to exciting stories, and imagining that they are floppy relaxed dolls or favorite characters with special magic powers (McGrath, 1990).

Progressive muscle relaxation is a specific training procedure, in which children are taught to tighten and relax various muscles, progressing gradually from readily observable body regions (e.g., the leg, foot, toes, fist) to more specialized areas (e.g., temporalis muscles for tension headaches). Many of the progressive relaxation procedures used for children are revisions of the technique developed for adults by Jacobsen (1938), in which adults learn to recognize and control even slight muscle contractions. Usually, children receive some concrete cognitive suggestions to assist them, such as imagining themselves in a past situation in which they felt completely relaxed. There have been no studies evaluating the efficacy of relaxation training alone to control children's pain. Yet, it is probable that relaxation in the absence of an overall cognitive-behavioral approach has some limited value for children.

Biofeedback

Biofeedback, in which a typically unobserved activity of the body is amplified and translated into salient auditory or visual signals, is a very useful technique for pain management (for review Jessup, 1984; Turk, Meichenbaum, & Berman, 1979; Turner & Chapman, 1982). Biofeedback is especially appropriate in pediatrics because children can receive immediate and direct feedback about the state of their bodies. Thus, biofeedback is a concrete tool that assists children to distinguish easily between relaxed and tense body states and facilitates training in how to achieve relaxed states. Although biofeedback has been used to treat many pain conditions in adults, it has been primarily used to treat headaches in children. Electromyogram (EMG) activity in the frontalis muscle is monitored to provide patients with feedback about the efficacy of different muscle relaxation strategies.

Biofeedback has a special advantage for use with children whose pain is caused or exacerbated by physiological changes associated with stress. Attanasio et al. (1985) cite eight advantages for biofeedback with children in comparison with adults: (a) children are more enthusiastic, (b) children learn more quickly, (c) children are less skeptical about self-control procedures, (d) children have more confidence in special abilities, (e) children have more psychophysiological ability, (f) children have had fewer failures with treatment, (g) children enjoy the practice sessions, and (h) children are more reliable at symptom monitoring. My observations from the use of biofeedback for children referred to the Pain Clinic, Children's Hospital of Western Ontario (CHWO), support these advantages.

Although children's relatively brief attention span, their limited understanding, their potential fear of the electronic equipment, and the lack of standardized sites for electrode placement have been cited as potential disadvantages for the use of biofeedback, these difficulties are not insurmountable (Attanasio et al., 1985). Biofeedback may be used successfully with very young children, who are likely to understand the rationale if it is presented as a special game. The major contradiction for biofeedback-assisted pain reduction is for children whose pain is related to their expectations for unreasonably high levels of performance in all their activities. They can become more stressed by their need to achieve dramatic reductions in their EMG levels, with subsequent increases in the intensity or frequency of their pain.

Modeling

Modeling refers to a method in which children learn vicariously by observing an individual's behavior in a particular situation and passively acquiring that new behavior. Modeling may lead to further learning when children imitate the observed behavior, without necessarily receiving direct instructions about the reasons for the model's actions. Modeling procedures have been shown to reduce many fears and avoidance behaviors in children (Melamed & Siegel, 1980). As an example, children may observe another child receiving a painful immunization injection. The child model calmly participates in the procedure by choosing an arm, cleaning the area with an alcohol swab, and then counting "one, two, three, now" with the nurse. The observer child may be less anxious and fearful after watching the manner in which the model has successfully coped in a potentially aversive situation.

Much research has been conducted to identify the critical components of modeling that ensure optimal learning. Participant modeling or modeling with guided practice consists of guided practice with the observer after he or she has watched the model (Bandura, 1976). Children practice the modeled behaviors in progressively more realistic circumstances, with the therapist providing consistent encouragement and assistance as the child attempts to imitate the model's performance. In our pain clinic, modeling can effectively reduce pain for children requiring invasive medical and dental procedures, particularly for young children, retarded children, and children who do not understand English. Most admission preparatory programs for children's hospitals include modeling procedures using films, puppets, and active teaching sessions with Nursing, Child Life, or Psychology staff.

Modeling can reduce the anxiety, fear, overt distress, and pain associated with finger pricks, injections, lumbar punctures, bone marrow aspirations, portacatheter care, and dressing changes. However, as with other behavioral interventions, the specific efficacy of modeling alone has not been adequately demonstrated. Instead, modeling is often used in conjunction with operant conditioning principles and desensitization techniques, and includes a cognitive aspect in which children receive a more realistic and accurate understanding of the pain source. More research must be conducted to identify the best models for children in terms of perceived similarity, the numbers of behaviors modeled, initial anxiety level of the model, and the general effectiveness of the modeled coping behaviors. The best model for teaching a child how to reduce pain presumably depends on the child's age, sex, cognitive level, previous experience, fear, anxiety, and the nature of the pain (McGrath, 1990).

Desensitization

Desensitization is a procedure in which individuals are gradually exposed to an anxiety-producing object or situation in a hierarchical sequence so that their conditioned anxiety is eventually deconditioned. The anxiety-arousing stimulus is systematically paired with a response that is incompatible with anxiety, such as relaxation (Wolpe, 1982). Children, who develop conditioned fears and anxiety about pain related to repeated invasive treatments, have been shown to benefit from systematic desensitization (McGrath, 1990; McGrath & deVeber, 1986).

During an initial pain assessment (that ideally includes structured interviews with parents and child and an observation of the child receiving the treatment) the specific anxiety-producing components of the treatment are identified. Then, a program is structured to expose the child gradually to the less anxiety-inducing components while teaching them coping strategies to help them relax, increase their control, improve their understanding of the treatment, and reduce the aversiveness of the situation. The child learns to relax and cope with each aspect of the procedure. Progressively more realistic practice sessions are scheduled, which include a successively greater number of the identified anxiety components, as the child learns to adjust to each one.

In summary, behavioral therapies increase adults' physical activity levels, decrease their medication use, and reduce their pain behaviors (for review, Turner & Chapman, 1982). Although the specific analgesic efficacy of exercise, operant conditioning, relaxation, biofeedback, modeling, desensitization, and art or play therapy has not been studied comprehensively for children, these behavioral therapies can increase children's physical activity, decrease their fear and anxiety, decrease their reliance on medication or on parents for pain relief, reduce maladaptive pain behaviors, and reduce their pain. Most behavioral therapies may be used to control pain for children of all ages from toddlers to adolescents. However, the selection of a particular method depends on the age of the child, the nature of the child and the family's behaviors, the child's pain coping abilities, the child's emotional state, and whether the pain represents an acute, recurrent, or chronic problem. Method selection is based primarily on clinical practice, since there have not yet been systematic evaluations of which behavioral methods are most effective for children according to the relevant factors that influence their pain. Table 4.3, which lists the various behavioral methods that are commonly used with children, indicates which methods have been most beneficial for the children referred to the Pain Clinic, CHWO.

In general, play therapy is the only behavioral method that is restricted to younger children. All other methods may be used with children of all ages from toddlers to adolescents. Yet, as shown by the + + symbol in Table 4.3, certain behavioral methods seem most appropriate for different age groups. Similarly, certain methods are more appropriate when children exhibit overt distress during painful treatments or painful episodes, when parents have unintentionally reinforced maladaptive pain behaviors or pain complaints, or when children have become conditioned to a variety of pain triggers. The type of pain, alone, is insufficient to determine a particular method for pain intervention. Although desensitization is usually used only for acute pain, several other behavioral methods are equally beneficial. Therefore, there are no simple rules that determine which method is best for which child simply based on age or pain complaint. Instead, method selection is guided by a careful and thorough assessment of the situational, familial, emotional, and

TABLE 4.3. Behavioral methods used at the Children's Pain Clinic, Children's Hospital of Western Ohio.

	Exercise	Operant conditioning	Relaxation	Biofeedback	Modeling	Art, play	Desensitization
Child's age							
2–6	+	++	+	+	++	++	++
7–11	++	++	++	++	+	+	++
12–16	++	+	+	++			+
Behavioral factors							
Child's overt distress	++	+	+	+	++	+	+
Parents reward pain behaviors		++					
Learned pain triggers		++		++			
No pain coping ability		++			++		
Fear, anxiety	+	++	+		+	+	++
Pain category							
Acute	+	++	+		++	+	++
Recurrent	++	++	++	++		+	
Chronic	++	+	++	+	+	+	

Symbols: Clinical impression that method is appropriate (+) or very appropriate (++) for this category.
From *Pain in children: Nature, assessment and treatment* (p. 158) by P. A. McGrath, 1990, New York: Guilford. Copyright 1990 by Guilford Publications, Inc. Reprinted by permission.

behavioral factors relevant to a child's pain to determine which of the available methods will modify those factors and reduce pain.

The diverse array of behavioral interventions constitutes a versatile repertoire of "tools" that can be incorporated into pain management programs for children who experience any type of pain. Many of these methods share a common focus in that children's physical activity and control increases, their pain behaviors decrease, fear and anxiety are reduced, and parental responses become more consistent. Children become more physically and mentally relaxed. Thus, although children's behaviors are specifically targeted for modification, there are concomitant positive changes in children's attitudes, expectations, and control. Pain reduction is probably achieved by a combination of physiological mechanisms due to increased physical activity, reduced postural restrictions, decreased muscular tension, and altered cognitive factors.

Cognitive Approaches

Many different cognitive interventions have been used successfully to reduce acute, chronic, and recurrent pains in children (McGrath, 1990). These interventions include simple distraction and attention, visual imagery, thought stopping, hypnosis, music therapy, and psychotherapy. Most cognitive methods share a primary objective, in which patients become completely and selectively focused on a thought or image so that they are unlikely to attend to or perceive sensory events (such as pain level) at their usual intensity. Patients' selective mental concentration blocks or lessens the perception of pain. Although there is considerable overlap among the different cognitive interventions, each method has unique characteristics.

Children have effectively used cognitive coping strategies to reduce acute pain evoked by the normal bumps and scrapes of childhood, acute pain evoked by invasive medical or dental treatments, recurrent headaches, abdominal pains, limb pains, phantom limb pain, arthritic pain, and cancer pain. Like behavioral interventions, the particular cognitive intervention selected depends on a child's age, cognitive level, previous pain experience, history of pain control, parental attitudes, and the nature of the pain. Although most cognitive methods are necessarily limited to children who are able to communicate verbally and express their ideas, some methods may be used with all children.

Distraction and Focused Attention

Distraction is undoubtedly the most common cognitive method used by parents and health professionals to alleviate children's suffering. When an infant is hurt and cries in pain, parents often provide comfort and reassurance after attending to the cause of the pain. They then attempt to distract the infant and divert attention away from the pain. When young children fall, bump their heads, or scrape their knees, parents usually try to focus their children's attention on an interesting topic or game after they have medicated the wound and comforted the child. Distraction does not passively divert children's attention away from pain, but actively alters their perception. The more absorbed they are by an event, the more they can reduce their pain.

The scientific rationale as to why distraction reduces the intensity and unpleasantness of children's pain has only recently been recognized. The child's active absorption or concentration may be the key factor for triggering an internal pain-suppressing system to block pain, so that cognitive interventions may directly attenuate the neuronal impulses evoked by a noxious stimulus. Distraction has been incorrectly perceived as a simple diversionary tactic in which children are passively placed in a situation where they do not attend to pain. The implication is that the pain is still there but the child is momentarily focused elsewhere, however, this interpretation is inaccurate because children do not simply ignore the pain but actually reduce it. Our revised understanding is derived from animal studies in which the neuronal activity, evoked by a constant noxious stimulus, varies depending on the animal's attention (Dubner, Hoffman, & Hayes, 1981; Price, 1988).

The critical component for reducing pain by distraction is the ability of the child to attend fully and to concentrate on something else besides his or her pain. Therefore, the choice of a distraction is critical to the success of this cognitive intervention. The choice of a distraction will necessarily vary according to children's ages and interests. Infants and young children require concrete external events or objects to absorb their attention, such as interesting toys with optimally complex visual, auditory, or tactile dimensions. Older children can be distracted by both concrete and abstract activities. As an example, distraction was used to assist several children with cancer who had been referred to our pain clinic (McGrath, 1990). These children developed anxiety about weekly intravenous chemotherapy treatments, identifying days as "good" or "bad" treatment days depending on the type of drug they would receive. They exhibited sleeping, eating, and behavioral problems prior to the "bad" days and experienced much more nausea, vomiting, and pain during those treatments. Although some of the nausea was due to the type of drug, there was a possibility that children's heightened anxiety contributed to some of their pain and distress. A trial program was designed in which children were encouraged to play video games, that required their complete attention to earn points, during the 3 to 4 hours in which the intravenous drugs were administered. This program was quite successful for 10- to 12-year-old boys. They were not allowed to play until they were already "hooked up" for treatment. They then played as long as they wanted, even though they vomited intermittently. Their weekly high points were recorded on a large poster in the clinic, along with the time at which they played. Prizes were allocated monthly.

Children became less anxious about treatments, vomited less during treatments, and resumed more of their normal activities after treatments than they had before using the video game as distractions. Children and parents recorded objective information about their progress and were guided to understand that the children's concentration, not the games, had truly reduced their distress and pain. The optimal use of distraction requires a creative and imaginative approach, so that staff select the most interesting available object or situation for each child. The current reasonable costs for microcomputers and the diversity of games and educational programs for children of all ages provides an extensive repertoire for choosing innovative and interesting distractions for children.

Imagery

Imagery refers to the process in which an individual concentrates intently on the mental image of an experience or situation. The image is not superficial, but involves a vivid and rich recall of all the sensations associated with the experience. Although the term *visual imagery* is used synonymously with imagery, true imagery should encompass more than visual perception. Imagery has been used frequently with children and adolescents to alleviate pain (for review, see Hilgard & LeBaron, 1984; McGrath, 1990). Often, children are guided to recall and vividly describe positive past experiences. They are asked to describe specific details — the colors, sounds, tastes, and feel — of the experience. They are asked about the reactions of others and are guided to become as immersed in their image as if it were occurring now.

Imagery, then, can be considered a specific method of distraction and focused attention. Yet, imagery can also be considered a specific method for producing physiological changes to relax the body. It is difficult for patients, adults or children, to control their physical state (heart rate or skin temperature) by simply concentrating on changing their state analogously to moving a limb. However, imagery can be used to induce these changes. For example, the vivid image of a frightening experience will accelerate heart rate. Similarly, the vivid image that your hand is placed against a hot surface can produce increases in skin temperature and blood volume. Even very young children can use imagery to produce dramatic physical changes. (Refer to McCaffery, 1979, for detailed description of the uses and effects of imagery for pain control.)

The manner in which imagery reduces pain or alters physiological systems is not yet understood, but the efficacy of imagery depends on the ability of the individual to select an appropriately vivid image and to concentrate fully on that image. Children generally have rich imaginations so that a diverse repertoire of potential images are available. Most of the images that are currently used in our pain program were developed from the children themselves. A young girl with cancer invented "magic sparklies," an invisible air to breathe in deeply prior to invasive procedures. The air helped to relax her and lightly numb her skin before medical treatments. Many other children have also chosen to imagine sparklies. They have been described variously as gold, silver, white, small stars, sunbursts, and speckles of rainbow. Although the images children choose change as they mature so that adolescents use more sophisticated images, imagery is a powerful tool that even children as young as 3 years of age can use to alleviate some of their pain.

Thought Stopping

Thought stopping is a process in which children, who anticipate pain either related to medical procedures or to diseases, learn to substitute positive thoughts for their negative ones. Ross (1984) developed this process for children to reduce their anticipatory anxiety and to increase their control during painful treatments. Children learn the positive and reassuring aspects associated with a feared event and condense this information into simple statements that they then memorize. Whenever children begin to think about the event, they are required to stop any activities and recite all the positive statements. Thought stopping has been used successfully to reduce anxiety in 6- to 9-year-old educable mentally retarded children during dental treatments and in hospitalized children who require repeated blood tests (Ross, 1984).

The procedure encourages children to develop some independent coping strategies. Children should always receive some positive and reassuring information about painful procedures or painful disorders, regardless of which pharmacological or nonpharmacological interventions are selected. Thought stopping may be a particularly useful therapy for children whose fear and anxiety represent conditioned emotional reactions.

Hypnosis

Since Mesmer's first magnetic treatments in 1794, the use of hypnosis for pain relief has gained both scientific credibility and popular appeal. A vast number of research studies have been conducted to identify the critical features in hypnosis and to understand how hypnosis can produce such diverse effects from curing warts to reducing chronic pain (for review, Fromm & Shor, 1979; Hilgard & Hilgard, 1983; Olness, 1981a, 1981b; Orne, 1983). Although some contradictory and controversial findings have emerged from the myriad of research on hypnosis, much knowledge has accrued about hypnotic analgesia in adults and children.

The major application of hypnosis in pediatrics has been to control acute pain related to invasive procedures for children with cancer. Several clinical studies have demonstrated unequivocally that hypnosis can reduce anxiety, discomfort, and pain evoked by chemotherapy, injections, lumbar punctures, and bone marrow aspirations in children and adolescents (Ellenberg,

Kellerman, Dash, Higgins, & Zeltzer, 1980; Hilgard & LeBaron, 1984; Katz, Kellerman, & Ellenberg, 1987; Kellerman, Zeltzer, Ellenberg, & Dash, 1983; LaBaw, Holton, Tewell, & Eccles, 1975; Olness, 1981b; Zeltzer & LeBaron, 1982). In addition, hypnosis has been used as the primary or adjunctive therapy for children with burns (LaBaw, 1973), migraine headaches (Olness & MacDonald, 1981), hemophilia (LaBaw, 1975; Varni et al., 1981), and sickle cell anemia (Zeltzer et al., 1979).

Hypnosis usually begins with an induction procedure, often involving relaxation exercises, in which the subject's attention is gradually focused on the hypnotist's suggestions. The induction is a simple procedure, which varies according to children's age and developmental level, as well as to children's interests. Children can be guided into a hypnotic state by instructing them to imagine vividly their favorite television shows, movies, books, or cartoon characters. As they imagine an activity, scene, or character, they can gradually receive suggestions for relaxation, reduced anxiety, increased control, and pain reduction. The therapist provides consistent positive suggestions, rather than authoritative commands. The emphasis is on the child's own natural abilities such as, "Notice that your back feels sleepy and my touch seems lighter than before; it seems as if you don't feel the hurt as much as before, you are learning how to turn off the pain switch."

Hypnosis provides both relaxation and cognitive pain coping skills for children. The responsibility for the success or failure of subsequent pain reduction is shared in that a child's ability to reduce pain is enhanced by the hypnotic process and not dependent solely on him- or herself. For children particularly, the assistance provides them with more mastery so that ultimately they can use self-hypnosis confidently without relying on a hypnotist.

In summary, many cognitive interventions such as hypnosis, visual imagery, distraction, and thought stopping share common principles of pain management. They modify relevant situational factors that have been shown in animal behavioral studies and human psychophysical studies to alter nociceptive responses and human pain perception. Like many nonpharmacological interventions, cognitive approaches provide patients with accurate information and realistic expectations about the noxious stimulus, improve the patients' perceived control over a noxious stimulus by teaching them specific coping strategies (relaxation, imagery, hypnotic suggestions, physical exercise), and reduce the aversive significance or meaning of the noxious stimulus.

Guidelines for Method Selection

In consideration of the diverse array of nonpharmacological interventions available for controlling pain, method selection is a special concern. Unfortunately, the choice of a method for pain control has often been based on the particular biases of individual health professionals, rather than on well-defined criteria. In fact, there has been a tendency to view pain as an entity distinct from the patient. As a consequence, certain interventions become matched to certain types of pain without attention to the patient who is experiencing the pain. For example, children with recurrent headaches often receive biofeedback and relaxation-based therapies for reducing the frequency and intensity of their headaches. However, usually no attempt is made to distinguish children on the basis of the relevant familial, situational, and emotional factors that contribute to the pain. Children are lumped together with the same pain diagnosis, recurrent migraine or tension headaches. Thus, the diagnosis represents the problem that requires treatment rather than the pain in relationship to the child and the context in which he or she is experiencing it.

This tendency has naturally evolved from the medical conception of pain as a symptom associated with disease. Disease treatment is consistent and usually determined solely by the disorder and its characteristics. However, many pains are not symptoms of underlying diseases, so that optimal management of these pains requires a different approach. Causative factors for the pain must be identified and managed to ensure effective and long-lasting pain control. Although all children with recurrent headaches may be generally labeled as having recurrent migraine or tension headaches, they may form special subgroups for which the etiology of their headaches is related to primarily emotional, primarily situational, or various combinations of factors.

Even when pain is a symptom of an underlying disease or is related to a well-defined noxious stimulus, the appropriate pharmacological or non-pharmacological interventions should be selected on the basis of the contributing factors, not simply on the basis of the pain type. More recently, attention is being focused on how to select a method for reducing pain, based on a careful evaluation of not only sensory attributes of the pain (quality, intensity, location, duration, and frequency) but also on the psychological and situational attributes of the patient. Clinicians and investigators are attempting to identify the relevant factors that may affect the patient's pain in order to select the method or combination of methods that most adequately modify those factors to attenuate pain. Children as young as 2 years old may benefit from a cognitive approach and adolescents with recurrent pain syndrome may benefit from a behavioral approach. Selection of the appropriate methods begins with a thorough and comprehensive pain assessment and the identification of all the factors that contribute to children's pain experience. An integrated multistrategy program is generally the most effective approach, because it provides a multidimensional modification of the many factors that are relevant to children's pain (multistrategy programs used in our pain clinic to alleviate children's acute, recurrent, and chronic pain are described in McGrath, 1990).

References

American Academy of Pediatrics, Committee on Drugs. (1977). Guidelines for the ethical conduct of studies to evaluate drugs in pediatric populations. *Pediatrics*, *60*, 90–101.

American Academy of Pediatrics, Committee on Infectious Diseases. (1982). Special report: Aspirin and Reye's syndrome. *Pediatrics*, *69*, 810–812.

Attanasio, V., Andrasik, F., Burke, E. J., Blake, D. D., Kabela, E., & McCarran, M. S. (1985). Clinical issues in utilizing biofeedback with children. *Clinical Biofeedback and Health*, *8*, 134–141.

Attia, J., Ecoffey, C., Sandouk, P., Gross, J. B., & Samii, K. (1986). Epidural morphine in children: Pharmacokinetics and CO_2 sensitivity. *Anesthesiology*, *65*, 590–594.

Bandura, A. (1976). Effecting change through participant modeling. In J. D. Krumboltz & C. E. Thoresen (Eds.), *Counseling methods* (pp. 248–265). New York: Holt, Rinehart and Winston.

Barr, R. G. (1989). Pain in children. In P. D. Wall & R. Melzack (Eds.), *Textbook of pain* (2nd Ed., pp. 568–588). Edinburgh: Churchill Livingstone.

Beers, R. F., & Bassett, E. G. (Eds.). (1979). *Mechanisms of pain and analgesic compounds*. New York: Raven Press.

Benitz, W. E., & Tatro, D. S. (1981). *The pediatric drug handbook*. Chicago: Year Book Medical.

Benson, H., Pomeranz, B., & Kutz, I. (1984). The relaxation response and pain. In P. D. Wall & R. Melzack (Eds.), *Textbook of pain* (pp. 817–822). Edinburgh: Churchill Livingstone.

Beyer, J. E., DeGood, D. E., Ashley, L. C., & Russell, G. A. (1983). Patterns of postoperative analgesic use with adults and children following cardiac surgery. *Pain*, *17*, 71–81.

Bromage, P. R. (1984). Epidural anaesthetics and narcotics. In P. D. Wall & R. Melzack (Eds.), *Textbook of pain* (pp. 558–565). Edinburgh: Churchill Livingstone.

Brown, R. E. Jr., & Broadman, L. M. (1987). Patient-controlled analgesia (PCA) for postoperative pain control in adolescents. *Anesthesia and Analgesia*, *66*, S1–S191.

Cohen, S. N. (1980). Ethics of drug research in children. In S. J. Yaffe (Ed.), *Pediatric pharmacology: Therapeutic principles in practice* (pp. 93–100). New York: Grune and Stratton.

Cousins, M. M., & Mather, L. E. (1984). Intrathecal and epidural administration of opioids. *Anesthesiology*, *61*, 276–310.

Diamond, S. (1979). Biofeedback and headache. *Headache*, *19*, 180–184.

Dodd, E., Wang, J. M., & Rauck, R. L. (1988). Patient controlled analgesia for post-surgical pediatric patients ages 6–16 years. *Anesthesiology*, *69*, A372.

Dubner, R., Hoffman, D. S., & Hayes, R. L. (1981). Neural activity in medullary dorsal horn of awake monkeys trained in a thermal discrimination task: III. Task-related responses and their functional role. *Journal of Neurophysiology*, *46*, 444–464.

Dundee, J. W., & Loan, W. B. (1983). Assessment of analgesic drugs. In N. E. Williams & H. Wilson (Eds.), *International encyclopedia of pharmacology and therapeutics: Sec. 112, Pain and its management* (pp. 79–88). Elmsford, NY: Pergamon Press.

Eland, J. M. (1974). *Children's communication of pain*. Unpublished master's thesis, University of Iowa.

Ellenberg, L., Kellerman, J., Dash, J., Higgins, G., & Zeltzer, L. (1980). Use of hypnosis for multiple symptoms in an adolescent girl with leukemia. *Journal of Adolescent Health Care, 1*, 132–136.

Finholt, D. A., Stirt, J. A., & DiFazio, C. A. (1985). Epidural morphine for postoperative analgesia in pediatric patients. *Anesthesia and Analgesia, 64*, 211.

Fordyce, W. E. (1976). *Behavioral methods for chronic pain and illness*. St. Louis: C. V. Mosby.

Fordyce, W. E. (1978). Learning processes in pain. In R. A. Sternbach (Ed.), *The psychology of pain* (pp. 49–72). New York: Raven Press.

Fromm, E., & Shor, R. E. (Eds.). (1979). *Hypnosis: Developments in research and new perspectives*. Chicago: Aldine.

Gladtke, E. (1983). Use of antipyretic analgesics in the pediatric patient. *American Journal of Medicine, 75*, 121–126.

Glenski, J. A., Warner, M. A., Dawson, B., & Kaufman, B. (1984). Postoperative use of epidurally administered morphine in children and adolescents. *Mayo Clinic Proceedings, 59*, 530–533.

Goodman, L. S., & Gilman, A. G. (Eds.). (1985). *The pharmacological basis of therapeutics* (7th ed.). New York: Macmillan.

Gross, S. C., & Gardner, G. G. (1980). Child pain: Treatment approaches. In W. L. Smith, H. Merskey, & S. C. Gross (Eds.), *Pain: Meaning and management* (pp. 127–142). Jamaica, NY: Spectrum Publications.

Gruner, O. C. (1930). *A treatise on the Canon of Medicine of Avicenna*. London: Luzac.

Hilgard, E. R., & Hilgard, J. R. (1983). *Hypnosis in the relief of pain*. Los Altos, CA: William Kaufmann.

Hilgard, J. R., & LeBaron, S. (1984). *Hypnotherapy of pain in children with cancer*. Los Altos, CA: William Kaufmann.

Huskisson, E. C. (1984). Non-narcotic analgesics. In P. D. Wall & R. Melzack (Eds.), *Textbook of pain* (pp. 505–513). Edinburgh: Churchill Livingstone.

Jacobsen, E. (1938). *Progressive relaxation*. Chicago: University of Chicago Press.

Jaffe, J. H., & Martin, W. R. (1980). Narcotic analgesics and antagonists. In A. G. Gilman, L. S. Goodman, & A. Gilman (Eds.), *The pharmacological basis of therapeutics* (pp. 245–283). New York: Macmillan.

Jay, S. M., Elliott, C. H., Ozolins, M., Olson, R. A., & Pruitt, S. D. (1985). Behavioural management of children's distress during painful medical procedures. *Behaviour Research and Therapy, 23*, 513–552.

Jessup, B. A. (1984). Biofeedback. In P. D. Wall & R. Melzack (Eds.), *Textbook of pain* (pp. 776–786). Edinburgh: Churchill Livingstone.

Katz, E. R., Kellerman, J., & Ellenberg, L. (1987). Hypnosis in the reduction of acute pain and distress in children with cancer. *Journal of Pediatric Psychology, 12*, 379–394.

Kellerman, J., Zeltzer, L., Ellenberg, L., & Dash, J. (1983). Adolescents with cancer. Hypnosis for the reduction of the acute pain and anxiety associated with medical procedures. *Journal of Adolescent Health Care, 4*, 85–90.

Krane, E. J., Tyler, D. C., & Jacobson, L. J. (1989). The dose response of caudal morphine in children. *Anesthesiology, 71*, 48–52.

LaBaw, W. L. (1973). Adjunctive trance therapy with severely burned children. *International Journal of Child Psychotherapy, 2*, 80–92.

LaBaw, W. L. (1975). Auto-hypnosis in haemophilia. *Haematologia*, *9*, 103–110.

LaBaw, W. L., Holton, C., Tewell, K., & Eccles, D. (1975). The use of self-hypnosis by children with cancer. *American Journal of Clinical Hypnosis*, *17*, 233–238.

Levine, M. N., Sackett, D. L., & Bush, H. (1986). Heroin vs. morphine for cancer pain? *Archives of Internal Medicine*, *146*, 353–356.

Masek, B. J., Russo, D. C., & Varni, J. W. (1984). Behavioral approaches to the management of chronic pain in children. *Pediatric Clinics of North America*, *31*, 1113–1131.

Mather, L. E., & Mackie, J. (1983). The incidence of postoperative pain in children. *Pain*, *15*, 271–282.

McCaffery, M. (1979). *Nursing management of the patient with pain*. Philadelphia: J. B. Lippincott.

McCaffery, M., & Beebe, A. (1989). *Pain: Clinical manual for nursing practice*. St. Louis: C. V. Mosby.

McGrath, P. A. (1990). *Pain in children: Nature, assessment and treatment*. New York: Guilford.

McGrath, P. A., & deVeber, L. L. (1986). The management of acute pain evoked by medical procedures in children with cancer. *Journal of Pain and Symptom Management*, *1*, 145–150.

McGrath, P. J. (1983). Migraine headaches in children and adolescents. In P. Firestone, P. J. McGrath, & W. Feldman (Eds.), *Advances in behavioral medicine for children and adolescents* (pp. 39–57). Hillsdale, NJ: Erlbaum.

McGrath, P. J., & Unruh, A. (1987). *Pain in children and adolescents*. Amsterdam: Elsevier.

McIlvaine, W. B. (1990). Spinal opioids for the pediatric patient. *Journal of Pain and Symptom Management*, *5*, 183–190.

Means, L. J., Allen, H. M., Lookabill, S. J., & Krishna, G. (1988). Recovery room initiation of patient-controlled analgesia in pediatric patients. *Anesthesiology*, *69*, A772.

Melamed, B. G., & Siegel, L. J. (1980). *Behavioral medicine: practical applications in health care* (Vol. 6). New York: Springer.

Melzack, R., & Wall, P. D. (1965). Pain mechanisms: A new theory. *Science*, *150*, 971–978.

Moulin, D. E., & Coyle, N. (1986). Spinal opioid analgesics and local anesthetics in the management of chronic cancer pain. *Journal of Pain and Symptom Management*, *1*, 79–86.

Olness, K. (1981a). Hypnosis in pediatric practice. *Current Problems in Pediatrics*, *12*, 1–47.

Olness, K. (1981b). Imagery (self-hypnosis) as adjunct therapy in childhood cancer: Clinical experience with 25 patients. *American Journal of Pediatric Hematology/Oncology*, *3*, 313–321.

Olness, K., & MacDonald, J. (1981). Self-hypnosis and biofeedback in the management of juvenile migraine. *Journal of Developmental and Behavioral Pediatrics*, *2*, 168–170.

Orne, M. T. (1983). Hypnotic methods for managing pain. In J. Bonica, U. Lindblom, & A. Iggo (Eds.), *Advances in pain research and therapy* (Vol. 5, pp. 847–856). New York: Raven Press.

Price, D. D. (1988). *Psychological and neural mechanisms of pain*. New York: Raven Press.

Rodgers, B. M., Webb, C. J., Stergios, D., & Newman, B. M. (1988). Patient-controlled analgesia in pediatric surgery. *Journal of Pediatric Surgery, 23*, 259-262.

Ross, D. M. (1984). Thought-stopping: A coping strategy for impending feared events. *Issues in Comprehensive Pediatric Nursing, 7*, 83-89.

Ross, D. M., & Ross, S. A. (1988). *Childhood pain: Current issues, research, and management.* Baltimore: Urban and Schwarzenberg.

Schechter, N. L. (Ed.). (1989). Acute pain in children. *Pediatric Clinics of North America, 36*, 781-1052.

Schechter, N. L., Allen, D. A., & Hanson, K. (1986). Status of pediatric pain control: A comparison of hospital analgesic usage in children and adults. *Pediatrics, 77*, 11-15.

Shannon, M., & Berde, C. B. (1989). Pharmacologic management of pain in children and adolescents. *Pediatric Clinics of North America, 36*, 855-872.

Shapiro, L. A., Jedeikin, R. J., Shalev, D., & Hoffman, S. (1984). Epidural morphine analgesia in children. *Anesthesiology, 61*, 210-212.

Swafford, L. I., & Allan, D. (1968). Pain relief in the pediatric patient. *Medical Clinics of North America, 52*, 131-136.

Turk, D. C., Meichenbaum, D., & Berman, W. H. (1979). Application of biofeedback for the regulation of pain: A critical review. *Psychological Bulletin, 86*, 1322-1338.

Turner, J. A., & Chapman, C. R. (1982). Psychological interventions for chronic pain: A critical review. *Pain, 12*, 1-46.

Twycross, R. G. (1978). Pain and analgesics. *Current Medical Research and Opinion, 5*, 497-505.

Twycross, R. G. (1979). The Brompton cocktail. In J. Bonica & V. Ventafridda (Eds.), *Advances in pain research and therapy* (Vol. 2, pp. 291-300). New York: Raven Press.

Tyler, D. C. (1987). Patient controlled analgesia in adolescents. *Pain*, (Suppl. 4), S236.

Tyler, D. C., & Krane, E. J. (1990). *Advances in pain research and therapy* (Vol. 15). New York: Raven Press.

Varni, J. W. (1981). Behavioral medicine in hemophilia arthritic pain management: Two case studies. *Archives of Physical Medicine and Rehabilitation, 62*, 183-192.

Varni, J. W., Gilbert, A., & Dietrich, S. L. (1981). Behavioral medicine in pain and analgesia management for the hemophilic child with Factor VIII inhibitor. *Pain, 11*, 121-126.

Wakeman, R. J., & Kaplan, J. Z. (1978). An experimental study of hypnosis in painful burns. *American Journal of Clinical Hypnosis, 21*, 3-12.

Wolpe, J. (1982). *The practice of behavior therapy.* Elmsford, NY: Pergamon Press.

Yaffe, S. J. (Ed.). (1980). *Pediatric pharmacology: Therapeutic principles in practice.* New York: Grune and Stratton.

Yaksh, T. L. (1981). Spinal opiate analgesia: Characteristics and principles of action. *Pain, 11*, 293-346.

Zeltzer, L. K., Dash, J., & Holland, J. P. (1979). Hypnotically induced pain control in sickle cell anemia. *Pediatrics, 64*, 533-536.

Zeltzer, L. K., & LeBaron, S. (1982). Hypnosis and nonhypnotic techniques for reduction of pain and anxiety during painful procedures in children and adolescents with cancer. *Journal of Pediatrics, 101*, 1032-1035.

5
Pediatric Pain Management: Professional and Pragmatic Issues

Jeffrey B. Gillman and Larry L. Mullins

The experience of pain is universal and is a part of the human condition from early in life until the moment of death (Mennie, 1974). Although the management of pain in adults has been studied and addressed by almost all medical specialties for many years, it is only within the last decade or so that similar work has been undertaken with children. It is quite evident to those who work with individuals who are experiencing pain, particularly those who work with pediatric populations, that the scientific and technical issues involved in pain assessment and management are extremely complex. The sources and mediating factors of a child's pain experience and its exacerbation may be numerous and interrelated. They are likely to include one or more of the following: physical and/or psychological trauma; an ongoing disease process; diagnostic procedures; therapeutic or treatment procedures; psychological distress resulting from disturbed family dynamics; anxiety; depression; fear regarding the etiology, prognosis, and treatment of a medical condition; and the child's cognitive/developmental level, previous history of pain experiences, and existing or previously developed coping skills. Although the assessment of these complex issues and the development of appropriate intervention strategies are more thoroughly discussed elsewhere in this volume, the focus of this chapter is on the professional and pragmatic issues involved in implementing a pediatric pain program.

As there are still relatively few medical or mental health professionals who have received specialized training in pediatric pain assessment and intervention, it can be logically suggested that those who have undergone relevant training in this area will frequently be called upon as consultants to work with medical staff, the child, and the family with regard to pain issues. Such cases are generally fraught with numerous and complex questions that belie the often posed and occasionally naively phrased referral question, "Please see this child for pain management."

By way of introduction to the complexity of pediatric pain issues, consider the following scenario:

Jenny is a 7-year-old girl who was admitted to the burn unit of a large pediatric hospital 10 days prior to the request for pediatric psychology consultation to aid in pain management. She had received third-degree burns over 40% of her upper body following an explosion in her home. The resulting fire had destroyed the majority of the family's belongings. A telephone conversation with the referring physician, a plastic surgeon, indicated that his primary concerns related to Jenny's panic and extreme combativeness during debridement and dressing change procedures. When not actually involved in medical procedures, she had been observed to be generally compliant, although quiet, withdrawn, and at times tearful. Furthermore, the medical staff had also expressed concerns regarding her ability to understand explanations of her current status and generally optimistic prognosis for survival and recovery. Upon meeting Jenny at bedside, she was observed to be swaddled in bandages from midtrunk to her shoulders as well as down her right arm. She presented as a sad and tearful child who avoided making eye contact with the examiner and who was generally unresponsive to concrete, informationally based questions.

Although this example may appear somewhat extreme in terms of the many questions raised and issues that need to be explored, this hypothetical case is not atypical. A comprehensive response in this case would include a detailed discussion with the referral source regarding his or her specific concerns and the level of consultant involvement sought, several interviews with the family regarding the child's preaccident functioning and subsequent behavioral changes, an assessment of current and previous family functioning, an interview and assessment of the child's cognitive/developmental and emotional status, behavioral observations of the child, discussions with pertinent medical staff, and a care planning conference of all care participants to develop and agree upon a pain management program. It has been our experience that the majority of pediatric pain consults are multidimensional, and not unlike this example. As such, they require much of the consultant in terms of the need for coordination of services among professionals, the necessity of frequent contact with the patient, family, and medical personnel, the related need for assessing both family system and medical system functioning, and the need for specifying and clearly differentiating boundaries of responsibilities for the provision of care. It is precisely because of this complexity that Bonica (1953) and more recently Berde, Sethna, Masek, Tosburg, and Rocklin (1989) have forcefully argued for the development of multidisciplinary pain management programs. Such complexity requires that a range of medical professionals work as a team in the assessment and development of pain management strategies for each pediatric pain patient.

Although a variety of professional disciplines may be called upon to assist the physician in evaluating and managing the child's pain, it is our position that the pediatric psychologist offers a unique perspective on a variety of salient issues related to childhood pain. As such, the ensuing discussion will primarily be addressed to professionals within this area. First, an overview of the unique aspects of pediatric pain intervention will be presented, including an emphasis on evaluating the child's cognitive/developmental level and typologies of children's pain. This will be followed by a discussion of the specific attributes and knowledge base that the pediatric psychologist brings to the area of pediatric pain and his or her consequently unique role. Attention will then be focused on the various models often used in addressing childhood pain. This will be followed by a comprehensive discussion of the dynamics of the consultation process from a practical standpoint, including an emphasis on the potential conflicts that may arise during the course of providing these services, as well as suggestions for circumventing such problems. Because the area of pediatric pain assessment and management is a relatively young subspecialty, at the present time there are no specific guidelines for training or credentialing in this area. Therefore, general recommendations for training will be offered. As in any area of medical and mental health service, a number of ethical issues will invariably arise, and several of the most important such issues will be discussed. Finally, we will offer a brief discussion of the future directions in the area of children's pain.

Developmental Issues and Typologies of Pain

The aforementioned example of the burned child illustrates the importance of evaluating the cognitive and developmental abilities of the child in pain. A number of papers (Broome, 1985; Bush, 1987; Gillman & Bush, 1991; Lavigne, Schulein, & Hahn, 1986; Ross & Ross, 1988) have discussed the necessity of considering the child's developmental level, both in terms of understanding affective and behavioral responses to the pain, as well as in the development and implementation of effective intervention strategies. Indeed, Roberts, Maddux, and Wright (1984) specifically state that " . . . more than at any other period of life, developmental changes in biological, physical status, cognitive and intellectual ability, and psychosocial behavior need to be considered in diagnostic evaluation and therapeutic intervention" (p. 56). This emphasis on developmental issues points to one of the major differences between clinical work with pediatric and adult pain populations: the significance of developmental factors as mediating variables in the child's perception of and behavioral presentation relative to pain.

As difficult as the evaluation of adult pain may be due to the numerous variables involved, the assessment of a child's pain is substantially more challenging, given the continual and rapid cognitive, affective, and physical changes in the child. Therefore, the methods used in the evaluation and treatment of adult pain cannot simply be applied in a blanket manner to children. As Eland and Anderson (1977) have pointed out, children are not merely miniature adults and therefore it is not appropriate to discuss pain experiences with children in the same fashion or at the same level as would be done with adults. When compared to adults, children possess not only less information about their pain experiences (as well as smaller vocabularies with which to describe these experiences), but the manner in which they comprehend this information is different and less sophisticated. As a result, the younger the child is, the more difficult it is to measure his or her experience of pain. Varni (1983) astutely points out that in order to appreciate and comprehend the child's pain experience fully, pediatric pain assessment should be multidimensional, interdisciplinary, and comprehensive. To accomplish such a goal, evaluative and interventive procedures should consider developmental, behavioral, cognitive, socioenvironmental, medical, and biological parameters, as well as the child's subjective experience. An assessment or intervention procedure that does not address the complexity of these factors is likely to yield less than optimal results (Thompson & Varni, 1986).

In addition to developmental factors, it is also crucial for the clinician working with pediatric pain patients to consider both the etiology and chronicity of the pain. The etiology of the child's pain may include observable physical injury or trauma, a disease state, medical procedures, or no identifiable disease process or physical trauma. Each of these etiological classes may be associated with different cognitive, affective, and behavioral manifestations. For example, in the scenario described earlier, the burned child may feel responsible for the explosion in her home. If so, she may experience feelings of guilt and remorse that may in turn be related to her affective presentation. In contrast, the patient who is experiencing recurrent abdominal pain (RAP) syndrome without any identifiable physical basis is likely to present a very different set of historical circumstances, as well as behavioral and emotional characteristics.

In terms of the chronicity of pain, the child may present with a history ranging from acute and time-limited pain (e.g., postsurgical pain, dental pain), to chronically recurring acute pain (e.g., migraine headaches), to chronic, progressive pain that is usually associated with an ongoing disease process (e.g., malignancies). Ross and Ross (1988) have pointed out that children who are experiencing chronic pain present different management issues than those experiencing acute pain. For example, it has been suggested that children who experience pain over a period of time have a greater opportunity to develop an understanding of the nature of their pain, display less behavioral distress in response to painful medical procedures, and certainly have more opportunity to develop effective coping strategies than do children who are experiencing acute pain (Beales, 1979; McCollum, 1981; Ross & Ross, 1982; Travis, 1969).

The Special Role of the Pediatric Psychologist

During the last decade or so, the role of the psychologist in the provision of comprehensive health care has greatly expanded, particularly since the inception of the biopsychosocial model (Engel, 1977; Schwartz, 1982). With this developing awareness and inclusion of social and psychological factors in the conceptualization of illness has come an increasing need for the pediatric health care provider to consult with pediatric psychologists in the care of their medical patients who have special psychological or emotional needs.

In the case of pain, the appropriately trained pediatric psychologist is uniquely prepared to offer a range of consultation services that focus on this aspect of the child's care. McGrath (1987) points out that,

since pain is not always a correlating symptom of disease or injury that diminishes progressively as the disease is treated or as the injury heals, it is necessary to objectively assess the emotional and situational factors that can exacerbate children's acute pain or that can contribute to the development or maintenance of recurrent or chronic pediatric pain. An evaluation of the factors that may modify children's pain, in addition to an assessment of the sensory dimensions of their pain, is an essential prerequisite for the design of effective pain management programs. (p. 147)

It is specifically in this regard that the pediatric psychologist is best equipped to help medical colleagues by virtue of his or her background and training in the assessment of and intervention with issues of cognitive, emotional, and personality development, parent-child relationships, family/systemic functioning, and the impact of chronic and acute illness on these variables. Green (1983) has discussed these more fundamental psychosocial variables, which, in addition to the specific medical factors, must be considered in working with pediatric pain patients. It is to this end that the pediatric psychologist may prove to be an invaluable resource in helping the physician and medical team identify specific variables that may in some way mediate, or on the other hand, be harnessed, to help diminish or manage a child's pain. In contrast, other members of the medical team (i.e., other physicians, nursing staff, occupational and physical therapists) tend to be predominantly trained in physiological aspects of pain assessment and treatment, and consequently emphasize biological and/or pharmacological methods of pain management.

The psychologist's role may be more specifically defined by the following: (a) educating the medical team regarding psychosocial factors and their impact on the child's pain; (b) clarifying for others the child's perceptions of the pain experience; (c) facilitating developmentally appropriate communication between the medical staff and the child; (d) helping the medical staff to communicate more clearly with the family, as well as with each other regarding the child's medical and pain condition; and (e) helping the child and family identify previously utilized resources and develop new coping and adaptation skills. Of course, the manner in which the pain consultant addresses these issues will vary, depending upon the type of setting, the nature of the referral question, the historical relationship that he or she has had with the referral source, and other particulars of the situation.

General Considerations in Pediatric Pain Consultation

Because pain has traditionally been considered to be a physiological phenomenon, it is reasonable to assume that virtually all pain complaints will initially be assessed by a physician. Many of these difficulties are rather easily addressed by the physician through the use of medications and/or simple behavioral instructions to the child and parent. However, when the pain is intense and unresponsive to such "first line" interventions, when it becomes chronic and interferes with normal development or daily functioning, or when the pain has no apparent medical basis, the physician may seek assistance. This often takes the form of a request for consultation from one or more medical specialists. In facilities that employ pediatric pain specialists or a well-developed pediatric psychology section, such professionals may also be called upon. However, it has been our experience that the pediatric psychologist is often viewed as the "last line of defense" and is generally summoned for assistance only when all other efforts have proven unsatisfactory. This places the psychologist in a delicate position. On one hand, the referral source, child, and family have probably developed a pessimistic outlook, given the lack of adequate pain control achieved by a string of previous experts. They may also be angry because of the perceived implication that the pain is "not real." On the other hand, the pediatric psychologist is in a position to "work magic" by assisting the physician in the development, organization, and implementation of a comprehensive approach.

With this background in mind, the consultant is faced with determining, in conjunction with medical colleagues, the manner in which the consult request can best be addressed. To provide a measure of organization to the level of consultation involvement sought by the consultee, Roberts (1986) has discussed three basic conceptual models for conducting pediatric consultations: the indirect psychological consultation model, the independent function model, and the collaborative team model. Roberts points out that flexibility in the use of these models is essential to the successful consultation response. The following sections will briefly discuss each of these models in the context of pain treatment.

Indirect Psychological Consultation Model

This model, also referred to as the resource consultation (Stabler, 1979), is generally used when the physician is seeking information or assistance in making decisions relative to a patient's care. For the pediatric psychologist, the focus is typically on helping either the consultee or the larger pediatric health care program address any of a number of child care issues. In the case of pain, questions may relate to whether a specific child's response to pain is developmentally appropriate, suggestions for simple and concrete pain management techniques, or a request for a brief general assessment of the child (e.g., an evaluation of intellectual functioning in order to facilitate appropriate explanation of medical information to the child). According to this model, it is assumed that the consultant's primary function is to serve as an information resource to the physician or program, but generally does not entail direct participation in treatment. It has been our experience that relatively few consultation requests of this type are made relative to pediatric pain. When such requests are received, many of them tend to develop quickly into more direct child care or team management of the child's pain. This is particularly true if the educational function of the pediatric psychologist is addressed appropriately.

Independent Function Model

This form of consultation is generally utilized when the referring physician is requesting that the consultant independently assess and manage a specific aspect of the child's care. Drotar (1978) refers to this as a "noncollaborative approach." Indeed, the potential for completely independent, noncollaborative, yet shared patient care does exist if the consultant is not sufficiently careful to maintain close and frequent communication with the physician.

The most effective form of this model occurs when the pediatric psychologist and the physician can cooperatively determine which specific issues can be addressed and managed by each party. In conducting this form of consultation it is incumbent upon the pediatric psychologist to ensure that he or she fully understands all medical aspects of the child's care. Similarly, it is crucial to educate medical colleagues regarding the specific nature and extent of pediatric psychology's work with the child and family, as well as all developmental and psychological information relevant to comprehensive intervention. It is in this regard that data relative to the efficacy of a team approach in addressing pediatric pain can be discussed. This, in turn, may lead to the implementation of the collaborative team model.

Collaborative Team Model

It is our opinion that the optimal situation exists when pediatric pain issues are addressed through the use of a comprehensive team approach. Roberts (1986) refers to this as the collaborative team model. As emphasized earlier, pain is a complex, multifaceted entity that is best approached by using an interdisciplinary team (Berde et al., 1989). As the name of this model implies, several professionals function on a team basis in which a collaboration of effort is fostered to address pain from multiple perspectives simultaneously. With this approach, the pediatric psychologist can be in a position to truly share patient care with the physician. Other disciplines that are generally most helpful to enlist in such a team effort include nursing, physical and occupational therapy, child life specialists, and nutritionists.

In the case of the burn patient discussed earlier, such a team venture might work as follows: With the physician taking major responsibility for the child's medical care, the pediatric psychologist may be delegated the responsibility of managing and organizing other team members in addressing pain management. The psychologist's role will obviously include an assessment component, teaching the child any of a variety of distraction and/or coping methods (e.g., progressive relaxation, guided imagery, hypnosis, focused breathing), psychotherapy related to changes in body image and psychosocial adjustment, and parent counseling that focuses on issues related to hospitalization in general and pain in specific. As the nursing staff tends to spend the greatest amount of time with the child, their observations of the child can and should be utilized in developing and implementing specific behavioral strategies for pain management. The physical and occupational therapists are likely to focus on developing activities to maintain and rehabilitate lost functioning. The child life specialist may be helpful in facilitating hospital adjustment through the use of play therapy.

In addition to the specifically patient-focused role, the pediatric psychologist may play a crucial role in helping to educate the other team members regarding developmentally appropriate communication with the child and family. The pediatric psychologist may also be helpful in orchestrating team functioning as it relates to pain management. This will entail defining the roles of each team member, as well as facilitating communication among team members. When such issues are not adequately addressed, turf issues, professional jealousies, and unfair expectations may arise. Needless to say, these difficulties must be minimized for the sake of the child and family as well as for the sake of professional cohesion.

Types of Settings

The pediatric pain specialist may practice in a variety of settings, each offering different types of professional opportunities. As such, the consultation process will differ. Although overlap exists between different settings, we have chosen to focus on four: the medical or health sciences center, the pediatric hospital, the outpatient setting, and the dental clinic.

The typical medical or health sciences center is a large tertiary care facility serving a major catchment area or population. Children's services are but one part of this large system, and can be comprised of inpatient services, outpatient services, or both. A broad spectrum of childhood pain problems may be seen, including severe burn injuries, recurrent abdominal pain, headache pain, and joint pain in children with juvenile rheumatoid arthritis. Medical centers tend to be affiliated with universities, and thus training becomes an additional objective of faculty and staff.

Because of the size and scope of such a setting, the roles (and hence the consultation process) of the pediatric pain specialist become complex and multifaceted. The pain specialist serves the role of educator, supervisor, coordinator of treatment services, and often researcher. Such role demands may be met simultaneously in the course of a short period of time. The psychologist may be treating one child individually for pain, supervising a predoctoral psychology intern on another case, educating the neurology clinic staff on treatment of headache pain, and lecturing to medical students about sickle cell pain, all in the course of a single week. Thus, the form of consulting in this setting may range from the independent function model, to the indirect model, to the collaborative team model.

Because of the size and complexity of this medical system, the psychologist is likely to have many different referral sources, some of whom he or she may never have met. Thus, although this setting is full of excitement and novelty, it is also fraught with numerous potential difficulties. Such difficulties range from coordinating the services of the many people necessary to implement a pediatric pain program, to meeting the service needs of several different departments simultaneously.

The pediatric hospital may demand any of the responsibilities and consultant roles listed above. Whether the pediatric hospital is private or affiliated with a teaching hospital will in part determine these responsibilities. Typically, however, large pediatric hospitals serve broad inpatient and outpatient populations with pain problems, presenting opportunities to utilize all three of the consultation models suggested by Roberts (1986). In general, the pediatric hospital may offer a smaller system with which to contend, and as a result, may yield to more comprehensive service delivery. Finally, it is quite likely that the medical staff of a pediatric hospital will possess greater awareness of and sensitivity to salient developmental issues, thereby simplifying the psychologist's educational role to some degree.

Outpatient settings can vary tremendously, ranging from large multispecialty clinics to private practice offices. Yet, because of the outpatient context of these settings, certain commonalities exist that affect the consultation process. First, an interdisciplinary approach will be more difficult. The independent function model will probably be the model not of choice, but of necessity. Coordinating treatment efforts is a more onerous task, and communication between team members is diminished. It may well be that in the outpatient setting, the practitioner must not only be more selective in terms of cases accepted, but also more responsible for maintaining communication without the benefit of close physical proximity or relationship to others.

The dental clinic lends itself to interesting consulting opportunities. Dental pain and distress have long been known to be common (Melamed, 1979) and are considered to be major problems by many parents and dentists. The literature strongly supports the use of psychologically based interventions for distress reduction in this setting (e.g., Klepac, 1975). In the dental clinic, the pediatric pain specialist has the opportunity to work on a collaborative team model basis and to teach the dentist various pain reduction skills.

The Consultation Process

Although the different forms and contexts of consultation provide a working structure for the psychologist, the process of consultation follows a more dynamic course. The manner in which one approaches the request for a pediatric pain management consultation will depend on a number of factors and will be guided by several basic principles. Primary among these is the specific nature of the referral question. The physician requesting consultation may simply be seeking information regarding developmentally appropriate pain behavior. In contrast, the consultant may be asked to take complete charge of managing the child's pain. It would certainly be inappropriate in the former case for the consultant to address the request in the same manner as would be done in the latter example. Beyond this consideration, the following general issues must be addressed before determining the level and type of involvement required:

1. the history of psychology's involvement within that setting;
2. the specific nature of the setting and organizational structure in which the consult is requested;
3. the nature of the relationship between the consultee and his/her physician colleague;
4. the availability of adjunctive support services; and
5. the specific needs of the child and family.

It is our strong belief that each request for a pain consultation requires a prompt response, preferrably within 24 hours for an inpatient consult. This emphasis on responding quickly serves several important functions. First, it is consistent with the medical model in which the physician functions. Prompt action on the part of the consultant therefore conveys a sense of common framework, as well as professional collegiality and commitment to patient care. Second, the request for consultation in the case of pediatric pain carries with it a sense of urgency that probably exceeds the immediacy required by other types of consult requests. The initial response may be conducted by telephone and should be used to clarify and refine the physician's referral question and provide information regarding assessment and intervention options. With regard to the latter, the psychologist should include very specific statements indicating that from a psychological perspective, pain management and control, not the curing of pain, is the ultimate goal. Furthermore, this discussion should be used to help the physician better understand the complex nature of pain, the important developmental issues involved in communicating with the child during assessment and intervention, and the suggestion that a multidisciplinary team approach is generally most efficacious if such an arrangement is possible. Stabler (1988) cautions that in sharing this material with the physician, care must be taken that the consultant conveys a sense of respectful collegiality. This is best done by prudently communicating patient-specific developmental and psychological information within an empirical framework.

History of Psychological Involvement

The process of pediatric pain consultation will certainly vary as a function of the history of psychological involvement in a particular setting. In some settings, psychologists initiated such services many years ago and are thus perceived as the primary referral source and coordinators of pain management services. In other settings, psychologists may never have had any role in pain management services, or have only been involved in more traditional treatment enterprises, i.e., psychotherapy. Some settings may never have had a psychologist on staff, much less a consultant available to provide psychological services. Thus, many different levels of involvement may pre-exist that, in turn, dictate how the consultation proceeds.

The ideal situation for the process of consultation exists when pediatric psychology has a long history of involvement in pain management, when clear lines of communication and role responsibility between disciplines have been established, and when pain management by psychologists has proven efficacy as perceived by other staff. In such a context, the consultation process can begin with the referral request itself. The psychologist can conduct the intake and initial assessment, proceeding with treatment as is deemed necessary.

Unfortunately, this ideal situation is probably still relatively rare, although one hopes that it is increasing in frequency. The more typical scenario is one in which (a) psychologists have never been utilized as providers of pain management services; (b) psychologists have only been utilized in other more traditional realms of care; or (c) psychologists have been utilized as providers of pain management services and such services were not well received.

In settings where pediatric psychologists have not previously been utilized in working with children in pain, the consultation process will begin with establishing professional relationships, delineating the nature of services that can be offered and their potential benefits, and creating the interdisciplinary team. Such an undertaking is best conceptualized as an educational process that can be quite time-consuming. This process generally begins with the medical staff. It must be emphasized that most pediatric psychologists depend upon referrals for their livelihood. Pediatricians hold the most powerful positions in many of the settings in which pediatric psychologists work; they also hold much of the medical and legal responsibility for the care of patients. Fortunately, most pediatricians are eager to help their patients in any reasonable way and openly welcome psychological involvement. Unfortunately, some psychologists approach the medical system with an antimedical-model stance, and are subsequently neutralized by not being referred patients.

Equally important is the education of ancillary staff, including physician's assistants, nurses, physical and occupational therapists, child life specialists, and others. Without their understanding and support of psychology's role in pain management, efforts at intervention will likely fail or be sabotaged. Given the importance of consistency in pain management efforts, the team's help is essential. Alienation of team members often results when they are perceived to be the "work horses" of the management efforts and given subordinate status. Although the psychologist may in fact hold a more powerful position on the team, it is crucial to respect the status and importance of other team members.

Occasionally, pediatric psychologists are called upon to implement pain management services in a setting where previous attempts to do so have failed. Rectifying such a situation may be difficult. However, a few suggestions in this regard may be offered. First, more likely than not, the preceding consultant may have made obvious "system errors," such as not appropriately establishing relationships with the pediatrician(s) and team members, not respecting interdisciplinary roles, not appropriately educating the key individuals, or not observing the norms of the medical culture. In other cases, the predecessor simply may not have used appropriate social skills or may not have been sufficiently knowledgeable about medical system issues. Such problems are often correctable by means of direct communication. Second, most facilities that treat pediatric pain patients truly desire means to decrease the pain experiences of children, and efforts to address these issues are generally appreciated.

Given these facts, it is generally most helpful for the practitioner to convey a sincere desire to work in collaboration with the physician in attempting to discern previous mistakes rendered, address latent systems issues, and work to correct or circumvent such difficulties in the future. A new consultant who makes genuine efforts to avoid previous mistakes may well lead to the establishment of successful pain management services.

The Assessment Phase

The purpose of this section is to outline professional issues involved in the assessment of the referral source's concerns, the system or program in which intervention will occur, and of course, the needs of the pediatric pain patient. The goal is not to provide a redundant overview of assessment technology and strategy. Other chapters in this volume eloquently discuss these issues. Rather, the goal is to capture and elucidate the pragmatic realities of actual clinical practice. Thus, this section will focus on the nature of the referral question, analysis of the various professional-client interrelationships, and multicomponent or multisystemic assessment.

Nature of the Referral Question

The formal assessment process begins with an analysis of the request for services. Referral requests may take many forms, e.g., "please see this child for pain management," "please keep this child from kicking and screaming during debridement," "please fix this kid," and are requested via different methods, e.g., letter, phone, personal contact. Common to many initially received referral questions is a relative lack of background information that provides a context for understanding the true reason for referral.

The vagueness behind many referrals may be explained by several factors, including the referring individual's lack of time to explain adequately the reason for referral, lack of available clinical information on the physician's part, or (as is often the case) a lack of understanding on the part of the referring individual as to *how* to phrase a referral. He/she may have little idea of what is actually needed, yet recognizes it is an issue that falls within the realm of psychological services.

Obviously, it is of critical importance to develop a common conceptual model with the referral source as to what the problem actually is, and to determine if pain management services are indicated. Thus, every referral needs to begin with an assessment of the reasons why a child is being referred. A general rule of thumb is to never accept a referral without interviewing the medical professional most familiar with the patient. That person may be a surgeon, pediatrician, resident, or nurse. Minimally, this individual should be posed the following questions:

1. What is the nature of the child's problem? In what specific ways is this manifested (e.g., behaviorally, affectively, cognitively)? Has an underlying physiological/medical etiology been identified? What has the child been told about the pain?
2. When did the problem begin? How was it that the child was referred now (and not earlier)?
3. For whom is it a problem? Is the child distressed, or is the staff distressed by the child?
4. Who is currently involved in the care of the child (e.g., staff, family, child life) and what steps have they taken to facilitate pain management? Will they be involved in the future?
5. What would the referral source like to see accomplished? Is the goal to achieve total remission of pain, to diminish pain, or to teach the child how to live with uncontrollable pain?
6. What level of responsibility is the psychologist being asked to assume? Is he/she to be the indirect consultant, team coordinator, or direct service provider?
7. Has the possibility of a pediatric pain consult been discussed with the parents? Have the parents offered consent?

In some cases, it will be abundantly clear that pain management services are indicated. In others, psychotherapy or behavior management may be more appropriate. Still other cases will be determined to be "dumps" or "turfs," that is, cases that are seen as overwhelmingly frustrating and resistant to treatment.

Apart from clinical significance, accurately understanding the referral question has additional ramifications. First, many ethical issues are involved in accepting certain kinds of referrals. Second, accurate conceptualization of the referral question has direct bearing on the relationship between the referral source and the psychologist. Recent research in pediatric psychology settings indicates that referral source satisfaction is often a function of congruence between the pediatrician's perception of the problem and feedback from the psychologist about the nature and treatment of the problem (Olson et al., 1988). A pediatrician who refers a child for pain management services, only to find 1 month later that the psychologist has referred the child to another practitioner for family therapy, may be quite dissatisfied with this response.

Assessment of the Medical Professional–Psychologist Relationship

Medical professionals vary tremendously in their sophistication regarding psychologically based pain management strategies. They also vary in terms of need for control over the care of "their patient," and in their attitudes toward interdisciplinary collaboration. In some cases, involvement of the referring physician and other medical personnel is not a necessary condition for effective treatment. Indeed, in outpatient settings, such involvement is often difficult to achieve. Given the complexity and nature of most pain problems, however, physician and interdisciplinary team involvement is highly desirable and may well be a requisite condition for pain management services to begin.

Because of their position as primary referral sources, physicians assume a prominent role in pain management. Therefore, it is important for the psychologist to establish from the time of referral the physician's expectation for his or her involvement, and to clarify the manner in which close communication can be maintained. In cases where management involves medical and/or surgical procedures (e.g., ulcerative colitis; burn debridement), establishing points of collaboration is a necessity. Equally important are those cases involving manipulative or "resistant" children and families, where all members of the treatment team must be consistent in their communications with the family. If initial assessment of the physician-psychologist relationship reveals little likelihood of close communication on such issues, then the psychologist can determine a range of alternative treatment options to circumvent the communication deficit. This may include (a) directly and assertively requesting such communication by providing a strong rationale for a close physician-psychologist relationship, (b) educating the physician about interdisciplinary treatment of pain problems, or (c) graciously declining the referral.

Nurses and other health professionals also assume prominent roles on the interdisciplinary team. Establishing and maintaining relationships with each of these professionals is often essential for successful treatment of the pediatric pain patient, particularly in inpatient settings. Each has his or her role and understanding of the rules of team functioning. Furthermore, just as family systems may become dysfunctional, so do interdisciplinary team systems. Team members can become "symptomatic" and begin to exhibit behavior that is inconsistent with quality patient care (e.g., they may become apathetic, angry, or depressed). They also may distort communications and sabotage team functioning. Many reasons exist for such dysfunction and can include power inequity, interprofessional rivalry, intrapersonal and interpersonal conflict, and organizational or financial pressures (Tefft & Simeonnson, 1979).

The psychologist, because of her or his specific training, is often in the best position to assess and address team relationships and functioning. The psychologist can help identify those team members who require additional education, role clarification, reassurance, or support. The psychologist should remain aware, however, of his or her own role as a treatment team member, and avoid becoming the psychotherapist for the team. Facilitating team functioning, while maintaining a team membership status, can often be a difficult and sensitive endeavor.

The Parent-Psychologist Relationship

Successful treatment of pediatric pain problems relies heavily on the implicit and explicit support, understanding, and active involvement of the child's parents. Drotar (1981) aptly noted the importance of a family-centered approach to treating the chronically ill child. In this regard, Munson (1986) has discussed the need for paying close attention to the dynamics of the child's family and the possible role that these dynamics may play in the development and maintenance of pain and illness, as well as their potential for facilitating "wellness." Others have documented the significance of more specific parent-child dyadic influences in the medical context (Bush, Melamed, Sheras, & Greenbaum, 1986; Peterson & Shigetomi, 1981). It is the parent who must consent to treatment and the parent who will communicate to the child various expectations and beliefs about the role of the psychologist in helping to manage pain. To the extent that a parent misunderstands the role of psychology in pain management, distrusts or dislikes the psychologist, or does not believe in the efficacy of pain management procedures, few treatment gains are likely. Furthermore, parents who are uninvolved in or uninformed about their child's care may manifest greater distress themselves, thereby increasing their child's distress. In contrast, when parents convey to the child a sense of trust in the psychologist and the pain management process, and when they model such confidence via active participation, the chances for success are greatly enhanced. It is therefore the responsibility of the psychologist to initiate a supportive and educative dialogue with the parents to facilitate this process.

In our experience, the lay person has little understanding of the role psychologists play in pain management. At best, parents understand that psychologists provide support and understanding to those in distress; at worst, they believe psychologists serve only the severely emotionally disturbed. Occasionally, parents have had negative experiences themselves or have known others who have had negative experiences with psychology. Parents may also have a conceptual model of their child's pain experience that does not include a psychological component. Such issues must be assessed as early as possible, so that the process of reeducation may begin. It is recommended that in initiating contact with parents the following information be discussed:

1. The psychologist has been asked by the physician to assist in reducing the pain experience of their child.
2. The psychologist is part of an interdisciplinary team that has been established to treat various pain problems.
3. Psychologists have many different roles and functions, not just psychotherapy or working in mental institutions.
4. The psychologist will be working closely with the parents to teach their child ways to cope with a stressful or distressing situation. Furthermore, the child's parents are recognized as experts with regard to their child's personality and coping style. As such, the parents will be enlisted as partners in the assessment and management of their child's pain/distress.
5. The focus will be on the acquisition of skills (not personality change) using procedures that are supported by scientific research.

Depending upon the particular concerns of parents, each of these issues can be discussed at greater length. Parents should always be asked directly about any concerns they might have about the psychologist's involvement; any identified concerns must then be directly and openly addressed. Such dialogue fosters trust and promotes the likelihood of a healthy relationship between parent and psychologist. Once this basis for psychological involvement has been established, the consultant can proceed with further data collection and assessment of the child as well as the family. Discussions should be held with the parents to elicit information regarding the child's normal, nonpain behavior, the child's history of pain and hospital experiences, other family members who have experienced pain or injury and who may serve as models for the child, the child's preferred methods of coping with illness and pain, and any specific concerns the parents may have regarding their child's emotional status relative to the pain. Furthermore, the sense of helplessness that most parents experience when seeing their child in pain should be addressed. It is often helpful for parents to know that they can and should be a part of the treatment process, as this tends to minimize their sense of helplessness.

The Psychologist-Child Relationship

Assessment proceeds with an interview with the child and subsequent development of the psychologist-child relationship. Just as parents may be puzzled, confused, or even angered by the psychologist's involvement, the child is likely to share such feelings. The child's response to the pain and the psychologist's subsequent involvement will in part reflect such parental responses and attitudes. Through observation of others, children learn about the nature of their pain problem, its etiology, and consequences of their reactions to the pain. The child's response will also be a function of many other variables including developmental level, perceived pain intensity, his or her conceptualization of the pain experience, and the expectations held by other medical personnel (Lavigne et al., 1986). Most children are quite frightened and distressed by the circumstances of their compromised health status, further influencing their emotional response to a new member of the treatment team.

Given the emotional distress experienced by the child in pain, the psychologist is encouraged to approach the new patient in a calm, warm, and supportive manner. Obviously, such an approach is warranted with any child, but should be particularly emphasized with the pediatric pain patient. To facilitate rapport building, it may be helpful first to establish a relationship with the parents and to subsequently have the parents introduce the psychologist to the child. The parents can also begin to help conceptualize the nature of the psychologist's presence and rationale for pain management for the child. This type of clinician-parent collaboration is crucial in fostering trust between the child and clinician.

As with the parents, it is also important to assess the child's understanding of what psychologists do and how they function. Older children and adolescents may have well-formed albeit distorted beliefs about mental health professionals. Such beliefs may range from "they're here because I'm crazy," to "they're here because they believe the pain is in my head," to "they're here because I'm out of control." Such cognitions can lead to an exacerbation of their distress. With more critically ill adolescents, the psychologist's presence may be construed as a message that the child is going to die and that the psychologist has been asked to engage the child in death and dying counseling. Although many children will not share such perceptions openly, a tactful and carefully worded initial interview will often elicit a description of such ideation.

The next phase of assessment should involve direct examination of the child. Using developmentally appropriate language, the child should be asked not only about his or her subjective pain experience, but also about his or her conceptual model of pain, coping resources, beliefs about the efficacy of controlling pain, previous experiences with pain, and use of coping strategies in such situations. This discussion not only serves the purpose of eliciting information necessary for teaching the child about pain management skills, but also communicates to the child that (a) the medical staff understands that the child is in pain, (b) the child's collaboration is crucial for successful intervention, and (c) the child has skills that will allow him or her to control the pain experience. Children are often able to share past experiences of coping with pain or distress on which the psychologist can capitalize when educating the child about pain, as well as in the development of management strategies. Additionally, this discussion should explore pleasant or comforting fantasies the child has so that these can also be incorporated in the development of the pain management program.

Aside from the direct interview with the child and parents, it is recommended that observations involving other medical professionals be utilized in assessing the child's pain from an objective, behavioral perspective. A number of standardized methods for observing and recording data about the child's pain have been developed (e.g. Jay, Elliott, Ozolins, Olson, & Pruitt, 1985; Katz, Kellerman, & Siegel, 1981). This method of assessing the child's pain presents an excellent opportunity for identifying and operationally defining specific behavioral manifestations of the child's pain that can be a focus for treatment.

The Intervention Process

Probably the most significant issue in the development of a pain management program is that of shared consent. By this we mean that all participants in this program must be in full agreement with its direction and specific parameters. In those situations in which one or more persons participating in the child's care either do not understand or are not in agreement with this program, the risk of sabotage arises. In other words, the program is likely to be undermined through either lack of consistency in conducting the program, or by engaging in aspects of care that are contraindicated by the plan. This may occur when a parent or health care provider feels sorry for the child and is unprepared to or does not understand the necessity of consistently carrying out behavioral contingencies. In another situation, the child may be excessively aggressive or hostile toward a particular staff or family member, resulting in this caretaker either withdrawing from the child or displaying reciprocal anger. Therefore, it is crucial that each person who will be caring for the child thoroughly understands and agrees to the plan so that it is implemented in a consistent manner.

To optimize the likelihood of shared consent, it is recommended that the development of the treatment plan be conducted using the input of all relevant participants. In developing the pain management program, it is important that each participant clearly understand the role he or she will play. Although there will often be a degree of overlap across roles, it is most helpful if each person involved has a clear sense of the specific contributions for which he or she is responsible. We have found that an initial care conference in which the parents, medical staff, and psychologist all participate is extremely beneficial in developing a comprehensive pain program upon which everyone agrees. This should be followed by regularly scheduled conferences that serve the purpose of reiterating goals and procedures, evaluating progress, and determining if changes are needed.

The efficacy of an intervention program is largely determined by the thoroughness of the assessment data upon which it is based. Therefore, it is recommended that the specific parameters of the program be operationally defined and based upon assessment data. All team members must understand these operational definitions, regardless of their training background. For example, if during the assessment phase the child is noted to become combative and hostile during a dressing change procedure, specific intervention strategies must be designed and agreed upon that address these particular behaviors. It is simply insufficient to state in the management program that "the child's aggressive behavior will be addressed." If this type of general (and in many ways meaningless) goal is offered, each caretaker may have a very different idea of what aggressive behavior is and how it should be managed. Instead, several specific and relevant behavioral contingencies should be decided upon. Similarly, plans for addressing the child's cognitive and emotional functioning should be defined and agreed upon.

Once a clearly defined program has been designed and shared consent has been obtained, we have found it to be quite helpful to type out and distribute to all participants a copy of this program. This not only increases the likelihood that each person will possess a clear understanding of the plan, but also increases the likelihood that it will be carried out as agreed upon. Parents, the physician(s), nursing staff, and all other health care providers should receive a copy of this plan. Additionally, it is helpful if a copy can be placed in the child's medical chart as well as at bedside if the child is hospitalized. Finally, it is imperative that close monitoring of the intervention be maintained, as well as a regular schedule for follow-up care. This follow-up contact should be made with the physician as well as the family to assure that progress is maintained over time and that all parties remain abreast of the child's status (Olson et al., 1988).

Training and Credentialing

At present, no formalized training structures, curricula, or credentialing process exists for pediatric psychologists who choose to spend part or a majority of their time working in the area of pediatric pain. Indeed, this area of focus is both so new and highly specialized that it is difficult to describe a single set of academic and clinical experiences that adequately provide basic training. Furthermore, there is a lack of widely accepted guidelines or standards for training in the practice of either child clinical psychology or pediatric psychology (Tuma, 1985b), much less that of a clinical psychologist whose specialty is the treatment of children's pain.

To address this problem, a number of proposed guidelines have been offered in recent years. They include the Guidelines for Training Psychologists to Work with Children, Youth and Families (Roberts, Erickson, & Tuma, 1985), as well as the recommendations of the Conference on Training Clinical Child Psychologists (Tuma, 1985a). In addition, other individuals have focused attention on training guidelines for the practice of pediatric psychology (Stabler & Whitt, 1980). Despite this progress, development of widely accepted guidelines for clinical child psychology and pediatric psychology remains in the early stages. Furthermore, the dynamic nature of both subspecialty fields makes it unlikely that any recommended guidelines will remain the same for long. The current consensus appears to be that for the child clinical psychologist or pediatric psychologist, the roles and responsibilities subsumed are so extensive that one particular training program cannot adequately cover the skills and provide the experiences necessary for successful service delivery (Drotar, 1985). In light of the absence of standardized curricula in these areas, it is incumbent on the individual psychologist to practice within the limits of his/her training and abilities, as per the American Psychological Association's (1981) Ethical Principles of Psychologists and individual state licensing laws.

General Training Experiences

As is apparent in preceding chapters, the area of pediatric pain is extremely complex and multidimensional in focus. Competent and successful implementation of pediatric pain services requires a plethora of skills and abilities. Acquisition of these skills requires a developmental sequence of training experiences, beginning with those general in scope and proceeding to the more specific.

First, it would seem apparent that the pediatric pain specialist requires broad-based training, preferably in a general clinical psychology program that adheres to a scientist-practitioner model. This type of program would provide the basic foundation of the requisite knowledge in theory and applications of basic psychological principles. Such principles include learning theory, life-span development, social processes, biological or physiological psychology, the assessment and treatment of a variety of behavioral disorders, as well as the professional and ethical conduct of clinical practice. Although it can be argued that other training programs such as school or developmental psychology may provide similar experiences, it is reasonable to expect that a general clinical psychology degree most comprehensively addresses the minimum training needs for the practice of psychology in applied medical settings. Furthermore, a scientist-practitioner model of clinical training should lead to an acquisition of both research skills and an orientation toward empirically based practice. Such skills are highly valued in the arena of pediatric pain management, and can facilitate the psychologist's acceptance by medical colleagues (Peterson & Harbeck, 1988).

A number of additional points should be emphasized. In the course of general training, it is essential that the pediatric pain specialist receive training in child clinical psychology and developmental psychology. Peterson and Harbeck (1988) have aptly noted that clinical child psychology is the preferred specialization for the practice of pediatric psychology, an idea supported by other experts in the field (Drotar, 1977). Developmental psychology, typically an integral aspect of the clinical child curriculum, has strong bearing on numerous aspects of pediatric pain practice. Most children referred for pain problems fall well within the normal limits of psychological development. Therefore, pediatric pain specialists must possess a basic understanding not only of child behavior problems and abnormal development, but also normal child development and children's responses to abnormal or stressful situations. Additionally, familiarity with biopsychosocial models of health and illness is critical (Drotar, 1985). It is gradually becoming more apparent that a comprehensive perspective that examines the interplay among biological, psychological, and environmental variables is necessary for understanding the etiology and treatment of childhood disorders within a pediatric context. Students can and should be introduced to this model at an early point in their training, thereby establishing a heuristic model for future study in pediatric pain.

Specialized Training Experiences

It is the acknowledged bias of the current authors that special emphasis should be placed upon pediatric psychology training experiences and/or child health psychology experiences at the internship and postdoctoral level. Pediatric psychology is, by definition, a specialty area that would prepare an individual for dealing with the many complex issues involved in pediatric pain assessment and treatment. Pediatric psychology involves a primary focus on the interrelationship between health and behavior in the pediatric context (Walker, 1979), with a service delivery focus on younger children with health related problems, chronic illness, and psychosomatic disorders (Roberts, 1986; Wright, 1977). Pediatric psychologists work in a variety of health-related settings, including pediatric hospitals and clinics, multispeciality medical clinics, health maintenance organizations, and health science centers. Because few training programs currently offer pediatric psychology practica or experiences in the university setting, it is typical that such experiences are obtained at the internship or postdoctoral level. Pediatric psychology is a rapidly growing specialty area, and numerous internship and postdoctoral fellowship programs now exist that can offer such specialized training (Tuma, 1987; Tuma & Grabert, 1983).

On a more specific level, it is recommended that the pediatric pain specialist receive organized training experiences in pain assessment and treatment
in the context of a designated and accredited setting. Such a setting can take
many forms, including inpatient pediatric hospitals, health sciences centers,
and outpatient clinics. It is essential that such training be closely supervised
by an individual experienced in treating pediatric pain. This type of training
experience would also help the pediatric pain specialist begin to understand,
at both a theoretical and practical level, the complexity of medical systems.
The practice of pediatric psychology takes place in an emotionally laden
system that is heavily influenced by the medical and hospital culture (Drotar,
1981). Unfortunately, few graduate programs in clinical psychology offer
didactic work that facilitates understanding the practical use of systems
theory vis-à-vis the institutional setting, nor is attention focused sufficiently
on the medical culture and the norms and realms of practice of pediatric
psychology. Yet, the practicing psychologist must understand the system in
which he or she operates in order to function effectively (Mullins, 1989).
Both the explicit and implicit rules of the institutional system should be
carefully examined and taken into account in the practice of pediatric pain
consultation. In other words, the psychologist must understand the complex
professional boundaries and territories that exist. A strong mentor-student
relationship can help assure that such a training experience is successful in
this regard.

Ethical Issues

The scope of ethical issues in the practice of pediatric psychology or pediatric pain is so immense that we cannot begin to cover all the salient concerns
in this chapter. The readers are referred to the excellent article by Weithorn
and McCabe (1988) for a thorough discussion of the many ethical issues
involved in the practice of pediatric psychology in general. We will focus on
issues of most concern to the pediatric psychologist dealing with pain problems. Various methods of addressing these situations will also be suggested,
taking into account that it is ultimately the responsibility of the individual
psychologist to make complex ethical decisions. The Ethical Principles of
Psychologists (American Psychological Association, 1981) should serve as
superordinate principles and be strictly adhered to in the course of practice.

Referral for Pain Services

Ethical dilemmas frequently arise early in the referral process for pain problems. More often than not, pain patients are referred by other professionals.
Such referrals are rarely accompanied by a wealth of pertinent medical and
psychological history. As mentioned earlier, the most important initial questions to address in accepting a referral involve clarifying the true reasons for
the request for services. Oftentimes, children are referred not because of

pain problems per se, but because these children are painful to staff. In other words, the child who is referred may be sullen, irritating, assaultive, or simply obnoxious. It is essential that the pediatric psychologist assess this issue as quickly as possible so as to intervene or not intervene as necessary. Most medical staffs probably have a set of explicit as well as implicit rules that guide their referrals. As Greist, Wells, and Forehand (1979) have pointed out, children are not always referred because their behavior is problematic, but sometimes because of factors specific to the referral agent.

In this regard, it is critical to work closely with treatment teams to help them identify which children are most likely to benefit from pain management services, which children are not likely to benefit, and which children need different forms of intervention, e.g., behavior management or psychotherapy. Unfortunately, the child who withdraws or regresses in response to pain, displays symptoms of clinical depression, or perhaps covertly becomes suicidal, may well be the child that is ignored and not referred. In contrast the tantrum-prone, combative, or arrogant child is quickly brought to the psychologist's attention. Both children may well be in need of psychological services, but the assessment and treatment of pain may not be the real issue. In this regard, the first ethical issue raised upon receiving a consult request for pain management services is that of clarifying the referral question and determining if pain management per se is the most appropriate form of intervention. Should this issue not be addressed early, the clinician may find himself in the ethical dilemma of being asked to provide services that are either unnecessary or inappropriate.

Informed Consent

In keeping with the ethical principles for psychologists, informed consent must be obtained in order for treatment to proceed. As it concerns children and adolescents, the right of consent largely falls to the parents or legal guardian. This form of "proxy" consent necessitates obtaining informed consent from the parents before any treatment can proceed. Most states have specific statutes for informed consent, denoting the age at which a child gains the right of consent. It should be pointed out that there are also limits to parental rights and discretion, such as in cases of neglect or abuse when parental rights are temporarily or permanently revoked by the state. In such cases, the need for providing informed consent is no less important, but the party who offers consent may be someone other then a parent, such as a guardian appointed by the state.

In the case of pediatric pain, it is essential that parents be informed about the nature of the psychologist's involvement in the assessment and treatment process. It is crucial that the pediatric psychologist be specific about the reason for referral and rationale for intervention, outlining the nature of the procedures, potential benefits, alternative procedures, and any risk that might result from psychological interventions. The reasoning behind this recommendation for specificity is multifold. As mentioned earlier, most lay people have a poor understanding of what psychologists actually do in the course of professional practice, much less in the specific case of pain management. Given that in a medical context most people feel the need to be conciliatory and deferential to authority, they may never question the reason for the referral. It should also be taken into account that many parents may be in distress at the time of referral, being concerned about their child's health status, and they may not understand specifically why pediatric psychology is involved. Finally, parents need to be fully informed so that they can help in the pain management process. Many times the success of a pain program hinges on parental compliance with various regimens, e.g., reinforcing well behaviors and ignoring attention-seeking forms of pain behavior. To the extent that the parents do not understand the rationale for treatment, the likelihood of active participation diminishes. In all of these regards, it is imperative to take time with parents to discuss adequately the rationale behind the recommendation for psychological intervention.

It is similarly important to obtain actual consent from the child. Although parents may hold the right of legal consent, it makes little sense either from an ethical or a treatment standpoint not to obtain specifically the child's consent to treatment, even with younger children. It has been documented that children ages 3 to 14 have the ability to comprehend and help make reasonable treatment-related decisions in the legal context (Weithorn & Campbell, 1982). Pain management strategies, by their very nature, require the active participation and cooperation of children; should they choose not to participate in such interventions, it is quite likely that such interventions will fail.

Finally, it should be taken into account that parents who have been referred by a physician or other medical personnel may already have been given inappropriate information about the reason for the referral. It is suggested that the pediatric psychologist ascertain what has been shared, given that any incongruence between the parents' initial understanding from the referral source and the psychologist's rationale may result in equivocation or ill feeling.

Systems Issues

Once a child has been evaluated for a pain problem, it is important that the nature of treatment be further explained to the child and family. Ideally, each family member should understand the complex relationship between pain and psychologically related issues and share a common conceptual model with the pediatric psychologist (Turk, Meichenbaum, & Genest, 1983). This includes an understanding of how emotional states affect pain, how distress behaviors, muscular tension, and stress can exacerbate pain, as well as how operant conditioning serves to alter manifestations of pain. In addition, families may need to understand how dysfunctional family patterns, roles, and behaviors can affect the pain experience. Discussing these issues with the family can, therefore, be a delicate matter vis-à-vis informed consent. The case of recurrent abdominal pain (RAP) may highlight this issue.

In certain cases of RAP, the pain experienced by the child can be conceptualized as resulting from their internal distress over family dysfunction, e.g., marital conflict, sexual abuse, or alcoholism. Heightened levels of family stress may exacerbate the pain experience, and yet the family remains relatively unaware of the relationship between their systemic functioning and the pain symptomatology. The recommendation may then be made for family therapy as the most appropriate form of intervention. This may sharply contrast with the family's expectation for individually oriented pain management services. This discrepancy may in turn elicit anger and guilt in the family. It is important that the pediatric psychologist explain such issues in a way that allows for understanding and subsequent intervention, without "blaming" and alienating family members.

In an inpatient setting, the unit staff members also compose a system. In some cases, this system of individuals does not fully understand the nature of the psychologist's involvement and oftentimes must be educated about the nature of his or her services. Often they do not understand the limits of confidentiality. Most medical personnel are accustomed to open and frank discussion of the various aspects of cases from a medical perspective. They may approach the psychologist requesting information about the psychological status of an individual, apart from pain-related issues. The psychologist must walk a thin line between disclosing what is necessary for the successful management of the patient, which of necessity requires the team approach, and avoiding disclosure of issues that have no bearing on the patient's health or pain status. Similarly, chart notes often pose an ethical dilemma for the pediatric psychologist. Although chart material is considered confidential, it has been our experience that the medical chart in a large hospital is virtually a public record, in that any number of staff members have access to this information. It is our recommendation that only material specifically relevant to pain management be shared and that other psychological information not be disclosed unless it pertains to the health status of the child.

Use of Medications

It is probably safe to say that clinical psychologists in general, and pediatric psychologists specifically, have a particular bias about the use of pain medications. Most graduate programs teach the budding clinical psychologist to avoid the medical model, both in theory and in practice. For this and other reasons, there tends to be a strong bias against the use of pain medications. Indeed, some medications have negative side effects and remove a sense of control from the individual in pain. It should be pointed out that such a bias against the use of pain medications with children also apparently extends to physicians who do not understand, or who have distorted perceptions of, the child's pain experience (Eland & Anderson, 1977). Schechter and Allen (1986) surveyed physicians from a number of specialty areas and found that exaggerated fears of children becoming addicted to pain medications still exist. Surgeons, as compared to pediatricians, tended to be even less generous with postsurgical analgesics. The authors expressed concern that although there seems to be a growing recognition that children experience pain similarly to adults, children continue to receive less pain medication than adults who were experiencing similar medical conditions (see chapter 3).

The reality is that many children present to pediatric psychologists not just in mild or moderate pain, but in *severe* pain. The tendency is to offer those children our armamentarium of skills to decrease pain including relaxation strategies, cognitive coping strategies, hypnosis, and behavioral programs. It takes only one visit to a inpatient burn unit to observe a 9-year-old child with a 60% total body surface area second/third-degree burn to understand that such interventions may have the total impact of reducing distress behaviors by 5 to 10%, at best. This may be referred to as the "shooting elephants with BBs" phenomenon. Furthermore, it appears that for some children the presence of a trained coach is necessary to insure utilization of the coping skills (Elliott & Olson, 1983). The financial cost of this coach, if billed, is likely to be $50 to $100 per hour. On the other hand, the available literature would suggest that indeed, psychologically based strategies can significantly reduce the emotional and behavioral distress of some children with certain kinds of injuries and certain levels of pain.

Thus, a number of ethical questions arise. Does the presence of the psychologist imply to medical staff that little or no pain medication is needed? Do psychologists tacitly approve of a low dose of, or no, pain medication? Does the psychologist have the ethical responsibility to monitor the use of pain medications by the physician, taking into account that the practice of medicine falls entirely within the physician's domain? There are no easy answers to these questions. The ethical imperative does seem to exist, however, for the psychologist to define clearly for the physician the limits of efficacy of psychologically based pain management interventions. The imperative also exists to inform the physician when typically efficacious strategies are not working. Similarly, it is appropriate for the psychologist to inform the physician of the literature suggesting that children indeed have significant pain experiences, and that research does not support the often held medical belief that children become easily addicted to narcotics or experience adverse psychological reactions when receiving pain medications (e.g., Eland & Anderson, 1977, Porter & Jick, 1980). One must avoid any implicit or explicit recommendations against medication use. New and more sophisticated pain medications with fewer side effects are becoming available that seem to decrease the pain experience of children (Forlini, Morin, & Treacy, 1987).

From an ethical standpoint, we must ask ourselves whether our psychological interventions are superior or inferior to medical interventions, or if some combination leads to the most efficacious results. Research may provide us with answers to this dilemma and work is in progress in this critical area (Jay, Elliott, Katz, & Siegel, 1987).

Child Abuse

Although current research evidence is relatively sparse concerning the relationship between childhood pain and abuse, clinical experience warrants comment on this issue. In large tertiary care settings, it is not uncommon to receive referrals on children with vague somatic complaints, oftentimes with a primary complaint of pain. After reasonable medical examination has ruled out a physical etiology, the pediatric psychologist is advised to include as a working hypothesis that sexual or physical abuse may be a precipitating or causative factor in the child's pain experience.

Obviously, the psychologist must be careful not to jump to conclusions before carefully scrutinizing the data. The base rate of child abuse is sufficiently high in certain settings that it makes diagnostic sense to maintain such a working hypothesis. From a clinical standpoint, it makes sense that children who are being abused but are fearful of the consequences of disclosure to legal officials may access a medical system via manifestation of a physical complaint, e.g., pain. At times, their conflict and turmoil may actually result in the experience of pain, such as gastrointestinal upset or headache. Although research is necessary to analyze more clearly the relationship between pain problems and child abuse, it is appropriate that we remain sensitive to this issue until such data are available.

Future Directions

It is only within the last decade or so that serious scientific endeavors have been undertaken to study pediatric pain. This is particularly true with regard to examining developmental factors as they relate to pain behaviors and the child's understanding of pain, objective and subjective methods of assessing the child's pain, and measurement of both the qualitative and quantitative aspects of a child's pain experience. With this gradually broadening knowledge base has come an appreciation of the tremendous complexity of pain in general and its impact on children and their families in particular. Indeed, Chapman and Bonica (1983) have suggested that pain is possibly the most complex of human stressors.

Throughout this chapter we have attempted to emphasize this complexity, while at the same time focusing on the pragmatic issues involved in working as a consultant with children who are experiencing pain. To this point, the discussion has dealt with two of the three major functions of pediatric psychologists within this area, notably the provision of direct clinical service and the education of medical professionals and families. Since this is a relatively new area of specialization, it has only recently begun to be recognized for its potential to improve the health care of children. However, as has been cogently discussed by others (Eland & Anderson, 1977; Ross & Ross, 1988), a serious sparsity of empirical data exists regarding virtually all areas of pediatric pain. This leads us to suggest that the third, but certainly not least important, area of involvement for the pediatric pain specialist is that of research. Because the progress and success of any applied science is based on a foundation of empirically sound basic, and clinically applied, research, this need is equally strong in the area of pediatric pain. Given the scientist-practitioner model espoused earlier, the pediatric pain clinician is in an optimal position to respond to this third imperative by systematically addressing the many questions raised throughout this volume.

Although a great deal of knowledge and information on pediatric pain has been obtained during the last decade, the study of pediatric pain is still at an early stage of development, with numerous questions and issues awaiting investigation. We believe that it is incumbent upon pediatric pain clinicians to pursue these issues within the setting in which they function. A first step in this process might be the education of physician colleagues so that they better appreciate the salience of such investigation and therefore support it. Ross and Ross (1988) point out that in order for this to take place,

the clinician should be willing to invest some time and energy in ensuring that existing information and new findings relevant to intervention are presented in a form sufficiently detailed to foster their use in pediatric settings. Research papers should include statements on the rationale, applicability, effectiveness, side effects (if any), developmental level at which the procedures have proven useful, and specific steps for implementing it; they should then be published in journals that reach the pediatric community. (p. 312)

We would like to conclude by briefly turning to two additional areas. These relate to the improvement of clinical services in response to consultation requests for pediatric pain management, and the development of pain education programs. In regard to the former, we would propose that pediatric pain consultants engage in efforts to develop comprehensive interdisciplinary pain management programs similar to those described by Berde et al. (1989). Such a program could be comprised of several health professionals, each of whom shares a special knowledge of and interest in the treatment of pediatric pain. Among those affiliated with such an interdisciplinary program should be a pediatric psychologist, behavioral or developmental pediatrician, clinical nurse specialist, social worker, and both an occupational and physical therapist. This team's function is viewed as threefold. First, it would serve as an educational resource to others in the setting. It is likely that medical professionals will more frequently turn to and be trusting of similarly trained professionals for information. Related to this would be the modeling function served by such an interdisciplinary team. In other words, this format of education and service could provide a model of collaborative team functioning for other health care providers.

A second major function of this team would be to provide clinical service to inpatient and outpatient populations. With regard to inpatient services, a well-integrated team could help the referring physician to assess and develop a pain management program for the particular child. Although it would not be recommended that such a team take responsibility for provision of care, the team role would be akin to the process-educative consultation model described by Stabler (1988). The interdisciplinary team could also provide care to children in pain on an outpatient basis. This outpatient clinic would function similarly to other types of outpatient medical clinics, e.g., cerebral palsy clinics and child development clinics. In this type of setting the interdisciplinary team's role would be to assess and provide service to such non-hospitalized populations as children with recurrent abdominal pain, headaches, and other forms of chronic but benign pain.

Finally, the third major function of such a team would be devotion to the development of a comprehensive pediatric pain research program. Research collaboration would certainly be fostered by an interdisciplinary team devoted to the specific empirical research programs in this area.

Several potential concerns arise in developing an interdisciplinary pediatric pain program. Chief among these is cost-effectiveness. Although it is certainly true that a team approach to pain management might prove financially costly, most pediatric facilities operate one or more inter- or multidisciplinary programs that are not money-making ventures at the outset. Yet, when one considers the frequency of "doctor shopping" in which families engage when they experience dissatisfaction with medical services, a team approach such as that outlined above may prove to be more cost-effective over time. Research is necessary to bear this hypothesis out. Bloch (1986) addresses this issue at greater length in his discussion of the economics of health care organizations.

The second area of concern with regard to this type of program is that of acceptance by other hospital staff. It is easy to foresee the resentment that hospital staff might experience if a team of "experts" is called upon to deliver services to a particular patient, thus undermining the sense of competence and confidence of the professionals on a given medical unit. It is hoped that this could be circumvented by properly educating the entire medical staff regarding the true nature and purpose of the presence of an interdisciplinary team that is devoted to the assessment and management of pediatric pain.

Finally, we would like to briefly focus attention on the area of pediatric pain education. Ross and Ross (1988) have outlined a very intriguing two-pronged approach involving primary and early secondary prevention of chronic pain. They suggest the implementation of an educational program devoted to teaching elementary school children about various aspects of pain. Children could be provided with a greater knowledge base about pain etiology and treatment in general, and coping skills for managing pain and its correlates in particular. It is the position of Ross and Ross (1988) that such a program would provide a valuable method of preventing the development of chronic pain behaviors that may develop later in life. Ross and Ross have piloted such a program (1985), the results of which are quite encouraging in terms of children's ability to acquire a knowledge base of pain and change behaviors accordingly. This program provides an excellent example of the more broad-based educational programming that we foresee and advocate. Furthermore, it is indicative of the creative and exciting opportunities that are available for practitioners in the area of pediatric pain.

References

American Psychological Association (1981). Ethical principles of psychologists. *American Psychologist, 36*, 633–638.

Beales, J. G. (1979). Pain in children with cancer. In J. J. Bonica & V. Ventfridda (Eds.), *Advances in pain research and therapy* (pp. 89–98). New York: Raven Press.

Berde, C., Sethna, N. F., Masek, B., Tosburg, M., & Rocklin, S. (1989). Pediatric pain clinics: Recommendations for their development. *Pediatrician, 16*, 94–102.

Bloch, D. A. (1986). The family therapist as consultant to health care organizations. In L. C. Wynne, S. H. McDaniel, & T. T. Weber (Eds.), *Systems consultation: A new perspective for family therapy* (pp. 139–149). New York: Guilford.

Bonica, J. J. (1953). *The management of pain*. Philadelphia: Lea and Febiger.

Broome, M. E. (1985, June). The child in pain: A model for assessment and intervention. *Critical Care Nursing Quarterly, 10*, 47–55.

Bush, J. P. (1987). Pain in children: A review of the literature from a developmental perspective. *Psychology and Health, 1*, 215–236.

Bush, J. P., Melamed, B. G., Sheras, P. L., & Greenbaum, P. E. (1986). Mother-child patterns of coping with anticipatory medical stress. *Health Psychology, 5*, 137–157.

Chapman, C. R., & Bonica, J. J. (1983). *Acute pain*. Kalamazoo, MI: Upjohn.

Drotar, D. (1977). Clinical psychology practice in a pediatric hospital. *Professional Psychology, 8*, 72–80.

Drotar, D. (1978). Training psychologists to consult with pediatricians: Problems and prospects. *Journal of Pediatric Psychology, 7*, 57–60.

Drotar, D. (1981). Psychological perspectives in chronic illness. *Journal of Pediatric Psychology, 6*, 211–228.

Drotar, D. (1985). Integrating pediatric and clinical child psychology: Perspectives in clinical training. In J. M. Tuma (Ed.), *Proceedings: Conference on training clinical child psychologists*. Baton Rouge, LA: Land and Land.

Eland, J. M., & Anderson, J. E. (1977). The experience of pain in children. In A. K. Jacox (Ed.), *Pain: A source book for nurses and other professionals* (pp. 453–473). Boston: Little, Brown.

Elliott, C. H., & Olson, R. A. (1983). The management of children's distress in response to painful medical treatment for burn injuries. *Behaviour Research and Therapy, 21*, 675–683.

Engel, G. (1977). The need for a new medical model: A challenge for biomedicine. *Science, 196*, 129–136.

Forlini, J., Morin, D. M., & Treacy, S. (1987). Painless pediatric procedures. *American Journal of Nursing, 87*, 321–323.

Gillman, J., & Bush, J. P. (1991). Is there a general factor in children's pain responses? A multivariate study of three types of pain in children. *The Society of Behavioral Medicine Proceedings*, 124.

Green, M. (1983). Sources of pain. In M. D. Levine, W. B. Carey, A. C. Crocker, & R. T. Gross (Eds.), *Developmental behavioral pediatrics* (pp. 512–518). Philadelphia: Saunders.

Greist, D., Wells, K. C., & Forehand, R. (1979). An examination of predictors of maternal perceptions of maladjustment in clinic referred children. *Journal of Abnormal Child Psychology, 88,* 277–281.

Jay, S. M., Elliott, C. H., Katz, E. R., & Siegel, S. E. (1987). Cognitive-behavioral and pharmacologic interventions for children's distress during painful medical procedures. *Journal of Clinical Child Psychology, 55,* 860–865.

Jay, S. M., Elliott, C. H., Ozolins, M., Olson, R. A., & Pruitt, S. D. (1985). Behavioral management of children's distress during painful medical procedures. *Behaviour Research and Therapy, 23,* 513–520.

Katz, E. R., Kellerman, J., & Siegel, S. F. (1981). Behavioral distress in children undergoing medical procedures: Developmental considerations. *Journal of Consulting and Clinical Psychology, 48,* 356–365.

Klepac, R. K. (1975). Successful treatment of avoidance of dentistry by desensitization or by increasing pain tolerance. *Journal of Behavior Therapy and Experimental Psychiatry, 6,* 307.

Lavigne, J. V., Schulein, M. J., & Hahn, Y. S. (1986). Psychological aspects of painful medical conditions in children. I. Developmental aspects and assessment. *Pain, 27,* 133–146.

McCollum, A. T. (1981). *The chronically ill child.* New Haven, CT: Yale University Press.

McGrath, P. A. (1987). An assessment of children's pain: A review of behavioral, physiological, and direct scaling techniques. *Pain, 31,* 147–176.

Melamed, B. G. (1979). Behavioral approaches to fear in dental settings. In M. Herson, R. M. Eisler, & P. M. Miller (Eds.), *Progress in behavior modification* (Vol. 7). New York: Academic Press.

Mennie, A. T. (1974). The child in pain. In D. Burton (Ed.), *Care of the child facing death.* London: Routledge & Kegan Paul.

Mullins, L. L. (1989). Hate revisited: Power, envy, and greed in the rehabilitation setting. *Archives of Physical Medicine and Rehabilitation, 70,* 740–744.

Munson, S. (1986). Family-oriented consultation in pediatrics. In L. C. Wynne, S. H. McDaniel, & T. T. Weber (Eds.), *Systems consultation: A new perspective for family therapy* (pp. 219–239). New York: Guilford.

Olson, R. A., Holden, W., Friedman, A., Faust, J., Kenning, M., & Mason, P. J. (1988). Psychological consultation in a children's hospital: An evaluation of services. *Journal of Pediatric Psychology, 13,* 479–492.

Peterson, L., & Harbeck, C. (1988). *The pediatric psychologist: Issues in professional development and practice.* Champaign, IL: Research Press.

Peterson, L., & Shigetomi, C. (1981). The use of coping techniques to minimize anxiety in hospitalized children. *Behavior Therapy, 12,* 1–14.

Porter, J., & Jick, H. (1980). Addiction rate in patients treated with narcotics. *New England Journal of Medicine, 302,* 123.

Roberts, M. C. (1986). *Pediatric psychology: Psychological interventons and strategies for pediatric problems.* New York: Pergamon.

Roberts, M. C., Erickson, M. T., & Tuma, J. M. (1985). Addressing the needs: Guidelines for training psychologists to work with children, youth, and families. *Journal of Clinical Child Psychology, 14,* 70–79.

Roberts, M. C., Maddux, J. E., & Wright, L. (1984). The developmental perspective in behavioral health. In J. D. Matarazzo, N. E. Miller, S. M. Weiss, J. A. Heard, & S. M. Weiss (Eds.), *Behavioral health: A handbook of health enhancement and disease prevention* (pp. 56–68). New York: Wiley Interscience.

Ross, D. M., & Ross, S. A. (1982). *A study of the pain experience in children*, Final report, #1 ROI EID 13672–01. Bethesda, MD: National Institute of Child Health and Human Development.

Ross, D. M., & Ross, S. A. (1985). Pain instruction with third and fourth grade children: A pilot study. *Journal of Pediatric Psychology, 10*, 55–63.

Ross, D. M., & Ross, S. A. (1988). *Childhood pain: Current issues, research, and management*. Baltimore: Urban and Schwarzenberg.

Schechter, N. L., & Allen, D. A. (1986). Physicians' attitudes toward pain in children. *Developmental and Behavioral Pediatrics, 1*, 350–354.

Schwartz, G. E. (1982). Testing the biopsychosocial model: The ultimate challenge facing behavioral medicine. *Journal of Consulting and Clinical Pschology, 50*, 1040–1053.

Stabler, B. (1979). Emerging models of psychologist-pediatrician liaison. *Journal of Pediatric Psychology, 4*, 307–313.

Stabler, B. (1988). Pediatric consultation-liaison. In D. Routh (Ed.), *Handbook of pediatric psychology* (pp. 538–566). New York: Guilford.

Stabler, B., & Whitt, J. K. (1980). Pediatric psychology: Perspective and training implications. *Journal of Pediatric Psychology, 5*, 245–251.

Tefft, B. M., & Simeonnson, R. J. (1979). Psychology and the creation of health care settings. *Professional Psychology, 10*, 558–570.

Thompson, K. L., & Varni, J. W. (1986). A developmental cognitive-biobehavioral approach to pediatric pain assessment. *Pain, 25*, 283–296.

Travis, E. (1969). *The chronically ill child and his family*. New York: Holt, Rinehart, and Winston.

Tuma, J. M. (1985a). *Proceedings: Conference on training clinical child psychologists*. Baton Rouge, LA: Land and Land.

Tuma, J. M. (1985b). The Hilton Head conference on training clinical child psychologists: History and background. In J. M. Tuma (Ed.), *Proceedings: Conference on training clinical child psychologists* (pp. 1–5). Baton Rouge, LA: Land and Land.

Tuma, J. M. (1987). *Directory of internship programs in clinical child and pediatric psychology*. Baton Rouge, LA: Author.

Tuma, J. M., & Grabert, J. (1983). Internship and postdoctoral training in pediatric and clinical child psychology: A survey. *Journal of Pediatric Psychology, 8*, 245–260.

Turk, D. C., Meichenbaum, D., & Genest, M. (1983). *Pain and behavioral medicine: A cognitive-behavioral perspective*. New York: Guilford.

Varni, J. W. (1983). *Clinical behavioral pediatrics: An interdisciplinary approach*. New York: Pergamon Press.

Walker, C. E. (1979). Behavioral intervention in a pediatric setting. In J. R. McNamara (Ed.), *Behavioral approaches to medicine: Applications and analyses* (pp. 227–266). New York: Plenum.

Weithorn, L. A., & Campbell, S. B. (1982). The competency of children and adolescents to make informed treatment decisions. *Child Development, 53*, 1589–1598.

Weithorn, L. A., & McCabe, M. A. (1988). Emerging ethical and legal issues in pediatric psychology. In D. R. Routh (Ed.), *Handbook of pediatric psychology* (pp. 567–605). New York: Guilford.

Wright, L. (1977). Conceptualizing and defining psychosomatic disorders. *American Psychologist, 32*, 625–628.

6
Coping and Adaptation in Children's Pain

LAWRENCE J. SIEGEL AND KAREN E. SMITH

Children's responses to painful experiences range from adaptive coping efforts to severe maladjustment. A number of factors may mediate the impact of pain on a particular child's adjustment. Among these factors are the coping skills that children use in their attempts to manage the potential stress and discomfort associated with the pain that accompanies illness, injuries, and medical treatment. The coping skills in a child's repertoire are an important focus of study in our understanding of the individual differences observed in children's response to pain under comparable degrees of severity and type of painful condition. Children's typical modes of responding to stress influence their ability to manage painful events, and likely affect their ability to benefit from various intervention programs. In recent years, the study of coping processes in children has received greater emphasis. Researchers have begun to identify self-generated cognitive and behavioral coping strategies that children use in response to painful experiences (Siegel, 1988a, 1988b).

The focus of this chapter is on the coping strategies in children's repertoires that they use in their responses to painful events. Studies that have evaluated the efficacy of coping skills taught to children in the context of an intervention program are not discussed, as this literature is presented elsewhere in this volume (see chapter 4). This chapter focuses on methodological issues and research in assessment of children's coping with painful events. In addition, consideration will be given to the various factors that can influence children's use of coping skills and their adaptive responding to pain including type, duration, and frequency of pain event, the extent to which the pain is controllable, parental factors, and personal resources such as cognitive-developmental level, previous experience, and beliefs regarding the ability to manage the pain effectively.

Definition and Types of Coping

When considering strategies children use to cope with pain, it is important to understand what we mean by coping and the specifics involved in the painful event with which the child must cope. Pearlin and Schooler (1978)

149

have identified three basic functions of coping: (a) eliminating or modifying conditions that contribute to the problem; (b) perceptually controlling the meaning of the experience so that the situation is perceived as less of a problem; and (c) keeping the emotional consequences of the problem within manageable limits. When considering painful events experienced by children, it may be difficult to eliminate or modify the situation because it is not feasible for the child to escape or avoid the situation that gives rise to the pain. For example, children with severe burns must undergo debridement as part of the healing process (see chapters 11 and 15). In this and other situations pharmacological agents may be useful in modifying the experience of pain. In many pain situations we are left with helping children cope via the latter two functions.

Coping has been defined by Lazarus and Folkman (1984) as "constantly changing cognitive and behavioral efforts to manage specific external and/or internal demands that are appraised as taxing or exceeding the resources of the person" (p. 141). This definition implies an ongoing process that requires some degree of effort to deal with specific demands. In the context of dealing with pain, external demands would involve the painful stimulus itself and the context in which it is embedded, whereas internal demands would involve the perception of pain and the feelings generated by the painful situation.

Different coping strategies may be needed to deal with different types of demands, with some strategies more problem-focused and others more focused on regulating emotions (Lazarus & Folkman, 1984). It is possible that strategies used to regulate emotions may interfere with problem-solving strategies or vice versa. For some children, crying and screaming prior to a lumbar puncture is a way to "cope" with fears generated by the impending procedure. Yet this may interfere with the successful completion of the procedure. Conversely, a child may stoically undergo the lumbar puncture with little outward sign of behavioral distress only to have recurrent nightmares over the next several evenings. This example also points out that behaviors do not have to be "adaptive" or "successful" to be considered a coping strategy. Often what clinically appears to be "not coping" is better described as unsuccessful coping. Furthermore, successful coping may be "in the eye of the beholder" in that behaviors that result in avoiding a painful treatment may be viewed as unsuccessful by the medical staff, whereas the child may use the same strategy prior to subsequent procedures if it successfully resulted in avoiding the pain (e.g., eliminated the problem situation).

In summary, the definition of coping should be considered independent of a given outcome. A particular coping response is not inherently adaptive or maladaptive. Furthermore, a coping strategy that is effective in one situation or with one set of demands may not necessarily be effective in another situation or in coping with other aspects of the pain event.

Assessment of Coping Strategies

This section briefly reviews the research literature on children's coping with distressing and/or painful experiences in health care settings or in response to their illness or injury. Although this is a relatively new area of research with children, there is an extensive literature with adult populations that addresses coping styles and their impact on the effectiveness of pain and stress management techniques (Auerbach, Martelli, & Mercuri, 1983; Mullen & Suls, 1982; Roth & Cohen, 1986). The studies reviewed in this section are summarized in Table 6.1.

The majority of investigations have taken a process rather than a trait approach to measuring children's characteristic methods of coping with painful or stressful health care examinations and/or treatment. Therefore, children have been queried about coping strategies used to deal with specific painful situations or aspects of their illness rather than about how they cope with pain in general. An exception has been recent interest in a more global coping style of information avoiding versus information seeking; a concept that will be discussed more fully in a later section of this chapter (Miller & Green, 1985; Peterson & Toler, 1986).

Instead of using inventories or questionnaires to assess coping as in the adult literature, most of the studies that assess how children cope with painful events have used interview procedures and/or behavioral observations to identify children's coping strategies in specific health care settings. Data generated by the assessment of children's coping strategies using a structured interview that allows generation of responses methodologically is certainly more complicated to analyze. This format typically requires categorization of the children's responses using multiple coders to achieve some indication of the reliability of the categories used prior to any analyses of the data. This is in contrast to forced-choice questionnaires that require the child to indicate whether or not he or she has used a particular strategy and/or how much the strategy represented by each item has been used. Items on these scales may be grouped using factor analytic techniques to derive measures of different types of coping. Yet Ross and Ross (1984) provide data that indicate that different responses are obtained from children using these two different methods. These authors suggest that the interview method may more closely tap those coping strategies children have actually used to deal with pain. In addition, Ross and Ross (1984) sensitively discuss skills that should be used by the interviewer to encourage the child's participation in the interviewing process.

Siegel (1983) conducted an ecological assessment of self-generated coping strategies used by hospitalized children to determine if children who make an optimal adjustment to hospitalization for illness or surgery use different coping strategies than children who make a less satisfactory adjustment to the experience. Of particular interest was the assessment of specific cognitive and behavioral coping responses in which children engaged during stressful and painful medical procedures. A multidimensional assessment approach was used to evaluate the anxiety level and response to pain of 80 children, 8 to 14 years old, who were hospitalized for minor elective surgery. In addition, the evening before surgery and following several potentially stressful and/or painful procedures (e.g., blood test, preoperative injection), a structured interview was conducted with the children to evaluate their typical coping responses to painful and anxiety-provoking experiences both in and out of the hospital. An example of one of the questions was: "Pretend your best friend has to go to the doctor for a blood test like the one you just had. What advice would you give so that your friend would not be worried about it so much or so it would not bother him (or her)? Did you do any of those things or think about any of those things when you had your blood test?"

In this study, children were classified as successful copers if they were consistently rated by a nurse or physician as cooperating with the procedures, showing low anxiety, and manifesting high thresholds for physical discomfort. On the other hand, unsuccessful copers were defined as uncooperative, showing high anxiety, and manifesting low tolerance for discomfort. The results indicated that successful copers had more accurate information about why they were in the hospital and asked more questions about the hospital than unsuccessful copers. Successful copers also reported using a greater number of different strategies for managing stressful and painful experiences than unsuccessful copers, such as imagery-based rehearsal in which they planned how they might confront a stressful or painful event prior to its occurrence. Unsuccessful copers, on the other hand, reported using significantly more negative self-statements regarding their ability to tolerate discomfort, such as thinking about how much the needle was hurting, and reported thinking more often about past experiences where they were unable to tolerate effectively painful procedures similar to those encountered in the hospital. The number of different coping strategies used by the children accounted for most of the reasons for successful coping, followed by the accuracy of their knowledge regarding the reason for their hospitalization. A more detailed discussion of the definitions of the coping strategies developed by Siegel in conjunction with the Coping Strategies Interview are presented in Siegel (1988b) and Siegel and Smith (1989a).

Similar results were found in a study by Peterson and Toler (1986) that assessed information-seeking versus information-avoiding coping methods used by children undergoing stressful medical procedures during hospitalization for surgery. The child's cognitive coping style reflecting an information-seeking disposition was measured by the interview developed by Siegel (1983). A Coping Behaviors Scale was used to measure observable coping strategies used by the children during a blood test, during anesthesia induction, and in the recovery room following surgery. The behaviors assessed by this scale included positive assertion with the medical staff, level of activity during a medical procedure, verbal discussion of the procedure, watching the procedure, and asking questions concerning the procedure. In addition, the children's behavioral distress during the medical procedure was measured using the observational scale developed by Katz, Kellerman, and Siegel (1980).

The interview measure of coping was found to be associated with a number of general and specific coping behaviors measured by parents and observers. Furthermore, the child's response to medical procedures was influenced by the child's coping style as assessed by the interview. High information-seeking scores predicted lower rates of distress-related behaviors during various medical procedures and were associated with children who were better informed about the hospital procedures and surgery prior to admission to the hospital.

The coping strategies used by children undergoing routine dental treatment were investigated by Curry and Russ (1985). A Behavioral Coping Observation Scale was developed to assess children's coping behaviors during dental treatment. This scale consists of three basic behavioral categories, including information seeking, support seeking, and direct efforts to maintain control. In addition, a Cognitive Coping Interview was developed to assess the children's cognitions (i.e., thoughts, self-statements, wishes) during four major procedures of dental treatment (explorer exam, injection of anesthetic, placement of rubber dam, and cavity preparation).

The observational and interview measures were used to identify the cognitive and behavioral coping strategies employed by 30 children, 8 to 10 years old who were undergoing restorative dental treatment. The results indicated that coping responses used by the children were distributed across all of the coping categories assessed. Every subject reported employing at least two cognitive coping responses and was observed using at least one behavioral coping response. Older children used a greater number and variety of cognitive coping responses than the younger children. The scores from the behavioral and cognitive measures were not significantly correlated with each other, suggesting that there may be differential use of these strategies among children.

Knight et al. (1979) used a structured interview and Rorschach responses to categorize coping styles in children hospitalized for elective surgery. Urinary cortisol levels were used as a measure of physiological distress. Children who were rated as using the defensive styles of intellectualization or a mixed pattern of defenses had significantly lower cortisol production rates than children who were rated as using denial, displacement, or projection.

Hyson (1983) examined coping behaviors in children ranging in age from 6 to 60 months who were undergoing a routine physical examination. Coping behaviors were operationalized using White's (1974) strategies of adapta-

TABLE 6.1. Representative coping studies.

Study	Age of subjects (in years)	N	Setting	Coping measures	Results
Knight et al. (1979)	7–11	25	Hospital	Structured interview Rorschach responses	Urinary cortisol levels were highest in children using defensive coping style compared with children using denial, displacement, or projection.
Pidgeon (1981)	3–5	24	Hospital	Observations of question asking in structured and unstructured situations	Children's questions served as a means of managing novelty and incongruity and to establish social support.
Siegel (1983)	8–14	80	Hospital	Coping Strategies Interview	Successful copers had more accurate information, asked more questions, and used a greater number of different strategies than unsuccessful copers. Unsuccessful copers used more negative self-statements.
Curry & Russ (1985)	8–10	30	Dental	Behavioral Coping Observation Scale	Subjects used at least two cognitive and one behavioral coping response. Older children used a greater number and variety of cognitive coping responses.

Study	Age	N	Setting	Measure	Findings
Brown et al. (1986)	8–18	487	School	Cognitive Questionnaire	The number of successful copers increased with age as did the number of different strategies used. Positive self-talk was the most frequently reported cognitive coping strategy.
Peterson & Toler (1986)	5–11	59	Hospital	Coping Strategies Interview Coping Behaviors Scale	High information-seeking was associated with lower rates of distress-related behavior and children who were better informed about medical procedures.
Worchel et al. (1987)	6–17	52	Hospital	Questionnaire assessing behavioral, informational, and decisional control	Behavioral, cognitive, and decisional control strategies predicted emotional adjustment. The quality of behavioral control strategies was more important than the quantity of strategies used. Older children used more cognitive strategies than younger children.

tion, which include information seeking (looking, asking questions), comfort seeking (contact with mother, familiar objects), and autonomy (attempts to control, structure, or protest). In addition, the child's facial expressions of emotion were classified according to a system developed by Izard (1972) and Ekman, Friesen, and Ellsworth (1972). Behavioral observations were obtained using an elaborate procedure reported by Caldwell and Honig (1971) that results in a sequential and continuous record of behavior. The results indicated that information-seeking behaviors were the most common among children of all ages in the period just before the examination. Autonomy behaviors were the predominant coping responses during the actual physical examination, although age differences were noted in the specific type of autonomy responses that were exhibited.

Pidgeon (1981) studied the coping functions of questions asked by young hospitalized children. Question asking was viewed as a means of helping children to manage novelty and incongruity in their environment, to establish supportive social contacts with adults in a stressful situation, to influence the action of others, and to achieve cognitive clarity or reality testing. The spontaneous questions of children 3 to 5 years old were sampled in structured and unstructured situations during the first 2 days after admission to the hospital. Using Piaget's functional classification system, the largest number of children's questions (53%) were about the actions and intentions of hospital personnel regarding therapeutic activities, play and social activities, and routine care. The second largest number of children's questions were about the names of objects and persons in the hospital environment. These findings suggest that the preschool-age child maintains a vigilant orientation in the hospital and that preparation procedures should include information about the actions and intentions of hospital personnel and the identification of familiar and unfamiliar objects.

Using Lazarus's stress and coping paradigm, Caty, Ellerton, and Ritchie (1984) content analyzed the coping strategies reported in 39 case studies of hospitalized children 20 months to 10 years of age. The majority of behaviors reported in the case studies were classified in the action/inaction dimension (64.3%). The information exchange dimension accounted for 31.1% of the behaviors, and 4.6% were categorized in the intrapsychic dimension. Younger children displayed greater numbers of behaviors in the action/inaction dimension, whereas older children showed a greater tendency to exhibit behaviors that were information focused, reflecting their greater cognitive and verbal abilities.

Control strategies used by child and adolescent oncology patients to cope with medical treatments and daily activities, including painful events and procedures, were investigated by Worchel, Copeland, and Barker (1987). A questionnaire was used to measure control strategies in four categories: behavioral, cognitive, decisional, and informational. The results of this study indicated that specific behaviors that children engaged in during medical treatments such as holding parent's hands and deep breathing (behavioral), thinking and talking about one's illness and treatment (cognitive), and perceived control over activities, treatments, and meals (decisional) were significant predictors of emotional adjustment. In addition, the quality of behavioral control strategies were found to be more important than the quantity of strategies used. Adolescents reported using more cognitive control strategies than the child patients.

Brown, O'Keefe, Sanders, and Baker (1986) investigated coping and catastrophizing cognitions used by children 8 to 18 years old during painful and/or stressful situations. Coping was defined by these investigators as imagining events that are inconsistent with the experience of pain, stopping oneself from thinking of the pain, using self-talk to minimize the pain, or thinking about the experience in a problem-solving framework. Catastrophizing was defined as focusing on or exaggerating negative aspects of the situation, making negative self-statements, and thinking about escaping or avoiding the situation. The results indicated that the number of copers increased significantly with age, and positive self-talk was the most frequently reported cognitive coping strategy. In addition, the total number of different types of strategies that were reported increased with age. Catastrophizing cognitions were found to occur at a relatively high rate at all age groups and most frequently involved the use of negative affect.

Factors Affecting Use of Coping Strategies

As previously noted, coping has been defined as a dynamic process used to "manage specific external and/or internal demands that are appraised as taxing or exceeding the resources of the person" (Lazarus & Folkman, 1984, p. 141). This definition raises the point that the child's evaluation of the situation is important in determining how he or she will cope with a painful event. Although situations can be evaluated as benign, irrelevant, or stressful (Lazarus & Folkman, 1984), it is most likely that painful situations will be perceived as stressful. The degree of stress experienced will depend on whether the child appraises the situation as a challenge or a threat to his or her well-being, and on whether harm or loss has already occurred (Lazarus & Folkman, 1984). Children's evaluation of the pain experience will theoretically be influenced by a variety of factors including factors specific to the pain situation itself, level of control available and/or perceived, parental support and modeling, and personal resources. Important personal resources include a variety of factors such as cognitive-developmental level, meaning ascribed to the pain event, perceived ability to handle pain (i.e., self-efficacy), and previous experience. Moreover, other individual difference factors such as preferred coping style are beginning to be included in the conceptualization of how children cope with pain.

Specific Event Factors

Type, Duration, and Frequency

Varni (1983) has classified pain-related problems in children into four categories: (a) pain associated with a disease state (e.g., sickle cell disease, juvenile arthritis), (b) pain associated with an observable physical injury or trauma (e.g., fractures, burns), (c) pain that is not associated with a specific disease or identifiable physical trauma (e.g., tension headaches, recurrent abdominal pain), and (d) pain associated with medical and dental procedures (e.g., venipunctures, lumbar punctures). Although there is certainly overlap in that all involve the experience of pain, other specific situational factors need to be considered including the frequency and duration of the pain and how much control the child has over the pain experience.

Some pain events may be acute problems requiring a single or infrequent episode, as with fractures or injections for a typically healthy child. Other pain events may be acute but repeatedly experienced over time, such as sickle cell crises or invasive treatment procedures experienced by cancer patients. Still other types of pain may be more chronic than acute, requiring coping over longer time periods as with arthritis.

Controllability

The degree of control a child has over a painful event may also affect his or her experience of pain and strategies used to cope with the pain. Control may be defined as the ability to regulate or influence an intended outcome through selective responding (Baron & Rodin, 1978). Research has demonstrated that it is not essential that control actually be provided; it is important, however, that the control be perceived by the individual as available if it is to be an effective strategy (Averill, 1973). Perceived control refers to the expectation of having the ability to obtain a desired outcome (Baron & Rodin, 1978).

Although the findings reported in the literature are by no means consistent, there is evidence that both actual and/or perceived control over an impending aversive or painful event generally reduces its aversiveness for the individual and can increase the level of noxious stimulation that the individual is able to tolerate (Folkman, 1984; Thompson, 1981). Several factors have been hypothesized to account for the manner by which controllability influences tolerance of aversive or painful stimulation. One of these factors is predictability, which is presumed to reduce the ambiguity of the experience, thereby facilitating the individual's ability to effectively manage any aversive aspects of the situation. Controllability also may function by providing the person with a sense of mastery and competence (Thompson, 1981).

Folkman (1984) discussed the role of appraisal processes as important mediators of perceived personal control and responses to stressful experiences. She noted that there are two basic types of appraisals that can influence controllability. Primary appraisal refers to the individual's judgment as to whether a particular experience represents a threat (negative appraisal) or a challenge (positive appraisal). Secondary appraisal refers to the individual's evaluation of the demands required by a situation and his or her resources and abilities to implement the necessary coping strategies to confront these demands. Thus, in each situation, the person weighs the costs and benefits of engaging in control-related strategies.

Involving children in the decision making and actual treatment may help reduce combative and resistant behaviors (Melamed & Siegel, 1980; Shafir, Weiss, & Herman, 1988). Providing information may be another means of increasing a child's sense of control over a painful event, though there is some evidence that children vary in the amount of detailed information they feel is helpful in coping with a potentially painful event (e.g., minor surgery) (Peterson & Toler, 1986; Smith, Ackerman, & Blotcky, 1989). Further investigation of how children's temperament and preferred ways of coping interact with situational factors to determine the degree of pain experienced is certainly needed.

Parental Factors

Parents play an important role in facilitating their child's coping with pain (Dolgin & Phipps, 1989). Both social learning and operant learning processes have been examined as factors in children's acquisition of adaptive and maladaptive strategies for coping with pain within the family system.

Parental response to a child's verbal or nonverbal expression of pain can influence a child's experience and/or report of pain (Melamed & Siegel, 1980). Minor pains can become incapacitating and the reports of pain and/or pain behavior can last well beyond what is expected when given too much attention by caretakers (Fordyce, 1977). Parents and medical staff may unwittingly encourage the expression of pain by increased attention and decreasing the child's responsibilities (e.g., chores, going to school) during painful episodes, with less attention and resuming expectations when pain behaviors subside. For example, Dunn-Geier, McGrath, & Rourke (1986) found that mothers of poorly coping adolescents frequently discouraged adaptive responding with negative statements such as "Doesn't it hurt?" or "You must be exhausted." The difficulty is in determining what is "too much" attention, particularly when the child has a chronic disease requiring parental attention to the child's physical state.

There is considerable evidence to suggest that parental anxiety and distress can be transmitted to the child, resulting in maladaptive coping. This may be due in part to a child's attempt to elicit support and emotional comfort from a significant attachment figure during a stressful event, and/or that parental anxiety has been transmitted to the child through nonverbal means (Melamed, Siegel, & Ridley-Johnson, 1988). The tendency for more anxious mothers to have more distressed children has been shown primarily with younger children. This may be due to the fact that, as children get older, they generally develop greater independence from their mothers, thereby reducing the influence of the mother's anxiety on the child (Siegel, 1988a).

Finally, social modeling has been examined as an important etiological factor in children's learning of coping responses to painful events. It is assumed that dysfunctional parental somatic responses in stressful situations are observed and later performed by the child (Sammons, 1988). A number of studies support the role of social modeling theory in children's coping with pain. Several reviews in this area strongly suggest that there are, in fact, "pain-prone" families (Payne & Norfleet, 1986; Turk, Flor, & Rudy, 1987). For example, studies have shown an increased incidence of pain complaints in children whose parents reported a history of similar pain-related problems (Apley, 1975; Oster, 1972, Violon & Giurgea, 1984).

The specific role of social modeling in children's coping with pain also has been investigated. Osborne, Hatcher, and Richtsmeier (1989) compared children with recurrent unexplained pain to children with recurrent explained pain due to sickle-cell disease. They found that children in the unexplained pain group had more models of pain and illness behavior in their environments. In addition, children with unexplained pain were able to identify more positive consequences of their pain behavior, whereas children with explained pain identified more negative consequences. Interestingly, the children perceived the frequency and intensity of their pain to be similar to their models. Furthermore, data regarding the location of pain suggest that children may model either general illness behaviors or exact pain-related symptoms.

Personal Resources

Cognitive-Developmental Level

An important variable that mediates a child's appraisal of a painful experience is his or her general level of cognitive development. Cognitive-developmental factors influence children's understanding of the causes of their pain and methods for its treatment. Although level of cognitive development is typically associated with a child's age, there is considerable variability in conceptual abilities at a given age.

Investigators have identified consistent developmental trends in children's understanding of illness, bodily functioning, and medical treatment (Bibace & Walsh, 1982; Campbell, 1975; Simeonsson, Buckley, & Monson, 1979). Children's developmental level of cognitive sophistication is associated with a progression in sophistication of their conceptualization of illness. The preschool-aged child tends to rely on global, undifferentiated conceptualizations of illness involving magical thinking and circular logic. Children in this period base their understanding of illness on external and observable cues. They are concerned with the outer surface of the body (i.e., what "looks" painful). Reassurance that painful experiences are usually temporary may not be effective with younger children because of their poorly developed sense of temporal relations. They are more affected by pain experiences in the immediate situation (e.g., painful events affect their ability to go outside and play).

Elementary school–aged children are better able than younger children to understand pain-related conditions. Because of their capacity for the reversibility of operations (see chapter 8), they have some ability to conceptualize the healing process. Reversibility involves the ability to reason about cause and effect relationships and to understand that some events that involve a change cannot be returned to their original state or are not reversible (e.g., death). Other events involving change can be returned to their original state (e.g., a broken leg can heal). Adolescents are generally able to comprehend abstract conceptualizations of illness including internal bodily processes. They can understand what causes pain under the body's surface. In addition, they can understand the multidetermined nature of painful events.

Meaning Ascribed to the Pain

The meanings ascribed to a disease-related pain versus a more acute trauma, like a fracture or injection, will differ and may affect a child's appraisal of the pain (Lazarus & Folkman, 1984). Children with chronic diseases must deal with such issues as loss (e.g., not having a healthy body), feeling different from peers, and perceived or real threats to one's life (Koocher & O'Malley, 1981; Zeltzer, 1980). These issues and the feelings they engender may affect the child's experience of pain. This may be particularly true for children who have a difficult time expressing feelings verbally, either because of developmental constraints (e.g., preschoolers have limited vocabulary to talk about feelings) or personality styles (e.g., children who are not comfortable with or have not developed adequate skills to talk about their feelings). As a result, the experience of pain and showing observable pain behaviors may become the means by which children express their emotional discomfort (Axline, 1947; Freud, 1965; Moustakas, 1953; Spinetta & Maloney 1978).

Beales, Keen, and Lennox Holt (1983) demonstrated the importance that the meaning and attributions children ascribe to painful sensations can have on children's responses to pain. They found that children between the ages of 6 and 17 years with juvenile rheumatoid arthritis reported similar qualities of sensations from their affected joints (e.g., burning, pinching, cutting). Despite these similar descriptions, the younger children (6 to 11 years) reported little or no pain, whereas the older children (12 to 17 years) reported high levels of pain severity. Perception of pain severity was found to be related to the attributions that children in each age group made in reference to the pain sensations. The younger children tended to view the pain sensations as separate from their illness and simply waited for them to go away. On the other hand, the older children, because of their higher level of conceptual understanding, tended to regard the pain sensations as reflecting internal pathology. In addition, the older group attributed greater significance to the sensations, because they were reminded of the limitations that were imposed by their illness.

Previous Experience

Previous experiences with pain events can have both positive and negative effects on subsequent coping. Prior experience can provide the opportunity to develop adaptive coping behaviors to minimize the experience of pain and to increase the child's confidence in dealing with painful events (Lazarus & Folkman, 1984). Inquiring about strategies children used to cope successfully with previous painful events may provide helpful information as to how to facilitate coping in the current situation.

Yet, previous experiences that are negative may actually sensitize the child, increasing his or her anxiety prior to subsequent similar procedures and events (Dahlquist et al., 1986; Faust & Melamed, 1984). Children's previous experience affects their expectations regarding their ability to cope and provides them with information about the controllability or lack of controllability of a given aversive situation. Prior experience also affects the parent's perceptions of how well the child will cope with the present stressor (Siegel & Smith, 1989b).

Perceived Self-Efficacy

Self-efficacy theory proposes that individuals' self-judgments of their capabilities can affect their performance, level of motivation, thought patterns, and emotional reactions in aversive situations. Specifically, self-efficacy is the belief that one has the skills to achieve the desired outcome (e.g., decrease pain or distress) (Bandura, 1977). The level and strength of one's efficacy expectations influence the extent to which a behavior will be attempted, how much persistence will be shown, and the eventual outcome. A particular coping response, therefore, should be effective to the extent that it enhances self-efficacy expectations for the individual.

An important distinction is made between judgments of self-efficacy and outcome expectations (Bandura, 1977). Although perceived self-efficacy refers to an individual's judgment of his/her ability to perform a particular response, outcome expectation refers to the judgment of the likely consequences of such a response.

Bandura (1986) has hypothesized further that one of the most important conditions for altering self-efficacy is the mastery of experiences that provide the individual with feedback that he or she has an effective repertoire of coping responses. Self-efficacy increases as a result of self-observations of improved performance and the perceived development of coping skills to manage stressful situations in the future.

A number of studies with adults have demonstrated consistently that individuals' beliefs that they have the ability to cope with or master a painful experience can facilitate increased pain tolerance (Litt, 1988; Vallis & Bucher, 1986). High self-efficacy beliefs appear to facilitate active coping efforts. In studies of behavioral approaches for pain management, self-efficacy expectations have been found to be related to experimental pain and acute and chronic clinical pain tolerance (Dolce, 1987; O'Leary, 1985). Research also has shown that increased self-efficacy is associated with lower levels of emotional arousal, increased efforts at pain control using cognitive-behavioral strategies, and reduced requests for medication to control pain (O'Leary, 1985).

Although the constructs of self-efficacy and perceived controllability would appear similar, research suggests that they are, in fact, distinct factors. Perceived control refers to perceptions of the availability of a response to influence an aversive event, whereas self-efficacy refers to the person's confidence in his or her ability to affect that response. Litt (1988) found that the highest levels of pain tolerance were achieved in individuals who perceived high control over the situation and who had the highest self-efficacy pertaining to their ability to use that control. Controllability, therefore, appears to be most salient for persons who are most confident in their ability to use controlling strategies (i.e., those highest in self-efficacy). In this regard, Schorr and Rodin (1982) have noted that although the opportunity to use control in a given situation may exist, the person may not have confidence in his/her ability to take advantage of that opportunity (see chapter 3). Similarly, a person may be confident in his/her ability to use controlling strategies, but the situation may not enable the person to use them. As a result, self-efficacy expectations may be a mediating factor in determining if providing control is effective for an individual in a given situation.

In sum, merely teaching children to use various strategies to cope with pain does not insure that the coping behaviors will be performed. Once the appropriate skills have been acquired, children need to be provided with successful experiences to strengthen their perceptions that their skills are, in fact, effective. Although additional research is clearly needed in this area, it is possible that the specific coping skills that children use are less important than their belief in the efficacy of the method to control pain.

Preferred Coping Styles

As more emphasis is placed on learning what strategies children use to cope with pain, several issues are raised. One issue, mentioned previously, is whether children have "preferred" coping strategies that are used across situations and over time or coping strategies that are more situation specific. The concept of a more global coping style (versus situation-specific coping strategy) emphasizes a cognitive process by which incoming stimuli are organized and translated into behavioral responses (Byrne, 1964; Goldstein & Blackman, 1978). This definition implies a consistency in responding to threatening or anxiety-provoking stimuli across situations, a trait notion rather than situational specificity in responses. In the adult literature, three coping styles — repression-sensitization, minimization-vigilant focusing, and distractor-monitor — have been described and seem to point to a similar construct (Byrne, 1964; Lipowski, 1970; Meichenbaum & Butler, 1979). People who are repressors, minimizers, and distractors seem to use selective inattention, denial, and avoidance of information when dealing with stressful events such as painful procedures. In contrast, people who are sensitizers, vigilant focusers, and monitors appear to actively seek information and details about the event in question. Some researchers suggest that rather than being one continuum, two constructs should be considered: an information-seeking style and an information-avoiding style (Miller & Green, 1985).

Though prior studies have been conducted primarily with adults (Andrew, 1970; Cohen & Lazarus, 1973; Mullen & Suls, 1982; Roth & Cohen, 1986; Shipley, Butt, & Horwitz, 1979; Shipley, Butt, Horwitz, & Farbry, 1978), this concept is gaining attention in research with children. Individual differences in how children cope with impending surgery were noted by Burstein and Meichenbaum (1979) who categorized children as "worriers" and "deniers" using a defensiveness scale developed by Wallach and Kogan (1965). Defensiveness in this study is conceptualized as a characteristic style of dealing with anxiety, with "deniers" reporting greater denial of imperfections and normal concerns usually seen in childhood compared to the "worriers." Children who were more defensive spent less time playing with hospital-related toys 1 week prior to hospitalization and were found to be more anxious 1 week after surgery. Follow-up interviews 7 months later revealed interesting differences between the two groups of children. Children categorized as "worriers" remembered more procedure-related hospital events, recalled more advice and preparatory statements from parents, and perceived the hospital experience as a series of threats to be handled with self-reassuring statements. Children categorized as "deniers" remembered more procedure-irrelevant events while hospitalized, did not recall any preparatory or advice-giving statements made by parents, and perceived the hospital experience as one undifferentiated threat. Though of interest, the follow-up data should be interpreted cautiously, as only a small subset of the original sample was able to be interviewed, raising the question of whether their responses are representative of the sample as a whole.

Other more recent investigations, which were reviewed in the section on assessment of coping strategies, have supported the concept of an information-seeking/information-avoiding coping continuum (Knight et al., 1979;

Peterson & Toler, 1986). Yet since few studies have assessed children's responses across a variety of stressful and anxiety-provoking situations, the question of whether children exhibit global coping styles that can be conceptualized under such labels as information avoiding or seeking remains an empirical one. As in other areas of psychological research of individual differences, the use of different assessment techniques to ascertain constructs that carry similar labels may create difficulties in comparing results across studies. Moreover, as research continues to explore this area, it will be important to determine if what is being assessed as information seeking or avoiding is independent of other more established constructs such as temperamental characteristics (e.g., general activity level and how children respond to novel situations or behavioral inhibition) (Chess & Thomas, 1986; Kagan, 1989) or correlated with other factors such as previous experience (Smith et al., 1989).

Whether children exhibit global coping styles or more situation-specific coping strategies, understanding more about what children perceive as their coping behavior raises another clinical question. Is it important to match behavioral interventions for pain management to children's preferred coping style or strategies used in the past? Will teaching new coping strategies inconsistent with a "preferred" coping style be less effective?

To address this question, Smith et al. (1989) examined the efficacy of matching coping styles with behavioral interventions in reducing anticipatory and procedure-related pain and distress in pediatric oncology patients undergoing bone marrow aspirations and lumbar punctures. Coping style was assessed as indicative of either information avoiding or information seeking, using the coping interview developed by Siegel (1983). Children were randomly assigned to either a sensory-information or a verbal-distraction group. Sensory information was conceptualized as more consistent with an information-seeking coping style and verbal distraction with an information-avoiding coping style.

Little support was found for the hypothesis that a greater reduction in measures of distress would be found in groups where intervention was consistent with coping styles. Interestingly, on the children's rating of perceived pain, information avoiders using distraction had significantly greater subjective pain ratings followed by information seekers provided information. Avoiders given information and seekers using distraction had the lowest subjective pain ratings. In this study, preferred coping style (e.g., information seeking or avoiding) was related to how long the children had their cancer, with avoiders tending to have been diagnosed 6 months or less. A tendency to use avoidance or denial during the early stages of a life-threatening illness has been found in other investigations (Levenson, Pfefferbaum, Copeland, & Silberberg, 1982; Spinetta & Maloney, 1978). Though these results are tentative, they suggest that children's experience with the procedure and the context in which it is embedded (e.g., a life-threatening illness) need to be considered. Furthermore, teaching children coping strategies that are not consistent with what they prefer to use may in some instances be effective.

Summary and Future Directions

The assessment of coping strategies used by children and adolescents is in its infancy, though some consistency has been found in the available literature. Studies suggest that children, on their own, utilize coping strategies when confronted with pain and stressful events and can report on the use of these strategies. Children and adolescents seem to use a variety of coping strategies during these events. Investigators appear to agree that it is important to assess both behavioral (what children do) and cognitive (what they think) strategies. The actual method of assessing coping strategies has differed somewhat, although learning about coping through interviews with children seems to be one component of most investigations. Some consistency has been found in that older children seem to possess a greater number of coping strategies in their repertoire and tend to use more cognitive strategies. These findings are not surprising given the differences in cognitive-developmental level as children mature. For example, older children have had more opportunities than younger children to "try out" different ways of coping with pain or stress. In addition, the thought processes of older children are more sophisticated than those of younger children.

Although studies of assessment alone are important, relating coping strategies to outcome in specific painful situations is needed to advance our understanding of which strategies are adaptive and which less helpful in "coping successfully." The present data would suggest that information-seeking strategies (e.g., asking questions about the procedure), and positive self-talk (e.g., telling oneself that a painful procedure is necessary in order to get well) are related to better adjustment based on behavioral observations. However, at least one study has suggested that a distraction strategy (e.g., talking or thinking about events unrelated to the procedure) may be helpful for at least some children. Future studies will need to use a variety of outcome measures including behavioral observations, children's subjective perceptions of pain, and emotional indicators (e.g., physiological arousal) since different coping strategies may result in different outcomes in these areas.

In addition, many studies have focused on children undergoing elective surgery with less consideration of strategies used by children who repeatedly experience pain. Little is known as to whether coping strategies change over time when similar types of pain are experienced multiple times. Very preliminary cross-situational data with some children who have cancer suggest this may be the case. As greater attention is paid to potential mediating factors such as self-efficacy, repeated exposure to similar events will be an important paradigm to study.

Future investigations need to include other factors that appear to affect the coping process. Such factors include the prior experiences of the child, cognitive level, social support, and the nature of the child's pain (e.g., acute versus chronic). Whether children have more global coping styles, such as information avoiding or information seeking, that are used across different types of situations remains an empirical question.

Given that a wide variety of behavioral interventions are available to help children minimize pain and emotional distress during stressful events, the ultimate goal of understanding differences in coping strategies that children use is to teach effective coping strategies and/or match interventions to children's preferred coping style. Very few currently available studies address this issue, and the one study reviewed (Smith et al., 1989) provided some interesting results with respect at least to subjective perceptions of pain experience. As the assessment of coping strategies becomes more systematic, it will be important to address the issue of providing the best intervention for a particular child within a specific situation that involves pain.

References

Andrew, J. M. (1970). Recovery from surgery, with and without preparation for invasive medical and dental procedures. *Journal of Behavioral Medicine, 6,* 1–40.

Apley, J. (1975). *The child with abdominal pain* (2nd ed.). Oxford: Blackwell.

Auerbach, S. M., Martelli, M. F., & Mercuri, L. G. (1983). Anxiety, information, interpersonal impacts and adjustment to a stressful health care situation. *Journal of Personality and Social Psychology, 44,* 1284–1296.

Averill, J. R. (1973). Personal control over aversive stimuli and its relationship to stress. *Psychological Bulletin, 15,* 286–303.

Axline, V. (1947). *Play therapy.* Boston: Houghton Mifflin.

Bandura, A. (1977). Self-efficacy: Toward a unifying theory of behavior change. *Psychological Review, 84,* 191–215.

Bandura, A. (1986). *Social foundations of thought and action: A social cognitive theory.* Englewood Cliffs, NJ: Prentice-Hall.

Baron, R., & Rodin, J. (1978). Perceived control and crowding stress. In A. Baum, J. E. Singer, & S. Valins (Eds.), *Advances in environmental psychology* (pp. 216–242). Hillsdale, NJ: Erlbaum.

Beales, J. G., Keen, J. H., & Lennox Holt, P. J. (1983). The child's perception of the disease and the experience of pain in juvenile chronic arthritis. *Journal of Rheumatology, 10,* 61–65.

Bibace, R., & Walsh, M. (1982). Development of children's concepts of illness. *Pediatrics, 66,* 912–917.

Brown, J. M., O'Keefe, J., Sanders, S. H., & Baker, B. (1986). Developmental changes in children's cognition to stressful situations. *Journal of Pediatric Psychology, 11,* 343–357.

Burstein, S., & Meichenbaum, D. (1979). The work of worrying in children undergoing surgery. *Journal of Abnormal Child Psychology, 1,* 121–132.

Byrne, D. (1964). The repression-sensitization scale: Rationale, reliability, and validity. *Journal of Personality, 29,* 334–349.

Caldwell, B. M., & Honig, A. S. (1971). APPROACH: A procedure for patterning responses of adults and children. *Catalog of Selected Documents in Psychology, 1*, 1.

Campbell, J. D. (1975). Illness is a point of view: The development of children's concepts of illness. *Child Development, 46*, 92–100.

Caty, S., Ellerton, M. L., & Ritchie, J. A. (1984). Coping in hospitalized children: Analysis of published case studies. *Nursing Research, 33*, 277–282.

Chess, S., & Thomas, A. (1986). *Temperament in clinical practice*. New York: Guilford.

Cohen, F., & Lazarus, R. S. (1973). Active coping processes, coping dispositions, and recovery from surgery. *Psychosomatic Medicine, 35*, 375–388.

Curry, S. L., & Russ, S. W. (1985). Identifying coping strategies in children. *Journal of Clinical Child Psychology, 14*, 61–69.

Dahlquist, L. M., Gil, K. M., Armstrong, D., DeLawyer, D., Greene, P., & Wouri, D. (1986). Preparing children for medical examinations: The importance of previous medical experience. *Health Psychology, 5*, 249–259.

Dolce, J. J. (1987). Self-efficacy and disability beliefs in behavioral treatment of pain. *Behaviour Research and Therapy, 25*, 289–299.

Dolgin, M. J., & Phipps, S. (1989). Pediatric pain: The parents' role. *Pediatrician: International Journal of Child and Adolescent Health, 16*, 103–109.

Dunn-Geier, B. J., McGrath, P. J., & Rourke, B. P. (1986). Adolescent chronic pain: The ability to cope. *Pain, 26*, 23–32.

Ekman, P., Friesen, W. V., & Ellsworth, P. C. (1972). *Emotion in the human face: Guidelines for research and an integration of findings*. New York: Pergamon.

Faust, J., & Melamed, B. G. (1984). Influences of arousal, previous experience, and age on surgery preparation of same day surgery and in-hospital pediatric patients. *Journal of Consulting and Clinical Psychology, 52*, 359–365.

Folkman, S. (1984). Personal control and stress and coping processes: A theoretical analysis. *Journal of Personality and Social Psychology, 46*, 839–852.

Fordyce, W. E. (1977). *Behavioral methods for chronic pain and illness*. St. Louis: CV Mosby.

Freud, A. (1965). *Normality and pathology in childhood: Assessments of development*. New York: International Universities Press.

Goldstein, K. M., & Blackman, S. (1978). *Cognitive styles: Five approaches and relevant research*. New York: Wiley.

Hyson, M. C. (1983). Going to the doctor: A developmental study of stress and coping. *Journal of Child Psychology and Psychiatry, 24*, 247–259.

Izard, C. (1972). *Human emotions*. New York: Plenum.

Kagan, J. (1989). Temperamental contributions to social behavior. *American Psychologist, 44*, 668–674.

Katz, E. R., Kellerman, J., & Siegel, S. E. (1980). Behavioral distress in children with cancer undergoing medical procedures: Developmental considerations. *Journal of Consulting and Clinical Psychology, 48*, 356–365.

Knight, R. B., Atkins, A., Eagle, C. J., Evans, N., Finkelstein, J. W., Fukushima, D., Katz, J., & Weiner, H. (1979). Psychological stress, ego defenses, and cortisol production in children hospitalized for elective surgery. *Psychosomatic Medicine, 41*, 40–49.

Koocher, G. P., & O'Malley, J. E. (1981). *The Damocles syndrome: Psychosocial consequences of surviving childhood cancer*. New York: McGraw-Hill.

Lazarus, R. S., & Folkman, S. (1984). *Stress, appraisal, and coping.* New York: Springer.

Levenson, P. M., Pfefferbaum, B. J., Copeland, D. R., & Silberberg, Y. (1982). Information preferences of cancer patients ages 11–20 years. *Journal of Adolescent Health Care, 3,* 9–13.

Lipowski, Z. J. (1970). Physical illness, the individual, and the coping process. *Psychiatry in Medicine, 1,* 91–102.

Litt, M. D. (1988). Self-efficacy and perceived control: Cognitive mediators of pain tolerance. *Journal of Personality and Social Psychology, 54,* 149–160.

Meichenbaum, D., & Butler, L. (1979). Cognitive etiology: Assessing the streams of cognition and emotion. In K. Blankstein, P. Pliner, & J. Polivy (Eds.), *Advances in the study of communication and affect: Assessment and modification of emotional behavior* (pp. 1–54). New York: Plenum.

Melamed, B. G., & Siegel, L. J. (1980). *Behavioral medicine: Practical applications in health care.* New York: Springer.

Melamed, B. G., Siegel, L. J., & Ridley-Johnson, R. (1988). Coping behaviors in children facing medical stress. In T. Field, P. McCabe, & N. Schneiderman (Eds.), *Stress and coping across development* (pp. 109–137). Hillsdale, NJ: Erlbaum.

Miller, S. M., & Green, M. L. (1985). Coping with stress and frustration: Origins, nature, and development. In M. Lewis & C. Saarni (Eds.), *Socialization of emotions* (Vol. 5, pp. 263–314). New York: Plenum.

Moustakas, C. (1953). *Children in play therapy.* New York: McGraw-Hill.

Mullen, B., & Suls, J. (1982). The effectiveness of attention and rejection as coping styles: A meta-analysis of temporal differences. *Journal of Psychosomatic Research, 26,* 43–49.

O'Leary, A. (1985). Self-efficacy and health. *Behaviour Research and Therapy, 23,* 437–451.

Osborne, R. B., Hatcher, J. W., & Richtsmeier, A. J. (1989). The role of social modeling in unexplained pediatric pain. *Journal of Pediatric Psychology, 14,* 43–61.

Oster, J. (1972). Recurrent abdominal pain, headache, and limb pain in children and adolescents. *Pediatrics, 50,* 429–436.

Payne, B., & Norfleet, M. A. (1986). Chronic pain and the family: A review. *Pain, 26,* 1–22.

Pearlin, L., & Schooler, C. (1978). The structure of coping. *Journal of Health and Social Psychology, 19,* 2–21.

Peterson, L., & Toler, S. M. (1986). An information seeking disposition in child surgery patients. *Health Psychology, 4,* 343–358.

Pidgeon, V. (1981). Functions of preschool children's questions in coping with hospitalization. *Research in Nursing and Health, 4,* 229–235.

Ross, D. M., & Ross, S. A. (1984). The importance of type of question, psychological climate and subject set in interviewing children about pain. *Pain, 19,* 71–79.

Roth, S., & Cohen, L. J. (1986). Approach, avoidance, and coping with stress. *American Psychologist, 41,* 813–819.

Sammons, M. J. (1988). Pain assessment in children II: Understanding recurrent abdominal pain. In P. Karoly (Ed.), *Handbook of child health assessment* (pp. 387–409). New York: Wiley.

Schorr, D., & Rodin, J. (1982). The role of perceived control in practitioner-patient relationships. In T. A. Wills (Ed.), *Basic concepts in helping relationships* (pp. 155–186). New York: Academic Press.

Shafir, R., Weiss, J., & Herman, O. (1988). Simple interventions — self treatment. *Pediatrics*, *81*, 710–712.

Shipley, R. H., Butt, J. H., & Horwitz, E. A. (1979). Preparation to reexperience a stressful medical examination: Effect of repetitious videotape exposure and coping style. *Journal of Consulting and Clinical Psychology*, *47*, 485–492.

Shipley, R. H., Butt, J. H., Horwitz, E. A., & Farbry, J. E. (1978). Preparation for a stressful medical procedure: Effect of amount of stimulus preexposure and coping style. *Journal of Consulting and Clinical Psychology*, *47*, 499–507.

Siegel, L. J. (1983). Hospitalization and medical care of children. In E. Walker & M. Roberts (Eds.), *Handbook of clinical child psychology* (pp. 1089–1108). New York: Wiley.

Siegel, L. J. (1988a). Dental treatment. In D. Routh (Ed.), *Handbook of pediatric psychology* (pp. 448–459). New York: Guilford.

Siegel, L. J. (1988b). Measuring children's adjustment to hospitalization and to medical procedures. In P. Karoly (Ed.), *Handbook of child health assessment* (pp. 265–302). New York: Wiley.

Siegel, L. J., & Smith, K. E. (1989a). Children's strategies for coping with pain. *Pediatrician: International Journal of Child and Adolescent Health*, *16*, 110–118.

Siegel, L. J., & Smith, K. E. (1989b, April). *Assessment of pain tolerance in children and adolescents*. Paper presented at the Florida Conference on Child Health Psychology, Gainesville, FL.

Simeonsson, R. J., Buckley, L., & Monson, L. (1979). Conceptions of illness causality in hospitalized children. *Journal of Pediatric Psychology*, *4*, 77–84.

Smith, K. E., Ackerman, J. D., & Blotcky, A. D. (1989). Reducing distress during invasive medical procedures: Relating behavioral interventions to preferred coping style in pediatric cancer patients. *Journal of Pediatric Psychology*, *14*, 405–420.

Spinetta, J. J., & Maloney, L. J. (1978). The child with cancer: Patterns of communication and denial. *Journal of Consulting and Clinical Psychology*, *46*, 1540–1541.

Thompson, S. C. (1981). Will it hurt less if I can control it? A complex question. *Psychological Bulletin*, *90*, 89–101.

Turk, D. C., Flor, H., & Rudy, T. E. (1987). Pain and families. I. Etiology, maintenance, and psychological impact. *Pain*, *30*, 3–27.

Vallis, T. M., & Bucher, B. (1986). Self-efficacy as a predictor of behavior change: Interaction with type of training for pain tolerance. *Cognitive Therapy and Research*, *10*, 79–94.

Varni, J. (1983). *Clinical behavioral pediatrics: An interdisciplinary biobehavioral approach*. New York: Pergamon.

Violon, A., & Giurgea, D. (1984). Familial models for chronic pain. *Pain*, *18*, 199–203.

Wallach, M. A., & Kogan, N. (1965). *Modes of thinking in young children: A study of the creativity-intelligence distinction*. New York: Holt, Rinehart, & Winston.

White, R. W. (1974). Strategies of adaptation: An attempt at systematic description. In G. V. Costello, L. Hamburg, & J. R. Adams (Eds.), *Coping and adaptation* (pp. 126–143). New York: Basic Books.

Worchel, F. F., Copeland, D. R., & Barker, D. G. (1987). Control-related coping strategies in pediatric oncology patients. *Journal of Pediatric Psychology*, *12*, 25–38.

Zeltzer, L. (1980). The adolescent with cancer. In J. Kellerman (Ed.), *Psychological aspects of childhood cancer* (pp. 70–99). Springfield, IL: Charles C. Thomas.

7
Developmental Issues: Infants and Toddlers

KENNETH D. CRAIG AND RUTH V.E. GRUNAU

The newborn emerges from the protective intrauterine environment well-equipped biologically to experience pain and display acute distress when tissue damage occurs. Pain will be a common experience for the infant and young child when physical development and socialization influences are occurring at a remarkable pace. Despite pain's dramatic and traumatic nature, our understanding of pain in the newborn and young child only recently has received concerted attention, and there have been serious misconceptions held by many practitioners and scholars. There also has been a substantial lag between our rapidly developing understanding of pain in the very young child and applications of this knowledge base in clinical settings.

Pain is virtually inevitable in current neonatal care as health professionals routinely engage in diagnostic tests, including heel lancing for phenylketonuria (PKU) blood tests, and perform prophylactic procedures, for example, injecting vitamin K. The likelihood of pain remains high thereafter. The diseases of childhood are a hazard for acute, recurrent, and painful conditions (McGrath & Unruh, 1987; Ross & Ross, 1988). Physical maturation (e.g., teething) or immaturity (e.g., colic, earaches) may yield acute and recurrent discomfort. Health professionals often must use invasive procedures for diagnostic, treatment, and preventive purposes. Less well documented, but crucial in terms of their impact on pain experience and expression, are those incidental and sometimes serious episodes of pain in the natural environment that do not come to the attention of clinicians. Parents soon may inflict pain for disciplinary or other personal and religious reasons, such as circumcision. And the slow onset of motor and judgmental skills inevitably leaves the infant and young child vulnerable to accidents and the suffering that only the trauma of lacerations, bruises, fractures, sprains, and burns of early childhood can bring. Pain is not always of severe and lasting proportion, but it can compromise the outcome of medical care and the long-term health of the child and leave enduring effects (Anand & Hickey, 1987; Anand, Sippell, & Aynsley-Green, 1987; Craig & Grunau, in press).

Although the infant and young child are vulnerable to many internal and invasive sources of pain, they are not devoid of either physiological or behavioral defenses for minimizing deleterious effects. Indeed, the massive physiological changes, behavioral reactions, and capacities to engage in self-regulatory behavior when the infant and young child are experiencing pain can be construed as self-protective behavior designed to reestablish homeostasis. Pain itself is recognized as often, but not invariably, serving valuable self-protective functions. The past several decades have seen striking advances in our recognition of the sensory, motoric, and social capabilities of the infant and young child (Hay, 1986; Reisman, 1987), but appreciation of the competence of the young child to respond to noxious events in an organized and self-protective manner has lagged behind. It is appropriate to construe the infant and young child as exercising their best efforts to establish and maintain control when in pain, rather than to view them as out of control. Any given child in a particular situation will display his or her maximal capability to minimize the harmful effects of tissue damage, albeit not necessarily effectively or efficiently. The limits of biological competency or environmental factors may prevent an optimal response, and caretaker intervention may be necessary to facilitate recovery to physiological and psychological homeostatic states.

Developmental Perspectives

Opportunities to intervene and to prevent pain differ with the age of the child. In consequence, it is important to know the unique features of the experience and expression of pain as they change throughout life (Craig, 1980; McGrath & Craig, 1989). In the young child, biological maturation is accompanied by rapidly developing behavioral competencies, many of which reflect socialization of the child. At a relatively rapid and inexorable pace, there are demonstrations of greater motor control; improved ability to handle sensory input; improved organization in behavioral states, including skills in moving through sleeping and waking states of consciousness; and enhanced skills for interacting with others. Paralleling these changes are systematic variations in the experience and behavioral response during pain at every stage of life. One could assume some continuity would appear as well as an orderly developmental sequence of changes or transformations in the nature of the experience. Unfortunately, few longitudinal studies are available to provide data for this proposition.

The broad characterization of cognitive development developed by Piaget (Piaget & Inhelder, 1969) has provided a constructive framework for understanding the differences between early childhood and later periods of life, as well as a context for appreciating the specifics of pain experience and expression during childhood (Gaffney & Dunne, 1986; Ross & Ross, 1988). From birth through 2 years of age has been characterized as the sensorimotor period. Associations between sensory events and motor actions acquired during active sensory exploration become established as perceptual schema that allow representation of events in the world when they are no longer present and are useful in recognizing situations. Limited language development takes place at this time, with children perhaps acquiring over time a receptive vocabulary of 300 words, and some children able to generate pain descriptors. The child will also learn to differentiate himself or herself from the environment, but only achieves a sense of an independent self in later stages of development. The infant would be unable to understand or to attach meaning to what is happening when in pain or to understand the causes of the distress. In consequence, the experience would seem to be affectively dominated, with raw distress and hurt preeminent. In the later stages of this period, with a vocabulary beginning to emerge, events can assume meaningful significance for the child, and causal explanations of a rudimentary nature may begin to be provided for painful experiences (Ross & Ross, 1988). By the time they are toddlers, children may have become capable of ignoring pain in the course of play, apparently because they are so heavily engaged or absorbed with the excitement of play that they do not have the time to attend to injury.

At approximately the age of 2, and continuing through to about the age of 7, the child has been described (Piaget & Inhelder, 1969) as entering the preoperational stage of cognitive development. The association of properties with situations permits the development of symbolic propositional thinking at this time and the child becomes capable of using symbols in talking and engaging in symbolic play (Olson, 1989). While thinking is concrete and the world is perceived in absolute terms (Gaffney & Dunne, 1987) concerning what the child can see, touch, or manipulate, rather than by verbal or more abstract terms, the capacity to impose meaning on events is emerging. Interacting with these perceptually dominant features would be the affective qualities of experience, with feelings of painful distress associated with the emotions of fear, unhappiness, and isolation. Social parameters also appear to become more salient. Children at this age have limited resources for self-management of pain. Although some coping behaviors are present, the child at this age frequently remains dependent upon parents and other caretakers to provide relief and support, and will turn to them when in distress. Development of the more sophisticated, abstract coping strategies older children employ (Branson & Craig, 1988; Brown, O'Keefe, Sanders, & Baker, 1986) seems to await further maturity.

Specific features of pain during this age span will be examined following discussion of additional contextual issues.

Outdated Perspectives on Pain in Infancy

Many early studies arrived at questionable conclusions about the nature of pain in infancy, arguing that newborns were relatively insensitive to pain.

The erroneous conclusions reflect methodological inadequacies of the early studies, including inadequate control of stimulus and measurement conditions, poor quality measurement, and the apparent imposition of the investigator's biases concerning what one would expect to observe (Grunau & Craig, in press). For example, McGraw's (1941, 1943) often cited observation that newborns from birth to 10 days of age made only diffuse body movements or did not react at all in response to a pinprick stands in contrast to more recent investigations that report that virtually all infants react vigorously to tissue damage, and suggests that either the pinprick was extremely mild, or that the assessment of reactions was so casual as to miss important qualities of the reaction pattern.

Until recently, this misunderstanding pervaded the scholarly and professional literature. A number of authoritative literature reviews and texts in the fields of developmental psychology and pediatrics have inaccurately asserted that newborns or young children were relatively insensitive to pain and rarely or never required analgesics (Bennett & Bowyer, 1982; Munn, 1965; Poznanski, 1976). For example, Sroufe (1979) concluded, "infants in the first 3 or 4 weeks of life are quite insensitive to noxious external stimulation" (p. 465). There were contradictory positions (Apley, 1975; Williamson & Williamson, 1983). For example, Swafford and Allan (1968) stressed the contradiction inherent in concepts of reduced sensitivity to pain during the first week of life when considerable restraint is required for alert newborns undergoing simple surgical procedures. Ritchie (1981) suggested that the protest may be to the restraint itself, a proposal that highlights the difficulties in distinguishing between observation and inference in studies of pain in infants. At the present time, the evidence, as reviewed here, makes it clear that newborns are sensitive to painful injury, display substantial distress vocally and in nonvocal behavioral reactions, and mount dramatic physiological stress responses as a consequence. Similar misconceptions of pain during the toddler and later childhood years are held, given that there has been a serious, systematic tendency to not prescribe adequate analgesics for toddlers in pain, and, when prescribed, adults consistently underutilize or fail to deliver appropriate medication (Beyer, DeGood, Ashley, & Russell, 1983; Eland & Anderson, 1977; Schechter, Allen, & Hanson, 1986).

Distorted perceptions of early childhood pain create serious potential for neglect and mistreatment of the child. In particular, there has been a long history of failure to prescribe analgesics or to use them adequately when prescribed, even though they are available, easy to use, and probably have fewer adverse effects than leaving the child in pain (Anand et al., 1987; Beyer et al., 1983; Schecter et al., 1986). It is also likely that health professionals use painful medical procedures unnecessarily and would hesitate to do so if they recognized the traumatic consequences for the child. For example, some clinicians would argue that routine blood drawing is overdone, and when it is necessary appropriate and known procedures for minimizing discomfort are not employed for venal punctures (Campos, 1989). McGrath and Unruh (1987, p. 140) review a variety of medical procedures that inflict pain and are done without due care (e.g., tracheal intubation) or are carried out without strong indications as to their necessity (e.g., lumbar punctures for septic workup).

There is also a likelihood of unnecessary surgery performed without proper consideration for the adverse effects of pain. This is certainly the case for circumcision. Although there are arguments in the professional literature concerning whether the surgery is painful or not (Craig, 1980), current accounts leave little doubt (Porter, Miller, & Marshall, 1986). For example, Bailey and Miller (1983) state that, "uncontrollable screams, clenched fists, and a flushed face indicate that the baby is in distress. Research corroborates these claims: sleep patterns are comparable with stress-induced ones, serum cortisol levels rise (a sign of stress) and the infants are generally awake and agitated after the procedure" (p. 30). Given that medical justification for circumcision is questionable (American Academy of Pediatrics, 1975; Bailey & Miller, 1983) and that personal values play an important role in determining if a boy will be subjected to the procedure, it is important that parents having the choice should be well aware of the humanitarian grounds for not using the procedure. Clinicians who have the professional responsibility to provide parents with information do not serve them or the newborns well if they argue that the newborn does not experience immediate pain or that it does not have persisting effects.

It is difficult to understand why there should be such a substantial discrepancy between empirical descriptions of infant and young children's reactions to tissue insult and authoritative accounts in the literature. It may have been adaptive at one time to ignore or minimize pain and suffering in young children given high infant mortality rates, and perhaps only now have greater survival rates left us capable of careful analyses of behavioral reactions. Only in recent times has the newborn and young child become recognized for their competence and individuality (Brazelton, 1984; McGrath & Unruh, 1987; Sammons, 1989). It is also the case that health care professionals tend to be preoccupied with life-threatening diseases in children and have overemphasized the potential for deleterious side effects, even though the latter are readily controlled (Schecter et al., 1986; Beyer et al., 1983). They often must administer painful diagnostic, treatment, and preventive procedures, and believe these are necessary, to the child's advantage in the long run, and probably easier to do if the ensuing pain is construed as minimal and the long-term effects inconsequential. In addition, the cues for pain may not be as clear as necessary. Some children are paralyzed and ventilated for surgical purposes. Under other circumstances, infants and young children do not have language available to verbalize distress (although they certainly can be vocal); behavioral reactions may be relatively brief and interpretable as unrelated to pain, particularly if the instigating event is difficult to identify.

Thus, misinterpretation of the infant or child's behavior may be easy. Mc-Grath and Unruh (1987) describe the capacity to inflict pain upon children as follows:

The denial of pain inflicted on children in medical procedures is made easier for a number of reasons. Children are not routinely asked if they are in pain. Younger children cannot say if they are in pain. Children's pain behavior can be physically controlled by restraint. The measurement of pain in children is not well developed. Children are unable to withdraw consent. They do not write letters of complaint; nor do they sue for medical malpractice; nor do they press charges for assault. In many cases of the most serious medically caused pain, parents are unaware of what is being done to their children. (p. 133)

There are also serious practical and ethical challenges to conducting even simple descriptive research in health settings where children can be observed in pain (Craig, 1989).

Adult Response to the Infant and Child in Pain

Infant and young children's expressions of painful distress fulfill important communicative and adaptive functions; they get the attention and sympathy of adults who are in a position to deliver relief and care. Adults may or may not elect to respond, with the substantial individual variability in response reflecting both child and adult characteristics, with some of the latter previously described. Caretakers can be objective, responsive only when necessary, and task oriented, or be hypersensitive to signs of distress, easily emotionally distressed, disorganized, and ineffective. Tendencies to be very solicitous of the infant are appropriate, given his or her vulnerability. Adults are more prepared to accept risk taking and tolerate more easily the ensuing minor injuries as children grow older and become less vulnerable to serious complications of injury or disease. If the tendency to be oversolicitous persists there may be a risk of abnormal illness behavior (Craig, 1986).

There is reason to believe that adults intimately associated with particular children become more adept in identifying subjective states, including pain. For example, Wasz-Hockert, Michelsson, and Lind (1985) claimed that parents can identify pain cries using specific acoustic features of the cry, and Sagi (1981) notes that mothers are able to distinguish the source of the cry. In contrast, Muller, Hollien, and Murry (1974) found that both mothers and other adult women had difficulty discriminating among pain, hunger, and startle cries. Given that intimate, prolonged experience with infants and children should enhance the capacity to perceptually discriminate fine differences in the sources of behavior, and that parents and other caretakers can be strongly motivated to do so, one would expect an emerging capacity to make the distinctions.

The importance of the transaction between the parent and child is apparent in Carey's model of colic in infants, in which he proposes the problem may be more likely to emerge among anxious caregivers who fail to soothe physiologically vulnerable infants (1983). However, colic is a complex phenomenon and numerous etiologies have been proposed (Barr, 1989a,b). Interpersonal dimensions may contribute to the problem for some subset of infants (Ames, 1985). In their informative analysis of colic, McGrath and Unruh (1987) note that the transactional model warrants assessment.

Assessment Issues

Parents, health care professionals, and other adults concerned with assessing pain in children confront a major challenge. Valid strategies for assessing pain are needed for early identification and treatment. At present, intuitive methods prevail, although standardized and validated measures are certainly preferable. Ultimately, the task for an observer involves integration of complex information. In most instances, the observer must assemble and integrate, when available, vocal and nonvocal behavioral, physiological information, and information concerning the physical and social context in which the pain is being experienced.

Although it can be difficult to decide if the infant is experiencing pain, it is clear that the response is organized and systematic, not random. The complex reaction pattern can be assessed in a multiplicity of ways. Fortunately, there have been sophisticated advances in multimodal behavioral measurement of pain in recent years, so the use of intuitive global judgments without reference to specific cues has become a questionable practice.

Before examining current approaches, it should be noted that questions remain concerning the measurement of chronic and recurrent pain in infants and toddlers. We know more about the assessment of acute pain, as current observational methods focus upon the initial reaction to the onset of phasic pain and seem less useful with tonic pain. At best with chronic pain, we rely upon clinical intuitions and general impressions. Children suffering from persistent pain likely will have built subtle and difficult to detect, but adaptive, reaction patterns into their lives, for example, not moving limbs when movement would induce pain, withdrawing socially, or retreating into sleep. Further, they may have become so accustomed to the pain that they do not complain. Persistent pain, and perhaps relapses, are most likely to manifest themselves in a general departure from normal living patterns for the individual child. Thus, persistent crying and irritability, and changes in mood states, in eating, sleeping, and motor patterns, and in activity levels are likely to be diagnostic. The child who becomes defensive about physical or social interaction, quiet, withdrawn, and cannot be attracted to activity is likely to warrant attention.

Throughout virtually all of the period of childhood under consideration, we cannot tap the child's unique view of painful experiences using verbal self-report. There remain three sources of information from which to infer the presence and nature of pain experienced by infants and toddlers: (a) observations of pain-related behaviors, vocal and nonvocal; (b) physiological events that are associated with pain-related behaviors and physical trauma; and (c) the presence of traumatic external events or disease states that produce tissue damage or stress and that would yield reports of pain and distress in older children and adults. In combination, information about these events permits inferences concerning what it is that the child is probably experiencing.

Nonvocal, Pain-Related Behavior

The use of nonvocal information to infer pain is time honored, but receives relatively minor attention compared to emphasis on verbal report in the scientific and professional literature (Craig & Prkachin, 1983). Physicians and others performing physical examinations provoke nonvocal behavior as they prod, squeeze, and manipulate their patients' bodies, carefully watching to see if they elicit any movements or physiological signs of pain (Pigeon, McGrath, Lawrence, & MacMurray, 1989; Purcell-Jones, Dormon, & Sumner, 1988). It is not difficult to demonstrate the newborn's capacity to experience pain; simply touching the child in the region of a wound will elicit withdrawal of the affected area. The behavioral response leads to the reasonable inference that the affected area is sore. Parents also know that children who are in physical discomfort become irritable, fuss, cry, and attempt to assume comfortable postures. Parents' unique appreciation of their children may be a crucial source of information about whether children are departing from typical styles of response. For example, their child may habitually be very stoic or reluctant to express himself or herself with strangers.

A limited number of standardized observational measures are now available for research or clinical assessment of pain in the age ranges of infancy or toddlers (Beyer & Wells, 1989; Craig, McMahon, Morison, & Zaskow, 1984; Grunau & Craig, 1987; Izard, Hembree, Dougherty, & Spizzirri, 1983; McGrath et al., 1985). Behavioral observation scales require observers to state if specific events, defined by objective descriptions of the behavior, have occurred within a specified time frame. The focus can be on vocal (e.g., language, cry, screaming) or nonvocal (facial grimaces, limb movements, torso movements) activity. Construction of the measures is constrained by the paucity of behaviors that are uniquely or invariably associated with the experience of pain (Craig & Prkachin, 1983), and the scales use behavior generated by other events as well. For example, Craig et al. (1984) trained raters to provide the incidence of the following: vocal actions (language, crying, screaming), facial activity (grimaces, eye orientation), torso positions (rigid, withdrawing), and limb positions (protecting, thrashing).

Some of the immediate reactions to acutely painful events probably qualify as unique markers of pain; for example, reflexive withdrawal from contact with an external stimulus would qualify. Further, there is enough consistency in the facial reaction elicited by noxious events at all ages (Craig & Patrick, 1985; Grunau & Craig, 1987, 1990; Johnston & Strada, 1986; LeResche & Dworkin, 1988; Patrick, Craig, & Prkachin, 1986) to suggest that a grimace of definable character qualifies as a marker of pain. Given that different facial displays appear to be associated with different emotional states, it may be possible to distinguish pain from other forms of distress (Ekman & Friesen, 1978).

Two different behavioral coding systems have been devised to study the facial display of pain in children (Grunau & Craig, 1990). Izard and his associates (Izard et al., 1983; Izard, Huebner, Resser, McGiness, & Dougherty, 1980) developed anatomically based photographic templates for configurations of facial activity that were inferred to be associated with specific emotional states in infants, namely interest, joy, surprise, sadness, anger, disgust, pain, and fear. Judges compare the facial display of an infant with the photographs to identify emotions that are being experienced. The second approach derives from the Facial Action Coding System (FACS) developed by Ekman and Friesen (1978) and revised for the study of babies by Oster (1978). This system provides a detailed account of all possible facial movements and does not use preconceived categories of emotion. Grunau and Craig (1987) developed the Neonatal Facial Coding System, based on the FACS approach and earlier work describing facial activity during pain in adults (Craig & Patrick, 1985; Patrick et al., 1986), but limited the actions to be identified to a subset likely to be elicited from infants in pain. Thus, coders look for brow bulge, eye squeeze, deepening of the nasolabial furrow, open lips, vertically stretched mouth, horizontally stretched mouth, lip purse, taut tongue, and chin quiver. Tongue protrusion was recently added because it was observed to be elicited by events when pain was not present (Grunau, Johnston, & Craig, 1990). Because facial expressions have this degree of specificity, they appear to have considerable potential as useful and convenient measures of pain in infants and young children.

Cry and Other Vocalizations

Crying, screaming, groaning, and other vocalizations provide an immediate source of information about the nature of the child's response to a variety of events (Lester & Zeskind, 1982; Levine & Gordon, 1982). Cry is highly salient and useful for adults concerned with a child's welfare. Despite its vivid qualities, cry is a very complex signal, comprising a mixture of temporal, frequency, and intensity characteristics. Sophisticated sound spectrographic and computer analyses are needed to reduce the physical patterns to constituent qualities.

Even then, its specificity to particular subjective states is questionable. To date, specific markers of cry that would differentiate pain from hunger, fatigue, fear, anger, or other subjective states have not been identified, although some discriminative features show promise (Fuller & Horii, 1988;

Johnston & O'Shaugnessy, 1988; Zeskind & Marshall, 1988). Wolff (1969, 1987) has characterized the pain cry as either an abrupt onset of loud crying or an initial long cry followed by an extended period of breath holding and, then, further cycles of more standard crying. The cycles eventually settle into a rhythm that is difficult to distinguish from other cries in the absence of contextual information as to instigating events. Murray (1979) has postulated that pain is associated with greater intensity of effort during crying. Hence, it is variations in crying along a continuum of intensity that would be of particular importance for observers.

In natural settings, adults are quite unlikely to be constrained to the exclusive use of cry in making judgments about pain in children. The cry may serve as a "biological siren" to signal alarm, but an attending adult will soon have behavioral observations, evidence of physical damage, and information about the context as a basis for judgment. When adults have both pain-induced cries and facial grimaces available to make judgments about pain in infants, their finer discriminations are based on facial actions (Craig, Grunau, & Aquan-Assee, 1988).

Physiological Measures

Tissue damage produces substantial metabolic, hormonal, and physiological change that is subject to objective measurement (Anand et al., 1987; Gunnar, Fisch, Korsvik, & Donhowe, 1981; Owens, 1984; Porter, Porges, & Marshall, 1988). As Ross and Ross (1988) note in their review of pain measurement in children, these changes offer considerable potential as indices of stress reactions induced by tissue damage, but they must be used with caution because nonpainful stress may elicit similar activity. Selye's (1976) distinction between stress, as a specifiable physiological response pattern instigated by various events, and distress, as the individual's emotional reaction to particular stressful events, is pertinent. These are not isomorphic states. The lack of correspondence between physiological measures and subjective states in adults suggests caution would be appropriate in interpreting their significance in children. Nevertheless, although the physiological changes may not be specific to pain, and there is often a lack of concordance between tissue damage and various measures of pain as well as discordance among the measures themselves, the absence of well-developed criteria for pain in young children will continue to make us dependent upon physiological measures.

In general, identifying the presence, severity, and nature of pain in infants and young children is a very complex task. Given evidence that they clearly have the sensory capabilities to experience pain, it may be reasonable to conclude that the deficits are in the child's ability to clearly communicate distress, so that observers may have difficulties unambiguously interpreting the significance of the children's behavior.

Determinants of the Child's Response to Noxious Events

Pain has complex origins and both predisposing and situational determinants can be identified in any child's reaction over and beyond the basic and fundamental tissue damage that provides the impetus for pain.

Predisposing Ontogenetic Factors

Inheritance provides the basis for the maturation of the biological systems responsible for nociception. These systems not only provide for predetermined biological development, but also are responsive to learning during pain experiences. A key issue concerns whether the brain is sufficiently mature at birth to provide the biological substrates needed for the experience of pain. There is now evidence to indicate that the nervous system is well developed at birth and neurologically capable of supporting pain experiences (Anand & Carr, 1989; Anand & Hickey, 1987). There is a substantial sensory receptive capacity to respond to painful stimulation, and even the fetus displays a remarkable ability to respond to many modalities of sensory input in utero, including touch, taste, and sound. In particular, the tactile system, which is sensitive to light touch, pressure, temperature, and pain, is well developed at birth (Gottlieb, 1971; Oppenheim, 1982). A capacity to respond to touch has been demonstrated at 6 to 8 weeks gestational age. Real-time ultrasound radiography has also made it possible to examine intrauterine fetal behavior patterns and to appreciate how early complex behavior is possible. Thus, detailed extremity movements become differentiated from 10 weeks on and include breathing, yawning, sucking, swallowing, hiccoughs, and bladder emptying. They become coordinated and organized into recognizable behavioral states toward the end of pregnancy (Whittmann & Ross, 1986), and the fetus can be characterized as a complicated and sophisticated organism. Further, intrauterine nociception appears to be demonstrated by invasive methods of assessment (e.g., fetal scalp blood sampling) that have demonstrable effects on fetal heart rate and behavioral activity. Volpe and Koenigsberger (1981) conclude that the premature of only 28 weeks gestation differentiate touch and pain. When empirical studies become available that have examined responses of premature infants born at even earlier gestational ages, this ability to differentiate between types of tactile stimuli will probably be found in even the most immature infant. What is missing is a detailed description of age-specific response patterns.

Biological maturation persists at a considerable pace following birth. All the biological substrates for the behavioral, affective, cognitive, and sensory systems that subserve pain are undergoing rapid development. The prospects for pain having a long-lasting impact are considerable. A research literature is emerging on subhuman species to suggest that postnatal physical trauma can have a substantial and enduring effect on further development of the brain (Campos, 1989; Franck, 1986).

Socialization

Concurrent with the innate unfolding of biological changes is the emergence of patterns of response to tissue damage that reflect the impact of the social environment on the child (Craig, 1983, 1986). The experiential and behavioral expression of pain comes to reflect the interaction between ontogenetic and learning factors. As the capacity to both understand and influence the environment increases, children learn through their own direct experiences with physically dangerous events and adults' attempts to influence them, as well as through vicarious experiences in which they observe others in similar situations (Craig, 1986). Through this process in these early years children learn to use familial and cultural behavior patterns to solve the problems of pain and illness.

Changes during socialization are not unidirectional; the infant and the parent are engaged in a reciprocal influence process. Parents tend to be sensitive to the capabilities of the child for minimizing distress and maintaining control. For example, Craig et al. (1984) noted that following immunization injections mothers' consoling efforts were related to the age of the child. Mothers of infants less than a year of age used more soothing and comforting vocalizations than did mothers of children in the 2nd year of life. The mothers attempted to verbally distract and used fewer soothing vocalizations with infants aged 13 to 24 months. Thus, the developmental process is based upon complex transactions.

Biological variations and the inexorable influences of socialization provide the grounds for the substantial individual differences and situational variability in behavior one observes early in life. Part of the variability is clearly intrinsic. Even during early blood lancing and injection procedures one can observe children who are quite unresponsive and others who react with striking vigor. Other differences reflect variations in the painful events children encounter, e.g., laboratory technicians vary in the amount of facial activity they generate after the heel lance during the "milking" process of extracting blood samples from the heel (Grunau & Craig, 1987). But social influences are increasingly evident. As children grow older, behavior becomes increasingly contingent upon the social context. It is not unusual to see a toddler sustain an injury, or simply be surprised by an abrupt event, check to see if a parent is present, and then express great distress and cry only if the parent is attending to what is happening. Availability of a parent has been shown to have a facilitating or attenuating effect upon a child's reaction to a potentially painful event. Ross and Ross (1988) review the complex and controversial systematic and clinical studies in the area and conclude that the child's reaction depends upon the nature of the mother's response. If she behaves in ways that are reassuring to the child, the effect is to diminish the child's fear and anxiety, with a concomitant decrease in pain reactivity and increase in manageability. In contrast, mothers or fathers may fail to behave in a reassuring way when they become unduly submissive, authoritarian, or unduly alarmed by what is happening to the child. This sensitivity to the social context provides the grounds for oversolicitous parents to reinforce excessive pain behavior (Fordyce, 1976) even at this early age, although empirical studies are lacking. It is noteworthy that the capacity to present oneself in a less than genuine manner emerges in the toddler years as children begin to engage in symbolic play, assume false roles, and pretend others and various situations to be something other than what they are (Chandler, Fritz, & Hala, 1989; Leslie, 1988). Possibly at this stage the capacity to suppress the display of pain or to malinger and fake pain begins to emerge, but evidence as to when this does occur is unavailable.

Developmental Transformations

The rapid biological changes that are patently obvious in the earliest months and years of life are paralleled by dramatic changes in behavioral and psychological capabilities of the infant and toddler. Although it is recognized that the relatively immature and reflexive reactions of the newborn to tissue insult become the coordinated patterns of experience and action of the adult, we are only beginning to describe the normative patterns one can expect at different ages. This section describes basic characteristics and key transformations in the expression of pain during the earliest stages of life.

The Neonate

The evidence is now clear that neonates respond both behaviorally and physiologically in a manner that unequivocally can be interpreted as pain. One can observe a well-integrated pattern of response that is present before it can have been shaped by the extrauterine environment. The healthy newborn's response to the sudden onset of painful events is, most often, a vigorous scream followed by crying, a dramatic facial grimace, abrupt jerking and stiffening of limb and body movements, including limb thrashing, tight clenching of the fists, and torso rigidity.

The cry can be characterized as having abrupt onset, rapid rise time, and substantial amplitude, with the initial cycle followed by a period of breath holding, and subsequent cycles following a more rhythmic pattern. There is debate in the literature as to whether the pain cry has a unique signature — either quantitative or qualitative characteristics that would distinguish it from cries instigated by nonpainful events. It may be that any sudden, disruptive event elicits essentially the same cry from the infant that is capable of generating the attention and alarm of other people present, with identification of the source dependent upon inspection of other features of the baby's response and circumstances.

Facial activity appears to provide the most substantial and specific information concerning the infant's painful state. Using an objective, anatomically based coding system we have observed facial grimaces of pain in newborns who were subjected to painful events in the course of normal nursery care. These included heel lances for blood sampling purposes (Grunau & Craig, 1987), and needle injections of vitamin K (Grunau, Johnston, & Craig, 1990). For comparison purposes, reactions to these events have been contrasted with responses to apparently innocuous events, including heel rubbing, swabbing the thigh, and application of dye to the residual umbilical cord.

Although there is substantial variability across infants, the display of pain most often observed (Grunau & Craig, 1990) consists, for most babies, of brow lowering and contracting, eyes firmly squeezed shut, the mouth open and stretched vertically, a deepening of the nasolabial furrow, and a taut tongue (a raised cupped tongue with sharp tensed edges). In a study contrasting the impact on the facial display of painful and nonpainful events, tongue protrusion, as if in the interests of sucking, was found virtually never to occur during a painful event, but appears to be a probable consequence of nonpainful physical contact, suggesting its usefulness as a discriminating variable (Grunau, Johnston, & Craig, 1990).

The general pattern of painful facial display was found to vary with the babies' state of sleeping and wakefulness (Grunau & Craig, 1987), with the most intense displays associated with a state of being awake and alert. This indicates that variations in the severity of pain are evident in the facial display. Further, the findings indicate that the severity of pain is modulated by ongoing variations in the central nervous system. Thus, pain in the newborn is substantially more complex than would be expected if it were simply a motor reflex unaccompanied by experiential states of distress.

One advantage to systematic study of the facial display is that it offers an opportunity to isolate different subjective states as components of the reaction to a noxious event. For example, different emotions are associated with different facial displays. Izard et al. (1983) examined the facial displays of infants during immunization injections at four different age groupings (mean ages were 2.1, 4.2, 8.1, and 19.2 months). They observed that responses of physical distress predominated in the younger infants, but these decreased with age, with the facial display of anger predominating later.

The limb and body movements of the newborn generated by an acute painful stimulus again tend to be abrupt, but they are relatively nonspecific and nonlocalized to the region of physical insult, suggesting a more generalized state of distress. McGraw (1943) concluded that newborns up to 10 days old either did not respond to pinprick or made only diffuse body movements, but the methodological limitations of this work, described earlier, and its inconsistencies with more recent studies make these conclusions questionable. Franck (1986) has reported that neonates subjected to heel lancing display active retreat from the stimulus and a tendency for the contralateral foot to swipe across, perhaps in a self-protective manner. The Brazelton neonatal behavioral assessment procedures (Brazelton, 1984) call for an analysis of behavioral reactions to repeated pinprick on the sole of the foot. One expects and observes in the healthy newborn initial generalized startle and diffuse reaction patterns, as well as localized withdrawal of the leg or extremities, which habituates or attenuates with repeated stimulation. It may be that more refined and detailed assessment procedures will yield further specificity to the reaction pattern.

The behavioral response is accompanied by substantial physiological changes. Williamson and Williamson (1983) and Owens and Todt (1984) report changes in blood oxygen levels and heart rate in response to circumcision and heel lancing, respectively. Anand and his associates (Anand & Aynsley-Green, 1985, 1988; Anand et al., 1987) report that neonates undergoing surgery mount a massive metabolic and endocrine response that can lead to postoperative complications unless adequate analgesia is used.

Variations in pain display within the first week of life are described in the literature, but the studies tend to lack methodological precision. For example, Lipsitt and Levy (1959) reported that declining intensities of electrical current were required to elicit withdrawal of a toe in infants over the first 4 days of life. This study has been widely cited as evidence of reduced sensitivity in newborns, but it is not clear that the apparently attenuated reactions to electrical shock at this age indicate reduced pain sensitivity. The authors themselves suggested their findings might reflect slow recovery from the effects of maternal anesthesia during childbirth, or possibly varying effects of childbirth anoxia.

There is little doubt about the capacity of the infant to experience pain following the neonatal period. Johnston and Strada (1986) provided a multidimensional description of 2- to 4-month-old infants' reactions to immunization injections that makes the distress reaction clear. They state:

The pattern that did emerge was characterized by an initial response: a drop in heart rate, a long, high pitched cry followed by a period of apnea, rigidity of the torso and limbs, and a facial expression of pain. This was followed by a sharp increase in heart rate, lower pitched, but dysphonated cries, less body rigidity, but still facial expression was of pain. Finally, in the second half of the minute's response, heart rate remained elevated, cries were lower pitched, more rhythmic, with a rising-falling pattern, and were mostly phonated, and body posturing returned to normal. Those faces that could be viewed also were returning to the at rest configuration. (p. 373)

Finally, it is appropriate to focus upon the capacity of the infant to engage in self-management of the disruptive effects of pain. The adult who carefully attends to the reaction pattern will not only see a conspicuous reaction to acute pain, but will observe the capacity of the child to reestablish comfort. In the newborn, this may be in the form of self-quieting or self-consoling behavior.

The First Year of Life

As the child grows older, one would expect greater competence in his or her response to painful events. Behavioral observations contrasting the first year of life with the second make the developmental process clear. Craig et al. (1984) reported contrasts of the reactions of infants in the first and second years of life to the physical insult of needle penetrations and hypodermic injections for the purposes of immunization. The children ranging in age between 2 and 12 months responded in a more global, diffuse manner, cried and screamed longer, did not appear to localize the region of distress, and did not engage in self-protective behavior. Not all forms of pain behavior change during the early months. Thoden and Koivisto (1980) did not observe changes in acoustically analyzed cry features in normal infants responding to a pinch of their arms in a longitudinal study at 1 day, 5 days, 3 months, and 6 months.

In this stage of life, the elements of the complex range of emotional states that accompany pain begin to manifest themselves. In the first few weeks of life, the capacity to self-calm when in distress begins to be obvious (Sammons, 1989). Between 6 and 8 months of age the child begins to display anticipatory fear (Levy, 1960) and may engage in rudimentary instrumental behavior designed to ward off what is perceived to be imminent attack. At this age, pain secondary to medical procedures is likely to be confounded with anticipatory and concurrent anxiety (Barr, 1989). The reaction to medically invasive procedures during the second half of the first year of life clearly demonstrates this. The observer sees a facial display of apprehension prior to the event, an immediate response of pain to the tissue insult, and often this is followed by a display of anger (Izard et al., 1980). It may be that at this time distraction with competing events would begin to serve as an effective intervention for attenuating infants' pain.

These changes reflect emergence of cognitive learning and memory. The capacity to anticipate pain clearly signals memory and can only reflect the accretion of perceptual schema that would have earlier origins. The newborn is clearly capable of learning (Rovee-Collier & Fagan, 1981), and thereby demonstrates a capacity for implicit memory. There has been little investigation of the persisting behavioral effects of pain in the newborn and infant, perhaps because pain has only recently been acknowledged.

The Second Year of Life

During the second year of life Craig et al. (1984) observed greater competence in the child's response to immunization injections. The children aged 13 to 24 months screamed and cried for a shorter period of time, visually scanned their mothers and the nurse prior to the injection, oriented toward the site of the injection, attempted to protect themselves with their arms and hands and by pulling their torsos away, displayed less torso rigidity in response to the injection, and were capable of using language to express themselves. Thus, the older children appeared to integrate their response to the injection into the ongoing flow of other events and situational constraints present at that time. They were sufficiently cognizant of what was happening to engage in voluntary, goal-directed behavior, including both verbal and motor activity. Their behavior also suggested a capacity for self-calming and quieting.

The toddler's response to pain-inducing events is more likely to be localized to the painful body region, to include purposeful efforts to relieve the pain, and to include essentially the same facial expression observed at earlier ages, but, in addition, there is more social meaning in the facial activity, including anger and perhaps disappointment, and the response includes specific verbalizations and demands as well as crying.

Ability to communicate distress improves with both age and experience, with the repertoire of verbal and nonverbal behaviors increasing and sometimes becoming more efficient. In general, as verbal skills for communicating painful discomfort become enhanced through maturation and experience, nonverbal manifestations of distress become more subtle and less vigorous.

Bridging to the Preschool Years

During these years the child truly becomes a socialized person with a capacity to communicate to others personal needs and desires and the skills necessary to respond to the demands of others and interact with them with some skill and effectiveness. Through direct personal experience and observation of others, children learn about potentially painful experiences, what personal reactions are likely to occur, and what skills are needed to cope with pain, using the child's own and others' resources (Craig, 1983). These skills include patterns of response to illness and pain that correspond to family and cultural expectations. The child must learn skills to effectively engage maximal cooperation from parents and other caretakers. The pressures to do so are strong; pain is compelling and commands action, others are capable of rescuing the child and providing relief and support. Failure to comply when there is a risk of physical injury can lead to swift punishment from caretakers, thereby ensuring that the response pattern conforms to familial and cultural expectations (Craig & Wyckoff, 1987).

As the child acquires the socialized patterns of pain and illness behavior, the capacity to express discomfort spontaneously in a manner that does not entirely correspond to the subjective state of distress begins to manifest itself. In the earliest stages of life, one would expect a high degree of fidelity between the subjective state of painful distress and the expressive display. Infants are not often suspected of guile or deceit. Later, the expectation would be that older infants and toddlers would not tolerate pain well and would exercise their ability to enlist the help of parents and others with minimal provocation; indeed, parents tend to be oversolicitous and encourage early communication of health risk or threat so that they can intervene even if there is minimal risk. But there also can be pressures to suppress spontaneous reactions. In some circumstances, children may learn to inhibit vocalizations, and the observer may have to attend to facial grimaces or muscle tension to detect distress. As children grow older and encounter the inevitable bumps and scrapes of childhood without serious injury or enduring damage, their parents become relatively inured to their crises and are likely to require that children withhold demands unless there are genuinely serious problems. In this manner, parents also promote the process of self-management and personal independence. This socialization process can also be construed as one that recognizes and promotes different communication styles as the child grows older.

Acknowledgments. The authors' work reported here was supported by grants from the Natural Sciences and Engineering Council of Canada and the Social Sciences and Humanities Research Council of Canada.

References

American Academy of Pediatrics (1975). Report of the ad hoc task force on circumcision. *Pediatrics, 56*, 610.

Ames, E. W. (1985). Mundus et infans. *Canadian Psychology, 26*, 262–274.

Anand, K. J. S., & Aynsley-Green, A. (1985). Metabolic and endocrine effects of surgical ligation of patent ductus arteriosus in the human preterm neonate: Are there implications for further improvement of postoperative outcome? *Modern Problems in Paediatrics, 23*, 143–157.

Anand, K. J. S., & Aynsley-Green, A. (1988). Does the newborn infant require potent anaesthesia during surgery? Answers from a randomized trial of halothane anaesthesia. In R. Dubner, G. F. Gebhart, & M. R. Bond (Eds.), *Pain research and clinical management* (Vol. 3, pp. 329–335). Amsterdam: Elsevier.

Anand, K. J. S., & Carr, D. B. (1989). The neuroanatomy, neurophysiology, and neurochemistry of pain, stress, and analgesia in newborns and children. *Pediatric Clinics of North America, 36*, 795–822.

Anand, K. J. S., & Hickey, P. R. (1987). Pain and its effects in the human neonate and fetus. *New England Journal of Medicine, 317*(21), 1321–1329.

Anand, K. J. S., Sippell, W. G., & Aynsley-Green, A. (1987). Randomized trial of fentanyl anaesthesia in preterm babies undergoing surgery: Effects on the stress response. *Lancet, i*, 243–268.

Apley, J. (1975). *The child with abdominal pains* (2nd ed.). London: Blackwell.

Bailey, C. R., & Miller, N. K. (1983). Routine circumcision of the male neonate. *Canadian Nurse, 79*, 28–31.

Barr, R. G. (1989a). Pain in children. In P. D. Wall & R. Melzack (Eds.), *Textbook of pain* (2nd ed., pp. 568–588). London: Churchill Livingstone.

Barr, R. G. (1989b). Recasting a clinical enigma: The case of infant crying problems (and colic). In P. Zelazo & R. G. Barr (Eds.), *Challenges to development paradigms: Implications for theory, assessment and treatment* (pp. 44–63). New York: Erlbaum.

Bennett, E. J., & Bowyer, D. E. (1982). *Principles of pediatric anesthesia.* Springfield, IL: C.C. Thomas.

Beyer, J. E., DeGood, D. E., Ashley, L. D., & Russell, G. A. (1983). Patterns of postoperative analgesic use with adults and children following cardiac surgery. *Pain, 17,* 71–81.

Beyer, J. E., & Wells, N. (1989). The assessment of pain in children and adolescents. *Pediatric Clinics of North America, 36,* 837–854.

Branson, S. M., & Craig, K. D. (1988). Children's spontaneous strategies for coping with pain: A review of the literature. *Canadian Journal of Behavioural Science, 20,* 402–412.

Brazelton, T. B. (1984). *Neonatal Behaviour Assessment Scale* (2nd ed.). Spastics International Medical Publications, Monograph #88. Philadelphia: J. B. Lippincott.

Brown, J. M., O'Keefe, J., Sanders, S. H., & Baker, B. (1986). Developmental changes in children's cognition to stressful and painful situations. *Journal of Pediatric Psychology, 11,* 343–357.

Campos, R. G. (1989). Comfort measures for infant pain. *Sensory Integration News, 16,* 2–8.

Carey, W. B. (1983). "Colic" or excessive crying in young infants. In M. D. Levine, W. B. Carey, A. C. Crocker, & R. T. Gross (Eds.), *Developmental-behavioral pediatrics* (pp. 517–521). Philadelphia: Saunders.

Chandler, M., Fritz, A. S., & Hala, S. (1989). Small scale deceit: Deception as a marker of 2-, 3- and 4-year-olds' early theories of mind. *Child Development, 60,* 1263–1277.

Craig, K. D. (1980). Ontogenetic and cultural determinants of the expression of pain in man. In H. W. Kosterlitz & L. Y. Terenius (Eds.), *Pain and society* (pp. 39–52). Dahlem Konferenzen. Weinheim/Deerfield Beach, FL/Basal: Verlag Chemie.

Craig, K. D. (1983). Modeling and social learning factors in chronic pain. In J. J. Bonica, U. Lindblom, & A. Iggo (Eds.), *Advances in pain research and therapy* (Vol. 5, pp. 813–828). New York: Raven Press.

Craig, K. D. (1986). Pain in context: Social modeling influences. In R. A. Sternbach (Ed.), *The psychology of pain* (2nd ed., pp. 67–96). New York: Raven Press.

Craig, K. D. (1989). Clinical pain measurement from the perspective of the human laboratory. In C. R. Chapman & J. D. Loeser (Eds.), *Issues in pain measurement* (pp. 220–230). New York: Raven Press.

Craig, K. D., & Grunau, R. V. E. (in press). Neonatal pain perception and behavioral measurement. In K. J. S. Anand & P. J. McGrath (Eds.), *Neonatal pain and distress.* Amsterdam: Elsevier Science.

Craig, K. D., Grunau, R. V. E., & Aquan-Assee, J. (1988). Judgment of pain in newborns: Facial activity and cry as determinants. *Canadian Journal of Behavioural Science, 20,* 442–451.

Craig, K. D., McMahon, R. S., Morison, J. D., & Zaskow, C. (1984). Developmental changes in infant pain expression during immunization injections. *Social Science and Medicine, 19,* 1331–1337.

Craig, K. D., & Patrick, C. J. (1985). Facial expression during induced pain. *Journal of Personality and Social Psychology, 48,* 1080–1091.

Craig, K. D., & Prkachin, K. M. (1983). Nonverbal measures of pain. In R. Melzack (Ed.), *Pain measurement and assessment* (pp. 173–179). New York: Raven Press.

Craig, K. D., & Wyckoff, M. G. (1987). Cultural factors in chronic pain management. In G. D. Burrows, D. Elton, & G. Stanley (Eds.), *Handbook of chronic pain management* (pp. 99–108). Amsterdam: Elsevier Science.

Ekman, P., & Friesen, W. V. (1978). *Facial Action Coding System: A technique for the measurement of facial movement.* Palo Alto, CA: Consulting Psychologists Press.

Eland, J. M., & Anderson, J. E. (1977). The experience of pain in children. In A. Jacox (Ed.), *Pain: A sourcebook for nurses and other professionals* (pp. 453–471). Boston: Little, Brown.

Fordyce, W. E. (1976). *Behavioral methods for chronic pain and illness.* St. Louis: Mosby.

Franck, L. S. (1986). A new method to quantitively describe pain behaviour in infants. *Nursing Research, 35,* 28–31.

Fuller, B. F., & Horii, Y. (1988). Spectral energy distribution in four types of infant vocalizations. *Journal of Communication Disorders, 21,* 251–262.

Gaffney, A. A., & Dunne, E. A. (1986). Developmental aspects of children's definitions of pain. *Pain, 26,* 105–117.

Gaffney, A. A., & Dunne, E. A. (1987). Children's understanding of the causality of pain. *Pain, 29,* 91–104.

Gottlieb, G. (1971). Ontogenesis of sensory function in birds and mammals. In E. Tobach, L. Avonson, & E. Shaw (Eds.), *The biopsychology of development* (pp. 67–128). New York: Academic Press.

Grunau, R. V. E., & Craig, K. D. (1987). Pain expression in neonates: Facial action and cry. *Pain, 28,* 395–410.

Grunau, R. V. E., & Craig, K. D. (1990). Facial activity as a measure of neonatal pain perception. In D. C. Tyler & E. J. Krane (Eds.), *Advances in pain research and therapy. Proceedings of the 1st International Symposium on Pediatric Pain* (pp. 147–155). New York: Raven Press.

Grunau, R. V. E., Johnston, C. C., & Craig, K. D. (1990). Facial and cry responses to invasive and non-invasive procedures in neonates. *Pain, 42,* 295–305.

Gunnar, M. R., Fisch, R. O., Korsvik, S., & Donhowe, J. M. (1981). The effects of circumcision on serum cortisol and behaviour. *Psychoneuroendocrinology, 6,* 269–275.

Hay, D. F. (1986). Infancy. *Annual Review of Psychology, 37,* 135–161.

Izard, C. E., Hembree, E. A., Dougherty, L. M., & Spizzirri, C. C. (1983). Changes in facial expression of 2 to 19 month old infants following acute pain. *Developmental Psychology, 19,* 418–426.

Izard, C. E., Huebner, R. R., Resser, D., McGiness, G. C., & Dougherty, L. M. (1980). The young infant's ability to produce discrete emotional expressions. *Developmental Psychology, 16,* 132–140.

Johnston, C. C., & O'Shaugnessy, D. O. (1988). Acoustical attributes of infant pain cries: Discriminating features. In R. Dubner, G. F. Gebhart, & M. R. Bond (Eds.), *Proceedings of the Vth World Congress on Pain* (pp. 336–340). Amsterdam: Elsevier Science.

Johnston, C. C., & Strada, M. E. (1986). Acute pain response in infants: A multidimensional description. *Pain, 24,* 373–382.

LeResche, L., & Dworkin, S. F. (1988). Facial expressions of pain and emotions in chronic TMD patients. *Pain, 35*, 71–78.

Leslie, A. (1988). Some implications of pretense for the development of theories of mind. In J. W. Astington, P. L. Harris, & D. R. Olson (Eds.), *Developing theories of mind* (pp. 19–46). New York: Cambridge University Press.

Lester, B. M., & Zeskind, P. S. (1982). A biobehavioral perspective on crying in early infancy. In H. E. Fitzgerald, B. M. Lester, & M. W. Yogman (Eds.), *Theory and research in behavioral pediatrics* (Vol. 1, pp. 133–180). New York: Plenum.

Levine, J. D., & Gordon, N. C. (1982). Pain in prelingual children and its evaluation by pain-induced vocalization. *Pain, 14*, 85–93.

Levy, D. M. (1960). The infant's earliest memory of inoculation: A contribution to public health procedures. *Journal of Genetic Psychology, 96*, 3–46.

Lipsitt, L. P., & Levy, N. (1959). Electrotactual threshold in the infant. *Child Development, 30*, 547–554.

McGrath, P. J., & Craig, K. D. (1989). Developmental and psychological factors in children's pain. *Pediatric Clinics of North America, 36*, 823–836.

McGrath, P. J., Johnson, G., Goodman, J. T., Schillinger, J., Dunn, J., & Chapman, J. A. (1985). CHEOPS: A behavioral scale for rating postoperative pain in children. In H. L. Fields, R. Dubner, & F. Cervero (Eds.), *Advances in pain research therapy* (Vol. 9, pp. 395–402). *Proceedings of the Fourth World Congress on Pain.* New York: Raven Press.

McGrath, P. J., & Unruh, A. M. (1987). *Pain in children and adolescents.* Amsterdam: Elsevier.

McGraw, M. B. (1941). Neural maturation as exemplified in the changing reactions of the infant to pin prick. *Child Development, 12*, 31–42.

McGraw, M. B. (1943). *The neuromuscular maturation of the human infant.* New York: Hafner.

Muller, E., Hollien, H., & Murry, T. (1974). Perceptual response to infant crying: Identification of cry types. *Journal of Child Language, 1*, 89–95.

Munn, N. L. (1965). *The evolution and growth of human behavior.* Boston: Houghton Mifflin.

Murray, A. D. (1979). Infant crying as an elicitor of parental behavior: An examination of two models. *Psychological Bulletin, 86*, 191–215.

Olson, D. R. (1989). Making up your mind. *Canadian Psychology, 30*, 617–627.

Oppenheim, R. W. (1982). The neuroembryological study of behavior: Progress, problems, perspectives. *Current Topics in Developmental Biology, 17*, 257–309.

Oster, H. (1978). Facial expression and affect development. In M. Lewis & L. A. Rosenbaum (Eds.), *The development of affect* (pp. 43–75). New York: Plenum.

Owens, M. E. (1984). Pain in infancy: Conceptual and methodological issues. *Pain, 20*, 213–230.

Owens, M. E., & Todt, E. H. (1984). Pain in infancy: Neonatal reactions to a heel lance. *Pain, 20*, 77–86.

Patrick, C. J., Craig, K. D., & Prkachin, K. M. (1986). Observer judgments of acute pain: Facial action determinants. *Journal of Personality and Social Psychology, 50*, 1291–1298.

Piaget, J., & Inhelder, B. (1969). *The psychology of the child.* New York: Basic Books.

Pigeon, H. M., McGrath, P. J., Lawrence, L., & MacMurray, S. B. (1989). Nurses' perceptions of pain in the neonatal intensive care unit. *Journal of Pain and Symptom Management, 4,* 179–183.

Porter F. L., Miller, R. H., & Marshall, R. E. (1986). Neonatal pain cries: Effects of circumcision on acoustic features and perceived urgency. *Child Development, 57,* 790–802.

Porter, F. L., Porges, S. W., & Marshall, R. E. (1988). Newborn pain cries and vagal tone: Parallel changes in response to circumcision. *Child Development, 59,* 495–505.

Poznanski, F. O. (1976). Children's reactions to pain: A psychiatrist's perspective. *Clinical Pediatrics, 15,* 1114–1119.

Purcell-Jones, G., Dormon, F., & Sumner, E. (1988). Pediatric anaesthetists' perceptions of neonatal and infant pain. *Pain, 33,* 181–187.

Reisman, J. E. (1987). Touch, motion, and proprioception. In P. Salapatek & L. Cohen (Eds.), *Handbook of infant perception* (pp. 265–303). New York: Academic Press.

Ritchie, J. A. (1981). Development of body concept and concepts of illness and wellness. In M. Tudor (Ed.), *Child development* (pp. 370–372). New York: McGraw-Hill.

Ross, D. M., & Ross, S. A. (1988). *Childhood pain: Current issues, research and management.* Baltimore, MD: Urban and Schwarzenberg.

Rovee-Collier, C. K., & Fagan, J. W. (1981). The retrieval of memory in early infancy. In L. P. Lipsitt (Ed.), *Advances in infancy research* (Vol. 1, pp. 226–254). Norwood, NJ: Ablex.

Sagi, A. (1981). Mothers' and non-mothers' identification of infant cries. *Infant Behavior and Development, 4,* 37–40.

Sammons, W. A. H. (1989). *The self calmed baby.* Boston: Little, Brown.

Schechter, N. L., Allen, D. A., & Hanson, K. (1986). Status of pediatric pain control: A comparison of hospital analgesic usage in children and adults. *Pediatrics, 77,* 11–15.

Selye, H. (1976). *The stress of life.* New York: McGraw-Hill.

Sroufe, L. A. (1979). Socioemotional development. In J. Osofsky (Ed.), *Handbook of infant development* (pp. 462–518). New York: Wiley.

Swafford, L. I., & Allan, D. (1968). Pain relief in the pediatric patient. *Medical Clinics of North America, 52,* 131–136.

Thoden, D., & Koivisto, M. (1980). Acoustic analysis of the normal pain cry. In T. Murray & J. Murry (Eds.), *Infant communication: Cry and early speech* (pp. 124–151). Houston, TX: College-Hill Press.

Volpe, J. J., & Koenigsberger, R. (1981). Neurological disorders. In G. B. Avery (Ed.), *Neonatology: Pathophysiology and management of the newborn* (pp. 910–963). Philadelphia: Lippincott.

Wasz-Hockert, O., Michelsson, K., & Lind, J. (1985). Twenty-five years of Scandinavian cry research. In B. M. Lester & C. F. Z. Boukydis (Eds.), *Infant crying: Theoretical and research perspectives.* New York: Plenum.

Whittmann, B. K., & Ross, A. G. (1986). Patterns of fetal activity and their relevance for the assessment of fetal wellbeing. In M. Hansmann, B. J. Hackeloer, & A. Staudach (Eds.), *Ultrasound diagnosis in obstetrics and gynecology* (pp. 6–9). New York: Springer-Verlag.

Williamson, P. S., & Williamson, M. L. (1983). Physiologic stress reduction by a local anesthetic during newborn circumcision. *Pediatrics, 71,* 36–40.

Wolff, P. H. (1969). The natural history of crying and other vocalizations in early infancy. In B. Foss (Ed.), *Determinants of infant behavior* (Vol. 4, pp. 81–115). London: Methuen.

Wolff, P. H. (1987). *The development of behavioral states and the expression of emotions in early infancy*. Chicago: University of Chicago Press.

Zeskind, P. S., & Marshall, T. R. (1988). The relation between variations in pitch and maternal perceptions of infant crying. *Child Development, 49,* 193–196.

8
Developmental Issues: Preschool and School-Age Children

Vivian Gedaly-Duff

The purpose of this chapter is to contribute to the study of pediatric pain through the understanding of preschool and school-age children's concepts of pain. The 2- to 12-year age range represents two cognitive periods in Piagetian theory: preoperational (2 to 7 years) and concrete operational (8 to 12 years). Research and clinical reports of children's experiences and descriptions of pain, as well as Piagetian theory, will be used to analyze concepts of pain during these two age periods.

To gain insight into how children perceive and experience pain, or the schema of pain, one must understand how children in each of these cognitive periods understand the world around them. A basic assumption is that children's reasoning (illogical or logical thought), world view (egocentric or objective), and ways of coping are different from adults and different at each developmental stage.

Pain, from the adult perspective, is (a) a universal experience; (b) experienced as a noxious sensation accompanied by negative affect; and (c) commonly associated with, or having the potential to cause, tissue damage. The general characteristics of each developmental stage color children's conception of the dimensions of pain such as location (space), intensity (number), duration (time), meaning (causality), and description (quality). Comparing preoperational and concrete operational children's general characteristics, as well as their understanding of each of these pain dimensions, will illustrate the ways in which the experience of pain remains constant and simultaneously changes as children develop.

This chapter contains five sections. First, principles of the Piagetian model of cognitive development and each of Piaget's developmental stages as they apply to the concept of pain are presented. The second section contrasts the characteristics of preoperational and concrete operational thought. The third section describes, from the preoperational and concrete operational child's view, each of the above-listed pain dimensions. Next, an examination of the research and clinical literature for the coping strategies observed in preoperational and concrete operational children is described. The chapter concludes with a discussion of the implications that this particular analysis suggests for clinical practice and future research.

Principles of the Piagetian Model

The Piagetian model proposes that adults and children have a system or structure that filters the experiences encountered in a real or imagined world. As we try to make sense of the world, we classify objects, events, and symbols into concepts. We classify them to particular instances and relate them to past and future events. Besides information about objects, finding meaning in an event that frightens or gives pleasure must also be interpreted in a systematic way. Humans use reasoning to make sense of the intellectual, social, and emotional aspects of their lives (Cowan, 1978; Piaget, 1972). Piaget did not research children's perceptions and cognition of pain; however, his conceptualization of genetic epistemology provides a model describing children's construction of knowledge. This framework may be useful in describing children's developing concepts of pain.

Acute pain may be defined as a "warning" of actual or potential tissue damage to the child, stimulating self-protective behaviors. Presumably Piaget, who prior to researching cognitive development was a biological scientist, would conceive a child's fight or flight action to pain as a human response of self-preservation. Over time, children's fight or flight actions become more complex; this complexity may be interpreted as children's developing comprehension of pain. From a Piagetian perspective, children's cognitive development is a form of human adaptation and survival.

The basic goal of Piagetian theory is to explain the nature and origins of knowledge. Children's making sense of the world may be construed to be the construction of knowledge. The fundamental structural element Piaget uses to explain children's developing knowledge is the schema. The structure or schema for pain is an organization of stimuli to which children will attend in a painful situation. The schema gives meaning to the experience upon which children will eventually act. The pain schema can include past experiences or memories associated with the painful situation. It binds or separates the emotional and sensory aspects of the painful experience (Leventhal & Everhart, 1979).

Pain schemas alter as children mature, experience the physical and social world, and adapt. Piaget uses three processes to explain a child's changing schema (or a concept such as pain): assimilation, accommodation, and equilibrium. A schema is a mental framework into which incoming sensory stimuli fit. When a child experiences a stimulus, the child fits the stimulus into an available schema. The stimulus will fit into what the child already knows or existing behavioral patterns: this is called assimilation. Alternatively, the stimulus will add to and change a reflexive behavioral pattern

or mental structure: this is called accommodation. Each stage of development has a period of equilibrium in which a major pain schema dominates.
Equilibrium is the balance between what is known (assimilation) and what is
new (accommodation) as the child interacts with his or her environment.
That pain schema and equilibration continue until it does not explain her or
his new experiences, then disequilibrium occurs and a new schema evolves
(Achenbach, 1978; Maier, 1978; Piaget, 1972).

Three basic assumptions of Piagetian theory that can be applied to children's understanding of pain are (a) the sensory/perceptual experience of
pain and the associated cognitive-emotional processes are continuations of
innate reflex processes; (b) the ways in which children organize, comprehend, and cope with pain is dependent upon past interactions with the
environment; and (c) each pain schema is integrated into the succeeding pain
schema as children develop. Consequently, development of the concept of
pain is neither purely social (stimulus-response) nor maturational (biological); rather it occurs through the interaction of the children and their environments. The understanding of pain is learned through the processes of
assimilation and accommodation and the stages of children's cognitive development (Maier, 1978; Piaget, 1972).

Processes of Assimilation and Accommodation

Children acquire dimensionalized concepts of pain through the adaptive
mechanisms of assimilation and accommodation (Piaget, 1972). Through
these two complementary processes, children progress in their ability to
organize, discriminate, and generalize information about pain. Assimilation
is the fitting of information to an existing structure or schema. It involves
the perception and interpretation of new information in terms of existing
knowledge and cognitive structures. Without assimilation, all stimuli would
be new and unintelligible. Accommodation involves modification of a structure or existing schema to incorporate a new experience. Accommodation is
the changing, discriminate side of intelligence whereas assimilation is the
stable, generalizing side (Cowan, 1978, p. 24; Flavell, 1963, pp. 47–50; Piaget
& Inhelder, 1969, p. 6).

A 9-year-old boy's behavior after surgery to remove a kidney as described
by Chapman (1984, p. 1265) may be explained by the processes of assimilation and accommodation. The boy, after recovering from anesthesia, was
transferred to his room. He was given no drugs for postoperative pain, in
accordance with his surgeon's normal practice. As part of an experiment
using transcutaneous electrical stimulation to reduce pain, electrodes had
been placed under his bandages before the child regained consciousness.
Throughout the day he was asked if he felt any pain in his belly. He repeatedly denied any pain, and everyone was impressed with the apparent success of
the intervention. When asked if there was anything he feared, he began to

cry and confessed he was afraid of the operation that would remove his kidney. His surprised nurse reassured him that the surgery had already been done, and not to worry. The boy shouted, "Its not true!" When asked why this could not be true, he replied, "Because I haven't got any bandages." He was asked to feel his belly, since his hands were outside his bedclothes. He broke out into tears, screaming, "It hurts! It hurts!" This behavior might be explained as demonstrating the process of assimilation. The noxious sensation the boy may have been feeling was not classified or assimilated initially into his pain schema because it lacked the criterion of "having a bandage." Because he did not see a bandage, he did not report having pain. Accommodation in the boy's pain schema will have occurred if in the future he includes the noxious sensation in his belly as pain even without the presence of a bandage.

Stages of Cognitive Development

Research studies, case presentations, and anecdotal descriptions using a cognitive developmental framework demonstrate that children's thinking and reports related to the dimensions of pain change qualitatively along with their cognitive level. In other words, a child's schema of pain accommodates, changes, to include another perspective. Piagetian theory (Piaget, 1972; Piaget & Inhelder, 1969) describes four major cognitive stages in children's development. Each stage is qualitatively different and is characterized by a particular type of schema, (a) sensorimotor or reflexive thinking, (b) preoperational or ego-centered thinking, (c) concrete operational thinking that includes the ability to take another's perspective, and (d) formal operational or abstract multidimensional thinking. The children move unidirectionally from one stage to another over a period of time; however, the ages identified for each stage of development are merely averages to be used as guidelines. For example, the concrete operational stage typically begins between 6 and 8 years. Although the focus of this chapter is on preoperational and concrete operational children, an overview of all four stages is presented. The infant's pain schema is the initial structure to which painful experiences are assimilated, and which changes (accommodation) as children develop.

Sensorimotor

Within the Piagetian framework, children's first experiences of pain would occur during the sensorimotor stage (0 to 2 years) of cognitive development, and are organized in genetic or reflexive schema. The reflexive schema, by the end of 2 years, evolve into primitive mental structures. The infant begins to perceive objects and himself as separate. McGraw (1941), through observations and motion picture film, studied 75 infants from birth to 4 years to examine the neural maturation and changing reactions of an infant to a pinprick. At approximately 200 days old, visual perception of the pin or the arm of the adult provoked fussing, crying, or withdrawal reactions in the child (McGraw, 1941, pp. 33,35). Levy (1960), using over 2,000 records of serial inoculations of infants and children 3 to 42 months old as well as observations and inquiry, investigated the infant's memory of inoculation by means of the infant's cry. Physicians recorded the infant's cry in relation to a sequence of events (entry into room, during physical examination, wipe before injection, after insertion of needle). Within the limitations of the study, Levy concluded that there was an increase in memory cries, starting at 1% at 6 months rising as high as 20% at 12 months (Levy, 1960, p. 36). In both the McGraw and Levy studies, infants and toddlers began to cry at the sight of a needle. The crying and fussing at the sight of a doctor's white coat or a needle can be equated to Piaget's description of children's early development of object permanence. Children respond to the signal on sight, but do not act without the object being present (Piaget, 1972, pp. 108–109). Although this behavior may also be explained by a competing hypothesis such as infants' stranger anxiety to unfamiliar routines, a Piagetian framework suggests that infants' reactions to potential pain are evoked when an object associated with pain is detected by sight or smell. Simmel (1962), after interviewing 116 young amputees about their phantom pain experiences, concluded that children 2 years old or younger experience phantom pain but do not necessarily remember it. Also, based on this data set, Simmel reported that children who had no sensory or motor function in their malformed limbs before amputation did not experience phantom pain. More current studies substantiate the behavioral (Craig, McMahon, Morison, & Zaskow, 1984; Johnston & Strada, 1986) and hormonal neurochemical changes associated with noxious stimuli (Anand et al., 1985; Anand & Hickey, 1987; Anand, Sippell, & Aynsley-Green, 1987) in infants. The Anand studies illustrate the reflexive schema associated with pain. Physiological responses in children 1 year and older manifest varied patterns that may be related to developmental and nociception patterns (Gedaly-Duff, 1989a). For example, palmar sweat patterns vary with age (Harpin & Rutter, 1982; MacKinnon, 1954).

Preoperational

The preoperational stage (2 to 7 years), which is further subdivided into the preconceptual (2 to 4 years) and intuitive (5 to 7 years) levels, is sometimes called the transition period leading from the sensorimotor to the concrete operational stage (Maier, 1978). During the preoperational stage the children use cause and effect sentence structures; however, perceptual egocentricity dominates their reasoning. For example, egocentric behavior is observed in hospital play: a group of 4-year-olds sit side by side each engrossed in their own hospital dolls or stuffed animals repeatedly giving shots, bandaging intravenous sites, and drawing blood. The children's parallel activity has no sharing of equipment or interactive play, which illustrates their absorption in only their own experience of pain. It often startles student observers to note that children imitate in detail the cleaning of the skin and elaborate taping of the punctured site. Children this age usually select the actual equipment to manipulate over other play materials such as drawing pencils. The handling of equipment enables the young child to experience and control the hurtful things.

Concrete Operational

During the concrete operational stage (7 to 12 years), children become able to take another person's perspective and construct mental symbols of the real and imagined world, but they still cannot hypothesize what "might happen." At the same hospital play session as the 4-year-olds, a group of 8- to 10-year-olds was observed by the author, each adding his/her favorite painful thing, gleefully drawing a gruesome picture of a generic patient receiving all the painful procedures each of them has experienced. These children could listen to their peers' tales of horror and symbolize the tales in a drawing. The drawing activity that concentrated on their actual experiences is indicative of this age's more present than future orientation.

Formal Operations

By 11 to 13 years or older, in the formal operations stage of cognitive development, adolescents and adults differentiate and identify multiple meanings and dimensions associated with the pain experience. The McGill Pain Questionnaire (Melzack, 1975; Melzack & Torgerson, 1971) is an example of an assessment instrument that reflects the complexity of the pain experience. The questionnaire is a four-part paper-and-pencil tool that asks patients (a) to locate their pain on a body outline; (b) to describe their pain, using a 77-item word list that categorizes pain according to three qualities: sensory (pressure, thermal, temporal), affective (fear, tension), and evaluative ("annoying," "miserable"); (c) to describe both the pattern of pain and information regarding what relieves or aggravates their pain; and (d) to describe the overall intensity of their pain. The complexity and different dimensions of the pain experience are reflected in this instrument.

Characteristics of Preoperational and Concrete Operational Stages

A detailed look at the characteristics of the thought processes of preoperational and concrete operational children illustrates how children's understanding of pain changes yet stays the same. Preoperational children's mental structures are characterized by (a) egocentrism, or viewing the world from only one's own perspective; (b) centering, or focusing exclusively on a single aspect of an experience; (c) concreteness, or focusing on external perceptual events; (d) irreversibility, or inability to think in reverse or to return to the starting point; and (e) transductive reasoning, or thinking particular to particular (sometimes called illogical or magical thinking) rather than inductive or deductive thinking. Concrete operational children's mental structures, in contrast, are characterized by the ability to (a) take another's perspective, or differentiate themselves from their own views of the world; (b) view multiple dimensions simultaneously; (c) conserve or think in reverse; and (d) engage in logical reasoning, thinking inductively and deductively (Piaget, 1972; Piaget & Inhelder, 1969).

Children frequently make correct statements as they explore and test out the world, yet it must be kept in mind that children's views are not adults' views. It is only inconsistently and under very limited conditions that young children's answers are truly logical, and it is through experience and biological maturation that the type of thinking that enables logical answers and adult-like reasoning is constructed.

The preconceptual substage of preoperational children's perceptions and explanations of pain is poorly understood. Most pain research in children has concentrated on infants and school-age children. Whereas infants are unable to perceive their actions as separate from their environment (a pinprick during diaper change, baby cry, and soothing cuddle are perceived as one experience), preoperational-preconceptual children have some mental images but still have not separated their thoughts and actions from external events. Preconceptual children are assumed to have the same but less developed attributes that characterize the preoperational-intuitive child.

According to Piaget's writings, the preconceptual period is included in the preoperational stage of development because these children are able to cognitively experience early mental images as exemplified by their use of language. Preconceptual children's (2 to 4 years) language is not symbolic but concrete. A child may say "owie" when he or she falls down or when her tower of blocks falls down. The meaning of the word changes with the situation; therefore the words have little social context and instead are quite personal (Cowan, 1978). Because of this, the preconceptual child's personal language has little or no meaning to the adult, and it may be more fruitful to use more direct, observational research methodologies. For example, physiological measurement and behavioral observations in relation to a pain stimulus, and play observations in which the actual instruments of pain are used by the child in a way meaningful to him are methods of investigating preconceptual children's pain that do not rely on a common language. Interview, drawing, or projective methods (having the research subject tell a story about a child in a picture) require a use of words or symbols understood by both the child and adult.

Both Mills (1989) and Taylor (1983) use behavioral observations to study toddlers' pain. Taylor reports on pain associated with surgical repair of an inguinal hernia in 20 children, age 18 months to 4 years with a mean age of 2 years, 5 months. This observational study of body movements and vocalizations indicated that grimacing, whining, and guarding of the wound in these children increased over the 3-hour period immediately after surgery. Restless generalized movement associated with recovery from general anesthesia was distinguished from pain associated with incisional tissue trauma. The children had more general restlessness with some guarding in the 1st hour; this pattern had reversed by the 3rd hour. Her findings leave little room for doubt that preconceptual children (1.5 to 3 years) were experiencing pain. Until behavior, play, observation, and Piagetian semiclinical method studies are done (Cowan, 1978; Flavell, 1963; Piaget, 1972), knowledge of the pain experience for the preconceptual age group will be based on extrapolation from the more researched sensorimotor infant (0 to 12 months) and preoperational-intuitive age groups (4 to 7 years).

Most of the pain research literature that illustrates preoperational developmental characteristics has focused on 4- to 7-year-olds, who are more representative of the intuitive than the preconceptual substage of the preoperational period. Children as young as 4 years are included in children's reports on pain; however, the findings of these studies represent mostly the views of older children whose language abilities provide more descriptive accounts of pain (Gaffney & Dunne, 1987; Lewis, 1978; Ross & Ross, 1988).

Egocentric Thinking Versus Taking Another's Perspective

The most dominating characteristic of preoperational thought is its egocentricity. It is not that the children are selfish, it is that the children's thought processes are not flexible enough to consider or even to recognize the existence of another's viewpoint or experience. An example of this egocentricity is reported by McCaffery (1977, p. 12) who described a 2-year-old girl who said her stomach hurt. When asked to point to the exact spot where she hurt, she lifted her skirt and in tone of disgust said, "There. Can't you see it?" The child's understanding is that since she felt the pain in her tummy, that her audience would also know where the pain was located. The child cannot differentiate herself or her thoughts from the external world.

In contrast, school-age children are reported to alter the description of their pain in relation to which audience they are addressing. For example, concrete operational children's pain descriptions to their parents were concise and unemotional, whereas to their friends they emphasized the discomfort of the pain, and to their doctors they described the pain in the most detail (Ross & Ross, 1984b).

Centering Versus Multiple Dimensions

Preoperational children center or focus on one aspect of an experience. Young children usually describe pain in general terms such as pain is "hurt."

Scott (1978) suggests that children, between 4 and 6 years, have a synaes-thetic perception of pain, meaning that all of the dimensions are perceived as one. These children cannot differentiate various dimensions of pain expe-rience, but can center only on its personally salient sensation of "hurt." The other aspects of pain such as color, texture, shape, and pattern, including other descriptions of the sensation of pain, are associated as one experience.

In contrast, concrete operational children describe several dimensions of pain (Abu-Saad, 1984a, 1984b; Abu-Saad & Holzemer, 1981; Ross & Ross, 1984a; Savedra, Gibbons, Tesler, Ward, & Wegner, 1982). Several research studies, although limited in number of subjects, report children, 7 to 17 years, not ill or hospitalized and with diverse pain experiences associated with chronic disease and surgery, are capable of rating the intensity of, localizing, and describing their pain.

Perceptual Concreteness Versus Experiential Concreteness

Preoperational children's reasoning is overwhelmingly influenced by what they perceive or see (Piaget, 1972; Piaget & Inhelder, 1969). Children believe that the way they see things, or the way they desire events to be, corresponds to the way things are. They attribute intentions and feeling to the thing, assuming that it operates like them and like people they know (Cowan, 1978, p. 11). Pain for preoperational children is reported predominantly as an external concrete event that the child has experienced such as "bumped my head," "banged myself," "eating too much," (Gaffney & Dunne, 1987, p. 95), or needles and blood (Eland & Anderson, 1977; Lewis, 1978; Prugh, Staub, Sands, Kirschbaum, & Lenihan, 1953). These children tend to de-scribe or attribute cause of pain to external events that can be seen.

Concrete operational children, like preoperational children, attribute pain to external concrete causes such as falls and needles. As a sign of their maturity, they also begin to associate pain with nonvisible physical and psychosocial variables. Nonvisible germs or psychosocial causes are mental constructs rather than visible entities. It is not until approximately age 9 years that children begin to state that pain is caused by disease, germs, malfunctioning body organs, and psychosocial experiences such as missing school or being teased (Abu-Saad, 1984a; Gaffney & Dunne, 1986, 1987; Savedra, Tesler, Ward, Wegner, & Gibbons, 1981; Schultz, 1971). Neverthe-less, concrete operational children refer to disease and illness in vague gener-al terms to describe pain. Although school-age children can differentiate between imaginative pretending and their feelings and thoughts, they are still concrete in needing to see and experience the actuality. Detailed and scientific terms that explain internal physiological functions related to pain do not usually appear until formal operations (11 to 18 years) (Bibace & Walsh, 1980; Gaffney & Dunne, 1986; Ross & Ross, 1984a). The pain schema for concrete operational children expands beyond external visible causes of pain such as injury, incorporates social-emotional causes of pain such as missing school, and yet cannot explain pain in neurochemical terms.

Centering Versus Decentering

Preoperational children do not have the mental capability to decenter, or in other words, to think objectively, to view a situation from varying points of view. This characteristic is affiliated with egocentric and irreversible thinking (Piaget & Inhelder, 1969). Because preoperational children are perceptually bound, the transformation of an object or substance from one state to another is understood by the child to be a fundamental alteration (as opposed to a change in appearance only). The classic example is the clay ball test: The child is shown two equal size clay balls. While the child is looking, one ball is rolled into a sausage shape. When the child is asked which clay ball is bigger, the child tends to point to the sausage shaped ball saying it is longer therefore bigger. The child misses the transformation process and reports what he considers the important outcome by reporting what he sees — using only one perceptually salient dimension (which in this instance is length) to influence his answer. In terms of a pain experience, a child who is informed that he will be getting a shot that is medicine to take his hurt away in 30 minutes is likely to fight the shot. He will be centered on the immediate outcome of the shot, which is "pain" and not the analgesic outcome that will occur 30 minutes later. The preoperational child cannot conceptualize the whole sequence of events and transformation, which is the gradually feeling better and then the pain-free state. It is as if preoperational children's mental images are like static snapshots rather than a movie show.

Concrete operational children have learned to decenter, to account for several aspects of a situation simultaneously, to distinguish between appearances and reality, and learned that there is permanence underlying apparent change (Elkind, 1974). Both clay objects have the same amount of clay although one ball has changed its shape. In the case of an analgesic injection, these children can decenter from the pain outcome of the shot, to the outcome of surgical pain relief. Another example is that concrete operational children can understand that the intravenous pain medicine is the same as the liquid pain medicine; the medicines are the same but their form has changed. Preoperational children, on the other hand, would understand them to be two separate medicines.

Transductive Versus Logical Reasoning

Preoperational children lack logical reasoning; rather, their reasoning is what Piaget calls "transductive" or particular to particular reasoning (Flavell, 1963; Piaget, 1972). This reasoning is most evident in the widely reported children's belief that their pain is punishment for their being bad

(Brewster, 1982; Freud, 1952; Gaffney & Dunne, 1987; Prugh et al., 1953). A child falls while crossing the street; since he had been told he was not to cross the street, he reasons that he is being punished. Empirical work by Gaffney and Dunne (1987) supports the assertion that preoperational children associate pain from needles and spankings as forms of punishment. The close association between their thoughts or behavior and the painful event lead, through particular to particular reasoning, to the conclusion that their pain was caused by their "being bad."

Preoperational children, due to their egocentric thinking, are prone to misattribute their own thoughts and activities as the causes of external events. The concept of chance, that something happens by accident, is not within their understanding. Although they are beginning to differentiate themselves from others, they have not learned that thoughts (subjective) and things (objective) are separate. In addition, when something cannot be accounted for within preoperational children's understanding, they resort to magical thinking. A child may explain the event within his wishes (e.g., the doctor has red hair like daddy, the doctor will be able to take away the hurt) or experience (e.g., people in white coats hurt children because they stick children for blood) (Cowan, 1978; Fraiberg, 1959; Lewis, 1978; Steward & Steward, 1981). Preoperational children's reasoning is imperfect. Their desire and egocentric perception, or their inability to consider another's view, lead them to erroneous conclusions. The children's conclusions about the cause of their pain may be wrong, but they do formulate a theory to explain their pain. One theory reported by a 7-year-old boy who had many blood tests was that "the doctors had decided that since he wasn't very sick his blood should be donated to other, very ill patients" (Lewis, 1978, p. 21).

In contrast, concrete operational children can take another person's perspective (nonegocentricity), differentiate between thoughts and things (objectivity), understand that even though medicine can change its form it is still the same (conservation), and realize that pain can be influenced by several factors (multidimensional). They can in a logical and concrete manner associate pain from injury and illness (Bibace & Walsh, 1980).

Dimensions of Pain

What can preoperational and concrete operational children understand about pain? Reports of preoperational and concrete operational children about their pain experiences is presented as each of the following dimensions of pain are discussed: (a) location (space), (b) intensity (number), (c) duration (time), (d) meaning (causation), and (e) description (quality, analogies).

Location

Identifying the location of pain aids in diagnosis and treatment. Goodnow (1977) proposes that children's drawings are "visible thinking." Being able to draw a human figure requires symbolizing the human figure and setting boundaries on space. Preconceptual children scribble and tell stories about their scribbles, they may not say anything, or they may acknowledge that the drawing does not look like anything (Golomb, 1974). From 2 to 6 years, children advance from spontaneous scribbling to drawing a person in six parts (Frankenburg & Dodds, 1990). Preoperational children's drawings of the body begin with circles for head and trunk with sticks for arms and legs (Golomb, 1974; Goodnow, 1977). Thus, it is not surprising that children as young as 4 years are reported to be able to locate their pain accurately on a body outline (Eland & Anderson, 1977).

In concrete operational age groups (Savedra et al., 1982; Savedra et al., 1981; Tesler, Ward, Savedra, Wegner, & Gibbons, 1983; Varni, Thompson, & Hanson, 1987), research has focused on developing paper and pencil assessment instruments. These investigators have developed instruments that include a body outline, which suggests that the children are able to locate their pain on a body outline. Respectable reliability and validity of the body outline has been reported (Savedra, Tesler, Holzemer, Wilkie, & Ward, 1989). A method of scoring pain from a body outline, currently used with adults, may prove useful with children. This involves a template of the body, with the figure divided into 45 anatomical regions (Margolis, Tait, & Krause, 1986).

Children do not appear to draw simplistic internal body parts such as bones, heart, and blood until approximately 8 years (Gellert, 1962; Smith, 1977); other major organs such as lungs, muscles, nerves, and stomach are not drawn until 10 to 11 years (Crider, 1981). In their drawings, children often view each organ in isolation, such as the heart pumps blood, the veins keep the blood, and the lungs breathe air. The relationships among these organs is not understood. These children frequently misname the organ and its functions. Their little understanding about the inside of their bodies, as reflected in their drawings, leads to the conclusion that children's understanding of internal pain will be even less understood.

Jeans (1983) asked 54 healthy nonhospitalized children, 5 to 13 years, to "draw a picture that shows pain." A person or part of a person was drawn by 90% of the children, followed in frequency by an animal in pain (4%) and abstract representations of pain (6%). Pain was localized in the limbs and head. Unruh and her colleagues (Unruh, McGrath, Cunningham, & Humphreys, 1983) asked 109 5- to 18-year-olds complaining of migraine headache or musculoskeletal pain, to draw a picture of their pain. Only 2% of the drawings were so nonspecific that the drawing could not be classified as representing some aspect of the child's pain. Both Jeans and Unruh et al. reported no developmental differences in the pain drawings; however, the methodological limitations, such as the small sample sizes within each age range and categorization systems that have not considered drawing abilities, may have prevented detecting developmental changes. It is intriguing that children who may not be able to report their pain verbally may be able to locate or draw it. Although children as young as 4 years may locate pain, representation of internal pain in drawings may not occur until approximately 10 years.

Intensity

Children's ability to report the intensity of their pain implies an understanding of classification, quantity, and numbers. Creative ways of measuring intensity of pain without using numbers such as color (Eland, 1981), describing their perception of one stimulus in terms of another in cross-modality matching (McGrath, deVeber, & Hearn, 1985), ranking pictures of pain situations (Lollar, Smits, & Patterson, 1982), and rating words (Tesler, Savedra, Ward, Holzemer, & Wilkie, 1989) have been developed for use with children. Rosch, Mervis, Gray, Johnson, and Boyes-Braem (1976) report that children as young as 4 years can pair up "basic" and "superordinate" categories. For example in the "basic" category, children were given three pictures, two different cats and one train, and asked "to put together the two that are alike." For the "superordinate" category, the children were presented with a cat, dog, and train; this time, to indicate similarity, the children would have to use the superordinate category (cat + dog = animal). Basic sorts for 3- and 4-year-olds were nearly perfect. Correct pair-up in the superordinate sorts occurred at more than 50% for the 3-year-olds, whereas the 4-year-olds were highly skilled. The ability to match the intensity of a pain sensation with a color, brightness, or picture employs the concept of classifying at a superordinate level.

Matching Negative Faces With Increasing Pain

A face, either a photograph or a cartoon line drawing, has been used to depict increasing negative affect associated with pain (Beyer, 1988; McGrath et al., 1985; Wong & Baker, 1988). The accurate association of facial expressions with pain implies an ability to conserve. Conservation requires ignoring inadequate or unstable cues and isolating the invariant cues associated with the affect. Negative affect is associated with pain, positive affect with no pain. Hester (1979), who identified negative facial expressions in the eyes, forehead, and jaw, reported behavioral observations with interrater reliability ranging from 75 to 81%. Children's accuracy in matching pictures of identical people with varying expressions of affect increases significantly with age, from 50% at 3 years to 83% at age 5 (Norbeck, 1981). The errors made by 3- to 5-year-olds were related to matching pictures for similar affect (but not the same person), or mouth configuration (amount of teeth showing in a smile or anger). Older children, who were more accurate, matched hair lines, thereby choosing a cue with less variability. Approximately one third of the children demonstrated mastery at age 4; a rapid rise in mastery was observed at 5 or older; and full mastery was demonstrated by age 7.

McGrath et al. (1985), using a sample of 40 3- to 15-year-olds (mean age = 9 years), including 20 healthy children and 20 oncology patients, quantified the affective dimension of pain represented in nine line-drawn faces of increasingly negative emotional expression. Two cross-modality matching responses, brightness matching and visual analogue scales, were correlated with the faces. The children rated the heaviness of five metric weights (objective stimulus), then the degree of the saddest and happiest faces (subjective stimulus), using both brightness matching and visual analogue scales. Children turned a dimmer switch to the brightness, or marked a 150-mm line, to match the perceived weight. They then matched faces with brightness and the visual analogue scale. Although seven children, with a mean age of 5 years, were not able to complete the study, the 5- to 6-year-olds had a respectable reliability correlation coefficient ($r = .70$), which increased ($r = .99$) for the 13- to 15-year-olds. It was assumed that if the children were consistent across objective and subjective stimuli that their brightness and visual analogue scale values accurately reflected their perceptions of the faces. Each face was presented four times in random order. The children's responses were averaged to obtain a mean affective value for each face. The faces were ranked happiest at the value of .08 to saddest imaginable at .97. The authors then used the faces and visual analogue scale to measure oncology children's affective and intensity responses to medical procedures.

Matching Numbers With Increasing Pain

Being able to classify is a conceptual component of being able to count. Children's ability to quantify pain includes the concept of "a lot or a little" and of numbers. Children at the preconceptual level cannot meaningfully count. Children at the intuitive level (approximately 5 to 6 years) can count but in a fragile form of one-to-one correspondence (Cowan, 1978, p. 154). For instance, intuitive 6-year-olds, given five blocks in two equally spaced rows, can count each row accurately. However, if the row of blocks is spread out or bunched together, intuitive children assert that there is no longer an equal number of blocks in each row. The children's perceptions that the row is now longer or shorter dominates their conceptual idea of equal numbers. For example, the shorter row of six blocks is identified as the row with less blocks. Toward the end of the intuitive substage, one observes the child carefully count, pointing a finger at each block in each row, then triumphantly announce that both rows are equal. Intuitive children achieve the correct answers through trial and error, by manipulating the materials. It is not until the concrete operational stage that children systematically and successfully count. De Avila and his colleagues, who have developed a Piagetian conservation scale, report that 60% of the children between 5 and 6 years can count to five and 100% of the children who take the test know the concepts of more, less, and the same (De Avila, 1980a, 1980b). Children as young as 2 to 3 years are reported to comprehend the concepts of more, less, and the same (Cowan, 1978, p. 123).

Children must be able to count and to grasp the concept of seriation (order from least to most) in order to quantify pain intensity. Intuitive children (4 to 5 years) are likely to arrange objects in random order or in small groups by size. Older intuitive children (6 to 7 years), after much trial and error, can match in one-to-one correspondence, for example, they can match the same-size stick with the same-size doll but if the dolls and sticks are placed close together, the perceptual closeness of one stick to a doll will destroy the seriation because the children tend to match the closer stick even though it is the shorter one (adapted from Cowan, 1978, p. 151). McGrath et al. (1985) concluded that children 5 to 15 years old can match pain symbolically and in a hierarchical manner in that the faces increase in negative expression with increasing intensity of pain. However, seven children (mean age 5 years; 17% of the sample) were not able to complete the study. One explanation for the failure of the children aged 5 years and younger to complete the study's tasks is that these young children were perceptually overwhelmed in the matching process. In addition, it is not known how many children were in the preoperational age range in the total sample; did the seven failures represent the majority of the preoperational age group? Preoperational children's fragile concept of quantity, which is so easily influenced by their perceptions, requires appropriate research methodologies and designs within their abilities in order for researchers and clinicians to better explore these children's perceptions of pain. Clearly, more research focused on preoperational children needs to be done before concluding that these children can match pain in a symbolic, hierarchical manner.

Beyer (1988; Beyer & Aradine, 1986) designed the Oucher to measure pain intensity in children 3 to 12 years. The Oucher consists of a numerical scale (0 to 100) for older children and a photographic scale of six faces (from a no-pain face to a most-pain face using a 3-year-old boy) for younger children. Beyer and Aradine (1988; Aradine, Beyer, & Tompkins, 1988) report that the mean age for the children who used the photographic scale of the Oucher was 5 years. In contrast, the mean age of the children who used the numerical scale was 9 years.

Hester (1979) measured preoperational children's reports of pain intensity. Four poker chips were used. Each poker chip equaled a piece of hurt: one chip represented a little bit of hurt, and four chips the most hurt. The poker chip tool (or a similar variant) has been demonstrated as a valid way to measure pain intensity in children in several studies (Aradine et al., 1988; Beyer & Aradine, 1988; Hester, Foster, & Kristensen, 1989; Molsberry, 1979; Wong & Baker, 1988).

Other measures of pain intensity that have shown varying levels of reliability and validity include the Pain Ladder (Hester et al., 1989); face scales (McGrath et al., 1985; Wong & Baker, 1988); the visual analogue scales (Abu-Saad & Holzemer, 1981; Scott, Ansell, & Huskisson, 1977); and the Glasses Scale (Wong & Baker, 1988). As would be expected, the reliability and validity of these instruments increase with age, consistent with children's advancing cognitive ability. Yet, several studies with children ranging in age from 3 to 18 have reported no such age differences (Beyer & Aradine, 1988; McGrath et al. 1985; Wong & Baker, 1988). In general, children of 5 years and younger have been reported to have difficulty completing various measures (Beyer & Aradine, 1988; McGrath et al., 1985). More research is needed before concluding that these modalities are appropriate measures of pain for this age group. Concrete operational children, on the other hand, seem to use these instruments readily.

Duration

The duration of the pain experience is related to the concept of time. Time is a cycle, such as the pain occurs at night time; time is a pattern, such as the pain is continuous or intermittent; time is an experience, such as the current joint pain means not walking in the future. The adult abstract concept of time is a slow, gradual, ontogenetic construction (Flavell, 1963). Adults think of time as a uniform movement that remains constant whether we are walking or driving. Preoperational children judge time by focusing on one dimension or another, but not both simultaneously. For example, Piaget (1971, p. 254) reports that preoperational children agreed that drawing lines quickly takes longer than drawing lines slowly, thus judging the duration by the results of the work and not by any kind of inner feeling. Children thought the work "short" as they drew the lines, but after completing the lines, judged the work "long," their answer depending on whether they focused on speed of work or its results. Between 7 and 8 years, children begin to understand time as a constant and to differentiate fewer lines when drawing slowly and more lines when drawing quickly. By 12 years, the children distinguished between "real time" and "inner feeling time," which may seem longer or shorter in relation to working slowly or quickly.

Cycle Time

Children's earliest experiences of time are related to bodily rhythms such as hunger. Other experiences basic to time are music and dance rhythms. Parents then impose breakfast time, nap time, bath time upon their bodily rhythms. Clock time is an event, such as 8 o'clock is bedtime. Parents and children have rituals that are related to time such as taking a bath, reading a story, and going to bed.

Calendar time is understood in terms of physical characteristics, such as being older is equated with being taller or having gray hair. For example, a child's father and grandfather are the same age because they are both the same size; however, the youngster realizes they are older than he is. The child knows he is in the younger place and father and grandfather are in the older place, but cannot tell which of them was born first. In contrast, concrete operational children can remember or anticipate an order of events without the confusion shown by the younger child. In addition, concrete operational children can arrange a sequence of pictures to correspond with previously experienced events (Cowan, 1978), such as ranking situational pictures related to pain (Lollar et al., 1982; McGrath et al., 1985). It should be noted, however, that Lollar et al. report the age range of their subjects as 4 to 19, but do not report the mean age of their sample. It appears that performance related to age was not obtained; therefore, it is not known if the 4- to 7-year-old children could rank the situational pictures consistently.

Children's understanding of time as an element of the pain experience has not been researched adequately. Ross and Ross (1988) hypothesize that the duration of time required for an invasive procedure, one that has been standardized, may serve as an index of children's perceptions of the magnitude of pain. This is based on their interviews with children who described the pain of shots as "torture" and estimated the duration of the time to administer a shot as longer than did those children who were more matter-of-fact about the pain. Piaget's (1971) differentiation between real time and inner time may be more salient than the length of time required to administer the shot. The child's inner time, centering on the intrusive pain, may dominate his perception of real time. Exploring how a child's temperament (Wallace, 1989) may be related to his inner time may shed some light on whether the actual length of time for an intrusive procedure or its "inner time" is related to reported pain intensity.

Clinically, the occurrence of pain in relation to activities (getting out of bed) and time of day (nighttime or after mother leaves) are routinely assessed. Preoperational children can often readily report these activities, perhaps because the questions are asked in the context of familiar events. Many clinical investigators have reported that young children, and even older children, will refuse to have a "shot" for their pain. This can be explained by their concept of time as a place or thing and their living in the "present" rather than the future. The adult sense of time has a past, present, and future, whereas children experience the "now." The event of relieving surgical pain is really a sequence of events made up of an analgesic injection, absorption of the analgesic from the muscle to the bloodstream, and pain relief. The unifying framework of each event is the passage of time from one event to the other. Because young children still experience time as a snapshot rather than moving pictures, they perceive only the immediacy of the pain of a shot. They cannot cross from the time of the immediate shot pain to the relief of surgical pain. This association is beyond young children's logic. Using nonpainful methods of giving analgesics is a more humane method of treating their pain.

Pattern

The pattern of pain, which might be considered a rhythm, is related to the time concept. This includes the continuous versus intermittent characteristics of pain, as well as the pounding rhythmic pattern. Scott (1978) used a sheet of paper with two rows of light bulbs to demonstrate an "off-and-on" quality. The continuous-pain row had all the bulbs colored yellow symbolizing "on"; the intermittent-pain row contained alternating lighted and unlighted bulbs. Ross and Ross (1988) suggest using musical instruments such as a whistle and drum (long unbroken whistle note to demonstrate continuous pain; stop and start drum beat to demonstrate intermittent pain). These concrete methods may prove fruitful in determining children's perceptions of the pattern of pain.

The Experience of Time

The experience of time, or the meaning of pain within a past, present, and future context, has not been extensively researched in children. Beales, Keen, and Lennox Holt (1983) interviewed 39 children, 6 to 17 years, diagnosed with juvenile chronic arthritis. These authors suggest that the meaning the children attributed to the sensations originating in their joints influenced the extent to which those sensations constituted pain. For concrete operational children, pain was more worrisome if it was seen as likely to interfere with their immediate ability to participate in physical activities. For formal operational children, on the other hand, the implications of the pain were interpreted in relation to more distal future activity, such as whether their current pain meant damaged joints leading to a future of being wheelchair bound.

Meaning

Preoperational and concrete operational children live more in the present than the past or future. They interpret their pain within their mental schemas. Tracing children's understanding of causality illustrates the meaning of pain within their schemas. Bibace and Walsh (1980) interviewed 24 healthy 4-year-olds who would be considered at the end of the preconceptual and beginning of intuitive understanding, and described these children's explanations of pain as prelogical. Either the children's reports were incomprehensible or they used immediate spatial or temporal cues to explain the pain

cause-outcome relationship. Unfortunately, Bibace and Walsh do not include pain examples in their paper; however, Gaffney and Dunne (1986)
report intuitive children stating that pain is a "thing," "it," or "something"
located in a body part such as the tummy. The pain is inflicted by an external
and concrete event such as a fall; the outcome is a "hurt." Interestingly,
Gaffney and Dunne (1987) suggest that children from the preoperational and
into the early formal operational stages reason that their pain occurred as
punishment for their transgressions, such as eating too much or breaking
rules. The continuation of transgressive thinking in older children is evident
in the Gaffney and Dunne study (1987), but becomes more complex as it is
linked with the physical and psychological causes of pain. Piaget's concept
of vertical *décalage* may help explain these observations. Vertical *décalage*
refers to repetition that occurs at different stages (Flavell, 1963). For example, the sensation of pain may be the same from one stage to another but the
pain is experienced from a new perspective. Concrete operational children
comprehend external causes such as falls, but their understanding later
expands to incorporate inner psychological and physical causes of pain such
as internal disease and moral transgressions. Although pain may be attributed to an internal disease in the stage-transitional child, it is described in
vague terms suggesting confusion about internal organs and functions
(Bibace & Walsh, 1980). The sensation is no longer just a "thing" as stated by
preoperational children, but is described as a "sore feeling," "a kind of
ache," "like a cramp" by concrete operational children (Gaffney & Dunne,
1986).

Description

Descriptions of pain follow a developmental pattern. Preconceptual children use global, private contextual words, that the adult has trouble interpreting. In fact, these children may not use words at all but run away, kick,
and cry. Intuitive children seem not to describe, but to name the sensation
such as "hurt." Concrete operational children actually call pain a "feeling"
such as a soreness.

Another example of concrete thinking in both preoperational and concrete operational children is the analogies used to describe pain. Children as
young as 4 to 7 years, when asked to describe a specific past pain experience,
have stated, "like a rock was bouncing round in my chest hitting the sides
hard" (a boy, 6 years, irregular painful heart beat), "like someone is biting
your ear . . . like a big volcano in your ear" (girl, 7 years, earache) (Ross &
Ross, 1988, p. 44). However, several studies report that children this young
rarely describe their pain this graphically, whereas older children (by grade
6) used an analogy 50% of the time to describe pain (Bibace & Walsh, 1980;
Gaffney, 1983). Ross and Ross (1984b) suggest that if a question is abstract
such as, What is pain?, the younger child is not likely to be specific. Instead,
if a question is anchored by asking, "Have you had pain? What was your

TABLE 8.1. Preoperational and concrete operational children's understanding of pain dimenions.

Pain dimension	Cognitive age		
	Preoperational-preconceptual (CA: 2-4 yrs)[a]	Preoperational-intuitive (CA: 5-7 yrs)	Concrete operational (CA: 8-12 yrs)
Location	Scribble (Golomb, 1974)	Mark on a body outline (Eland & Anderson, 1977)	Mark on a body outline (Tesler et al., 1983)
Intensity	Understand the concepts of more, less, and the same (Cowan 1978, p. 123; De Avila, 1980a, 1980b). Observation of body movements has been used as an indicator of degree of pain (Taylor, 1983).	Although children 5 years and younger have been included in pain studies rating pain intensity, they are generally reported as having difficulty doing the tasks. Reliability and validity increases with age. Young children have rated pain intensity by: (a) color (Eland, 1981; Scott, 1978), (b) faces scales (Beyer & Aradine, 1988; McGrath et al., 1985; Wong & Baker, 1988), (c) glasses scale (Wong & Baker, 1988), (d) poker chips: one chip is "a little bit of hurt," four chips is "most hurt" (Hester, 1979), (e) pain ladder (Hester, Foster, & Kristensen, 1989)	School-age children usually can rate pain using same measures as younger children as well as numbers and visual analogue scales. They have rated pain by: (a) color (Scott, 1978; Savedra et al., 1982), (b) numeric scales (Beyer & Aradine, 1988; Abu-Saad, 1984b), (c) visual analogue scales (VAS) (Abu-Saad & Holzemer, 1981; children younger than 3 years unable to use VAS (Scott, Ansell, & Huskisson, 1977).

214

Duration		
(1) Pattern	When concrete objects are used, continuous vs. intermittent patterns of pain are beginning to be reported (Ross & Ross, 1988; Scott, 1978). Beginning to be able to sequence pictures related to past pain experiences (Lollar et al., 1982).	Concerned with pain that threatens present activities rather than future abilities (Beales, Keen, & Lennox Holt, 1983).
(2) Time orientation	Immediate pain threat overwhelming; the future benefit of pain is not conceptually understood (Beyer & Byers, 1985).	
Meaning	Nonsense, prelogical, egocentric and synaesthetic meanings of pain are observed (Bibace & Walsh, 1980; Scott, 1978). Pain is perceived as an object, a "thing," "it," or "something" located in a body part (Gaffney & Dunne, 1986). Pain is understood to be caused by something external and visible such as a fall or cut (Gaffney & Dunne, 1986). Pain is understood to be punishment for transgressions (Gaffney & Dunne, 1987).	Confusion about the relationship of internal body parts and illness/pain exists (Bibace & Walsh, 1980). Pain is understood to be a "sore feeling, a kind of ache . . ." (Gaffney & Dunne, 1986). Pain is understood to be punishment but is also linked with physical and psychological causes (Gaffney & Dunne, 1987).
Description	Use the term "owie", run away, kick, cry, or limit movement of an injured body part (McGraw, 1941; Taylor, 1983). Pain is named as if an object (Gaffney & Dunne, 1986).	Pain is described as a feeling (Gaffney & Dunne, 1986). Analogies are used to describe pain, such as "like a lot of knives poking me one after another," most commonly by 6th graders (Ross & Ross, 1984a; Ross & Ross, 1988).

Note. Research referenced in this table is used to exemplify children's understanding of pain. This is not a complete list of children's pain research.
[a]CA = children's age ranges.

pain like?," a more concrete and descriptive answer might be obtained. For a summary of preoperational and concrete operational children's understanding of pain dimensions, see Table 8.1.

Coping

Pain is a psychophysiological experience (Fields, 1987; Leventhal & Everhart, 1979; Melzack & Wall, 1965; Price, 1988). The process of coping must engage pain in both its psychological and neurochemical aspects. From this perspective, children's cognitive schemas and pharmacological interventions are discussed as methods of coping with pain on these two levels.

This section is not an overview of children's coping mechanisms to reduce pain (see chapters 4 and 6), nor is it a review of medications that are available to treat children's pain (see chapter 4). Instead, we examine the innate schemas children have for building coping strategies and the developmental implications of giving medication.

Coping is defined as a process that involves cognitive and behavioral efforts to manage external or internal stimuli that are judged nociceptive and that exceed the established resources of the child; the child must have assistance in overcoming danger (Lazarus & Folkman, 1984). This definition implies that coping is an effort, in contrast to innate reflexes and automatized mastery. Adaptation implies that the individual has learned to act in an automatic manner and little effort is needed to accommodate to stimuli. The nervous system becomes exhausted after prolonged exposure to pain, which means that traditional physiologic changes, such as increased pulse rate, or behavioral actions, such as crying loudly, lessen. These children have not adapted, but are exhausted from pain. Children and families may adapt to chronic illness, but the pain is endured or redefined (Gedaly-Duff, 1989b).

A review of the pain research in children supports the thesis that there are two major schemas in children's experience of nociception. One is a grimace followed by a cry, and the second is a pulling away of the affected limb. The majority of children's pain research has focused on acute or time-limited pain in healthy children. Healthy children experience acute pain as a surprise and as resulting from an accident, a short hospitalization, or a medical/dental procedure. An examination of how these two major pain schemas change and stay the same in preoperational and concrete operational children's coping will begin to explain children's behavior in painful situations.

It is assumed that children with chronic illness experiencing repeated painful procedures or chronic disease pain begin with the same schemas as healthy children; however, the two basic pain schemas may be expected to have assimilated or accommodated nociceptive experiences in the context of the chronic illness experience. For example, Ross and Ross (1988, p. 66) report two concrete operational children diagnosed with leukemia: a girl age

7 recently diagnosed with leukemia described her finger sticks as "stab, stab, stab, sometimes a lot in one day," whereas a boy age 8 dismissed the pain of a venipuncture as minor and unimportant, "it's quick, like a cut, you go ouch, then it's finished." The pain is at first very bothersome, then becomes minor as the schema accommodates in response to discrepant experience. The concrete operational children experience repeated finger sticks, lumbar punctures, and bone marrow aspirations in the course of their treatment and monitoring of their illness. They learn that the pierce of a finger stick is short in duration and tolerable in comparison to a bone marrow aspiration. Their concept of pain accommodates to their various experiences.

The acute pain experience signals danger. The physiological responses of increased heart and respiratory rates and decreased salivary secretions ready the individual for "fight or flight" (Cannon, 1929). It is assumed then that pain alerts and motivates humans to escape or avoid danger from injury or disease (Izard, Hembree, & Huebner, 1987; Wall, 1979). The infant's schemas associated with pain are the foundations for preoperational and concrete operational schemas; therefore, a discussion of sensorimotor schemas is relevant.

McGraw's study (1941) of 75 infants from birth to 4 years examined the neural maturation and changing reactions of an infant to a pinprick. In this classic study, as in more current studies (Craig et al., 1984; Dale, 1986, 1989; Franck, 1986; Grunau & Craig, 1987; Izard, Hembree, Dougherty, & Spizzirri, 1983; Izard et al., 1987; Johnston & Strada, 1986; Owens & Todt, 1984; Porter, Miller, & Marshall, 1986; Rich, Marshall, & Volpe, 1974), three infant behavioral changes associated with nociceptive stimuli are described: (a) a specific facial expression, (b) generalized reflexive movement or withdrawing the affected part, and (c) a cry related to pain. The cry, which could be interpreted as the baby's signal of danger and need for help, has been documented to continue signaling pain but to change in proportion of pain and anger expressed associated with individual differences, age, sex, and time (Izard et al., 1987). Commonly, the first action of a caretaker to the baby's combined signal of pain/anger, after removing the noxious stimulus, is to soothe the baby by secure holding, soft murmuring, and human presence (Gedaly-Duff, 1988). Thus this first schema or action associated with pain, the infant's cry for help, can be classified as "turning to others" or "seeking social support" (Cohen & Lazarus, 1979; Lazarus & Folkman, 1984; Murphy & Moriarty, 1976). This "turning to others" schema becomes a coping mechanism that continues throughout the life span. Several researchers report children ages 5 to 15 seeking comfort and caring from others (Abu Saad, 1984a; Gedaly-Duff, 1988, 1989b; Hester, 1989; Ross & Ross, 1988; Tesler, Wegner, Savedra, Gibbons, & Ward, 1981).

Hester (1989) cautions clinicians about relying too heavily on children's developmental level as the determining factor in managing their pain. Even though concrete operational children have demonstrated their ability to use other coping methods such as "thought stopping" (Ross, 1984) or "distraction" (Tesler et al., 1981), they often prefer to be comforted by others. Bloome, Lillis, and Smith (1989), in their meta-analysis of 27 pain intervention research studies in children, point out that although preparation of children for painful procedures has a significant effect on children's physiologic, self-report, and behavior responses, these findings may be confounded by the presence of a supportive adult in 60% of the studies.

In an attempt not to be disrespectful of older children's ages by treating them like babies, caregivers may overlook the benefit comforting provides older children. An infant's helplessness is acceptable, the cry of pain is not readily ignored; yet the older child who may be afraid to ask for comfort needs comforting as well. Unfortunately, professionals may ignore pain particularly in painful procedures that the adult perceives as brief and insignificant. When others' initial efforts to ameliorate their pain fail, children usually must simply endure the pain. Children often request that their parents be with them. A girl, age 13, following an intravenous needle insertion stated, "I like to have somebody there just so I can look up to them and maybe see their face; it makes me not want to cry or it makes me feel safe. But when nobody's there, it makes me feel . . . kind of unsafe" (Hester, 1989, p. 17).

The almost simultaneous pulling away or striking out is the second important sensorimotor schema associated with nociception. Franck (1986) documents newborns age 4 hours actively drawing their legs away from the heel stick or "swiping" at the site of the noxious stimulation. She does not attempt to qualify if the movements are purposeful or reflexive. The action schema of the more generalized activity patterns of the infants developmentally progress so that by 2 to 4 years the children run away, kick, or protect the limb to be injected (Grunau & Craig, 1987; McGraw, 1941).

Caty, Ellerton, and Ritchie (1984) using the Lazarus stress and coping paradigm analyzed the coping behaviors in 39 published case studies of hospitalized children (20 months to 10 years) with chronic and nonchronic illness. The cases were categorized into three categories of coping: (a) information exchange, which was all verbal or nonverbal behavior of the child that sought to attain, clarify, confirm, regulate, or relate information; (b) action-inaction, which was all noncognitive behavior directed toward managing the self or the environment by either acting upon or holding back actions; and (c) intrapsychic mental processes designed to regulate emotions. Their findings revealed that the action-inaction coping category was dominant (72% for children 20 to 24 months; 68% for children 3 to 5 years; 57% for children 6 to 10 years), followed by information exchange (23%; 26%; 41%, respectively) and intrapsychic (6%; 7%; 2%, respectively). The limitations of the Caty et al. study make it imperative that these findings be viewed cautiously; however, their findings support several researchers' assertions that children who are experiencing pain may use activity as a means of coping (Eland & Anderson, 1977; Freud, 1952; Hawley, 1984; Mills, 1989; Ross & Ross, 1988).

The Lazarus paradigm includes inaction under the definition of the action category. Taylor (1983) and Mills (1989), in their surgical and burn/trauma samples of toddlers and preschoolers, describe the children increasing in vocalization and grimacing but lying still or protecting the traumatized area. Experienced clinicians often suspect children are in pain (a) when after trauma they are observed to be lying quietly in bed either from exhaustion or fear of causing pain (McCaffery, 1969), or (b) when they "hide" their pain in order to avoid an injection (Beyer & Byers, 1985).

Children learn by doing. Preoperational children's early symbols are words for things and it is the doing and the words that expand their ability to use their words as thoughts. In the concrete operational stage, they begin using their thoughts as they did their building blocks at the preoperational age. Thought processes can now be used as a means of coping. The action-inaction schema associated with pain is first observed as reflexive action in infancy, is changed to purposeful running away or fighting in the toddler and preschooler, and is inclusive of cognitive mechanisms in the school-ager. Although children are capable of using cognitive means, it is not clear if in painful situations these modalities can be called upon effectively.

The deeply embedded schema of the presence of a caring trusted person and avoiding or fighting pain may be more salient to children than using cognitive modalities in managing pain. The absence of sickness and pain in the child's everyday world, the surprise and transient nature of acute pain, limits children's practicing and playing pain. Children usually do not play "pain" or "needle play" except in hospital situations where hospital play is part of a child's day. In addition, pain in childhood has not been perceived as something a child can control. Rather children are expected to endure and cooperate during painful procedures; they are not taught ways of controlling their pain. The play activity and practicing of cognitive mechanisms that may reduce pain are important in preschool and school-age children who need concrete experiences to enhance their cognitive thinking. More importantly, it may not be the technique itself that is important but the distraction the technique provides the child (Bloome et al., 1989, p. 157).

Effective assessment of children's pain, perhaps the most difficult part of pain management, is beginning to be addressed by clinicians and researchers. The other side of the coin is managing the pain. Understanding how children conceive and cope with pain is important, particularly in assessing and evaluating efforts to ameliorate pain. Cognitive methods can reduce and in very flexible minds can block pain effectively. The idea of using cognitive methods with children is particularly attractive because of the plasticity of children's learning. To learn these methods, though, children must practice them. How and when to employ these methods is currently being researched (Caty, Ritchie, & Ellerton, 1989; Jay, 1989).

Equally important in managing pain is the use of medications in altering the physiopsychological responses to pain. Pain involves sensation. Pharmacologically altering nociception (primary afferent nerves with peripheral terminals), transduction (nerve activation), and transmission (relaying pain information) (Fields, 1987) are accepted methods of pain intervention in Western medicine. The combined use of cognitive-emotional and pharmacological modalities can be an even more powerful intervention (Abu-Saad & Tesler, 1986; Barr, 1989; McCaffery, 1979; Whaley & Wong, 1991). Administering medication in noninvasive ways such as liquids or chewable pills is highly desirable with children. However, there are times, such as when the child is vomiting or after surgery, that oral administration is not viable. Patient-controlled analgesia (PCA), self-administration of intravenous narcotics through an infusion pump, is a new method that has been shown to be safe and effective with adults (Atwell et al., 1984; Bollish, Collins, Kirking, & Bartlett, 1985; Kane, Lehman, Dugger, Hansen, & Jackson, 1988). PCA is being used with hospitalized children suffering from postoperative, cancer, sickle cell anemia, and burn pain (Shapiro & Cohen, 1989; see chapter 4, this volume). The goal of PCA is to maintain an even level of drug in the bloodstream that interrupts nociceptive transduction and transmission. This is accomplished by having the child press a button that releases the analgesic. The child has a concrete and easy to use device within his control. Clinically, it has been observed that some children under 10 years cannot grasp the concepts of using PCA. Webb, Stergios, and Rodgers (1989) corroborate this clinical observation. Two 11-year-old children at times were reluctant to self-administer their pain medication and needed encouragement from their parents and nurses to trigger the machine (Webb et al., 1989, p. 85). Anecdotal observations indicate that children do not press the button, may push the button when anxious and when in pain, or may push the button when an adult asks them if they have used the button. Speculation within the Piagetian framework can explain these observations. Preoperational children who may have the fine motor skills and imitative skills to handle a PCA device, do not conceptually link the nonvisible medicine with the button and with pain; each aspect is perceived individually. Concrete operational children are conceptually able to understand but the newness of the situation requires repeated experiences before fully grasping the sequence of events. In other words, their conservation ability enables their understanding of the PCA device, but they need repeated concrete demonstrations and experiences if they are to accommodate and assimilate the when and how of the situation. Another example supported by anecdotal observations concerns chronic disease pain in school-agers. These concrete operational children, who have endured chronic pain, push the button and do not get immediate pain relief, stop pushing the button. The repeated episodes of their pain and narcotic use most likely has led to a narcotic tolerance and the current dosage undermedicates their pain. Because their experience contradicts adults' statements, they may have developed a pain schema that combines nociception, helplessness, and depression. Verification through research is needed before these explanations can be accepted.

Clinical and Research Implications

Can chronological age rather than cognitive testing be used to designate children as being in preoperational or concrete operational stages of development? Only a few children's pain studies have actually measured cognitive development prior to analyzing the data within a Piagetian framework (Gedaly-Duff, 1984, 1988; Hester, 1979). All of the pain studies (unless specifically excepted) in this chapter have relied on chronological age and grade level to determine cognitive developmental status. Contradictory evidence exists for both sides of the question.

Brown and Kodadek (1987), who studied children's responses to lie scales and cognitive age, provide statistical evidence that age and developmental level are equivalent. Gaffney and Dunne (1986) and other investigators (Beales et al., 1983; Bibace & Walsh, 1980) found that children's definitions and meaning of pain are developmentally different as the children age. Other investigators found no age differences (Beyer & Aradine, 1986; McGrath et al., 1985; Ross & Ross, 1984a; Savedra et al., 1982). The inability to detect age differences may be explained by sample size and the uneven nature of development.

Studies that examined age and had sufficient subjects on either end of the cognitive age range have found age differences (Bibace & Walsh, 1980; Gaffney & Dunne, 1986). Lack of age differences, such as between preconceptual and intuitive preoperational children's responses to a dental injection, was probably because there were few 3- to 4-year-olds, mostly 5- to 7-year-olds, and a few 8- to 9-year-olds; the preoperational age group was not adequately represented (Gedaly-Duff, 1984, 1988).

The nature of the development of the concept of pain may also hinder detection of age differences. Pain has a generic definition that includes hurt and trauma that is reported by all age groups (Gaffney & Dunne, 1986). If the data collection utilizes short-answer interview or paper/test format, differences may not be detected. Vertical *décalage*, in the case of measuring pain intensity, may be operating. For example, the quantity of pain is understood fundamentally ("same," "more," or "less") by approximately 3 to 4 years; therefore, conceptually intensity may not demonstrate an age difference, even though the measurement instrument may vary from four poker chips to a 10-cm abstract line. Given the current status of children's pain studies, one cautious conclusion is that age and grade level can be used to differentiate cognitive age.

Children's understanding of pain dimensions changes qualitatively with age. Preconceptual children's knowledge of pain dimensions is unknown; speculation about their knowledge is based on sensorimotor infants and preoperational-intuitive children. The preconceptual or individualistic use of words (that is, a common meaning of a word is understood among a group), makes behavioral observation and play methodologies appropriate ways to study children at this age.

Preoperational children's knowledge of the dimensions of pain are (a) location is marked on a body outline (because their understanding of the inside of their bodies is diffuse or focused on food and elimination, pointing to internal pain on their bodies is suspect); (b) intensity is reported by pointing to a face (affect faces scale), poker chip counts, or using words ("a lot" or "a little"); (c) duration is reported with reference to an event such as "nighttime"; (d) meaning of pain is related a bump, a needle, a punishment, and a thing ("it just is"); and (e) description is expressed as a generic term, "hurt."

If preoperational children were asked, "Tell me about your pain," they would likely look at the questioner in confusion, since their synaesthetic perception encompasses all dimensions of pain as one. The children if focused (centered) on each dimension can reply; however, their answers may alter from moment to moment as the characteristics (perceptual, egocentric, undifferentiated) of their thinking suggest. Inconsistencies are to be expected in their pain reports. Children's answers to the caregiver's questions concerning their pain may not tell how things really are, but how the pain experience appears to them. Be cautious! Although children's changing answers about their pain may reflect the nature of their development, it can also be accurately indicative of the nature of their pain. Preoperational children can communicate about their pain; their replies are one piece of information that is evaluated along with other data such as their behavior, physical findings, and parental insights.

Concrete operational children's knowledge of the dimensions of pain are (a) location is marked on a body outline, the painful part of their bodies is pointed to or drawn free hand; (b) intensity may be reported by pointing to an affective faces scale, using a "0" for no pain to "10" as the worst pain scale, and using descriptive words or analogies; (c) duration is reported as an event such as "nighttime," as clock time if the cycle of time is understood, and as a pattern (continuous or intermittent); (d) meaning of pain is related to as a transgression (not following the rules), an accident, a disease, and a feeling (sadness); and (e) description is expressed as a generic term, "hurt," and as a feeling term such as "soreness."

Both preoperational and concrete operational children's schemas for coping are based on sensorimotor coping schemas. Clinical anecdotes and research report that the schemas of "turning to others" and "fight or flight" continue in the preoperational and concrete operational years (Gedaly-Duff, 1989b; Hester, 1989). The persons children turn to are their parents. A relatively unexplored area of research in children's pain is how the family is involved in childhood pain experiences.

It is not unusual to observe professionals usher a parent out of the treatment room during painful diagnostic or treatment procedures. Is this for the convenience of the professional because it is one less person to respond to in a stressful situation? Is it because children seem more cooperative with their parents absent? This may be the case because children may become passive when their "secure" person is removed. How does this affect the child's subjective experience and suffering? How does this affect the developing pain schema? Attention to supporting and teaching parents (or any trusted person) appropriate ways to help their children cope is an area that may enable children and their families to ameliorate painful experiences.

Summary

Children's understanding and ways of coping with pain change with age and experience (Bibace & Walsh, 1980; Gaffney & Dunne, 1986; Savedra et al., 1982; Tesler et al., 1981). Preoperational children's segmented (centered), present-oriented, and illogical (transductive) reasoning can make the experience of pain overwhelming. Concrete operational children perhaps are often prematurely held accountable for "grown up" behavior. The years from 6 to 9 are transition years; the old preoperational schema sneaks in while the child is learning a new concrete operational schema. These children should not be expected to use cognitive strategies with which they have not had adequate practice. The helping person, parent or professional, who knows how children understand and behave in painful situations, can facilitate children's capabilities in understanding and coping with pain.

References

Abu-Saad, H. (1984a). Cultural group indicators of pain in children. *Maternal-Child Nursing Journal, 13*, 187–196.

Abu-Saad, H. (1984b). Assessing children's responses to pain. *Pain, 19*, 163–171.

Abu-Saad, H., & Holzemer, W. L. (1981). Measuring children's self-assessment of pain. *Issues in Comprehensive Pediatric Nursing, 5–6*, 337–349.

Abu-Saad, H., & Tesler, M. (1986). Pain. In V. Carrieri, A. Lindsey, & C. West (Eds.), *Pathophysiological phenomena in nursing* (pp. 235–269). Philadelphia: W. B. Saunders.

Achenbach, T. M. (1978). *Research in developmental psychology: Concepts, strategies, and methods.* New York: Free Press.

Anand, K. J. S., Brown, M. J., Causon, R. C., Christofides, N. D., Bloom, S. R., & Aynsley-Green, A. (1985). Can the human neonate mount an endocrine and metabolic response to surgery? *Journal of Pediatric Surgery, 20*(1), 41–48.

Anand, K. J. S., & Hickey, P. R. (1987). Pain and its effects in the human neonate and fetus. *New England Journal of Medicine, 317*(21), 1321–1329.

Anand, K. J. S., Sippell, W. G., & Aynsley-Green, A. (1987). Randomized trial of fentanyl anaesthesia in preterm babies undergoing surgery: Effects of the stress response. *Lancet, 1*, 243–248.

Aradine, C. R., Beyer, J. E., & Tompkins, J. M. (1988). Children's pain perception before and after analgesia: A study of instrument construct validity and related issues. *Journal of Pediatric Nursing, 3*(1), 11–23.

Atwell, J. R., Flanigan, R. C., Bennett, R. L., Allen, D. C., Lucas, B. A., & McRoberts, J. W. (1984). The efficacy of patient-controlled analgesia in patients recovering from flank incisions. *Journal of Urology, 132*(4), 701–703.

Barr, R. G. (1989). Pain in children. In P. Wall & R. Melzack (Eds.), *Textbook of pain* (2nd ed., pp. 568–588). New York: Churchill Livingstone.

Beales, J. G., Keen, J. H., & Lennox Holt, P. J. (1983). The child's perception of the disease and the experience of pain in juvenile chronic arthritis. *Journal of Rheumatology, 10*(1), 61–65.

Beyer, J. (1988). *The Oucher: A user's manual and technical report* (2nd ed.). Author: University of Colorado Health Sciences Center, School of Nursing, 4200 East Ninth Avenue, Campus Box C-288, Denver, Colorado 80262.

Beyer, J. E., & Aradine, C. R. (1986). Content validity of an instrument to measure young children's perceptions of the intensity of their pain. *Journal of Pediatric Nursing, 1*(6), 386–395.

Beyer, J. E., & Aradine, C. R. (1988). Convergent and discriminant validity of a self-report measure of pain intensity for children. *Children's Health Care, 16*(4), 274–282.

Beyer, J. E., & Byers, M. L. (1985). Knowledge of pediatric pain: The state of the art. *Children's Health Care, 13*(4), 150–159.

Bibace, R., & Walsh, M. E. (1980). Development of children's concepts of illness. *Pediatrics, 66*(6), 912–917.

Bloome, M. E., Lillis, P. P., & Smith, M. C. (1989). Pain interventions with children: A meta-analysis of research. *Nursing Research, 38*(3), 154–158.

Bollish, S. J., Collins, C. L., Kirking, D. M., & Bartlett, R. H. (1985). Efficacy of patient-controlled versus conventional analgesia for postoperative pain. *Clinical Pharmacy, 4*(1), 48–52.

Brewster, A. B. (1982). Chronically ill hospitalized children's concepts of their illness. *Pediatrics, 69*(3), 355–362.

Brown, M. S., & Kodadek, S. M. (1987). The use of lie scales in psychometric measures of children. *Research in Nursing & Health, 10,* 87–92.

Cannon, W. B. (1929). *Bodily changes in pain, hunger, fear and rage* (2nd ed.). New York: Appleton.

Caty, S., Ellerton, M. L., & Ritchie, J. A. (1984). Coping in hospitalized children: An analysis of published case studies. *Nursing Research, 33*(5), 277–282.

Caty, S., Ritchie, J. A., & Ellerton, M. (1989). Helping hospitalized preschoolers manage stressful situations: The mother's role. *Children's Health Care, 18*(4), 202–209.

Chapman, C. R. (1984). New directions in the understanding and management of pain. *Social Science Medicine, 19*(12), 1261–1277.

Cohen, F., & Lazarus, R. S. (1979). Coping with the stresses of illness. In G. Stone, F. Cohen, & N. Adler (Eds.), *Health psychology* (pp. 217–254). San Francisco: Jossey-Bass.

Cowan, P. A. (1978). *Piaget with feeling.* New York: Holt, Rinehart and Winston.

Craig, K. D., McMahon, R. J., Morison, J. D., & Zaskow, C. (1984). Developmental changes in infant pain expression during immunization injections. *Social Science Medicine, 19*(12), 1331–1337.

Crider, C. (1981). Children's conceptions of the body interior. In R. Bibace & M. Walsh (Eds.), *New directions for child development: Childrens' conceptions of health, illness, and bodily functions* (no. 14, pp. 49–65), San Francisco: Jossey-Bass.

Dale, J. C. (1986). A multidimensional study of infants' responses to painful stimuli. *Pediatric Nursing, 12*(1), 27–31.

Dale, J. C. (1989). A multidimensional study of infants' behaviors associated with assumed painful stimuli: Phase II. *Journal of Pediatric Health Care, 3*(1), 34–38.

De Avila, E. (1980a). *Cartoon Conservation Scales (CCS): Administration manual.* Corte Madera, CA: Linguametrics Group.

De Avila, E. (1980b). *Cartoon Conservation Scales (CCS): Technical manual.* Corte Madera, CA: Linguametrics Group.

Eland, J. M. (1981). Minimizing pain associated with prekindergarten intramuscular injections. *Issues in Comprehensive Pediatric Nursing, 5*(5–6), 361–372.

Eland, J. M., & Anderson, J. E. (1977). The experience of pain in children. In A. Jacox (Ed.), *Pain: A source book for nurses and other health professionals* (pp. 453–473). Boston: Little, Brown.

Elkind, D. (1974). Of time and the child. In *Children and adolescents: Interpretive essays on Jean Piaget* (2nd ed., pp. 38–49). New York: Oxford University Press.

Fields, H. L. (1987). *Pain.* New York: McGraw-Hill.

Flavell, J. H. (1963). *The developmental psychology of Jean Piaget.* New York: Van Nostrand.

Fraiberg, S. H. (1959). *The magic years.* New York: Scribner.

Franck, L. S. (1986). A new method to quantitatively describe pain behavior in infants. *Nursing Research, 35*(1), 28–31.

Frankenburg, W. K., & Dodds, J. B. (1990). *Denver II screening manual.* Denver, CO: Denver Developmental Materials, Inc.

Freud, A. (1952). The role of bodily illness in the mental illness of children. *Psychoanalytic Study of the Child, 7,* 69–81.

Gaffney, A. A. (1983) *Pain: Perspectives in childhood: A study of the development of non-hospitalized children's verbally mediated ideas about pain between the ages of five and fourteen years* (Vol. 1, Vol. 2). Unpublished doctoral dissertation, University College, Cork, Ireland. [Note: also cited in Ross and Ross, 1988, p. 43.]

Gaffney, A. A., & Dunne, E. A. (1986). Developmental aspects of children's definitions of pain. *Pain, 26,* 105–117.

Gaffney, A. A., & Dunne, E. A. (1987). Children's understanding of the causality of pain. *Pain, 29,* 91–104.

Gedaly-Duff, V. (1984). Preparing the young child for a painful procedure: The dental injection (Doctoral dissertation, University of California, San Francisco). *Dissertation Abstracts International, 45*(2), 513B. (Michigan: University Microfilms No. DA 8411065.)

Gedaly-Duff, V. (1988). Preparing young children for painful procedures. *Journal of Pediatric Nursing, 3*(3), 169–179.

Gedaly-Duff, V. (1989a). Palmar sweat index use with children in pain research. *Journal of Pediatric Nursing, 4*(1), 3–8.

Gedaly-Duff, V. (1989b). [Family management of childhood pain. Phase 2: Parents' experiences in care of their children's repeated pain episodes associated with chronic illness such as juvenile rheumatoid arthritis.] Unpublished raw data.

Gellert, E. (1962). Children's conceptions of the content and functions of the human body. *Genetic Psychology Monograph, 65,* 293–405.

Golomb, C. (1974). *Young children's sculpture and drawing.* Cambridge, MA: Harvard University Press.

Goodnow, J. (1977). *Children Drawing.* Cambridge, MA: Harvard University Press.

Grunau, R. V., & Craig, K. (1987). Pain expression in neonates: Facial action and cry. *Pain, 28,* 395–410.

Harpin, V. A., & Rutter, N. (1982). Sweating in preterm babies. *Journal of Pediatrics*, *100*, 614–619.

Hawley, D. D. (1984). Postoperative pain in children: Misconceptions, descriptions and interventions. *Pediatric Nursing*, *10*(1), 20–23.

Hester, N. O. (1979). The preoperational child's reaction to immunization. *Nursing Research*, *28*(4), 250–255.

Hester, N. O. (1989, March). *Caregivers' responses to children's pain from the child's perspective.* Paper presented at national conference, Nursing Care of the Hospitalized Child, San Francisco, California, pp. 1–25. Adapted from Hester, N. O., Comforting the child in pain. In S. Funk, E. Tornquist, M. Champagne, L. Copp, & R. Wiese (Eds.), *Key aspects of comfort: Management of pain, fatigue, and nausea* (pp. 290–298, 1989), New York: Springer.

Hester, N. O., Foster, R., & Kristensen, K. (1989). Measurement of pain in children: Generalizability and validity of the Pain Ladder and the Poker Chip Tool. In D. C. Tyler & E. J. Krane (Eds.), *Pediatric pain (Advances in pain research and therapy*, (Vol. 15, pp. 79–84). New York: Raven Press.

Izard, C. E., Hembree, E. A., Dougherty, L. M., & Spizzirri, C. I. (1983). Changes in facial expressions of 2- to 19-month-old infants following acute pain. *Developmental Psychology*, *19*, 418–426.

Izard, C. E., Hembree, E. A., & Huebner, R. R. (1987). Infants' emotion expressions to acute pain: Developmental change and stability of individual differences. *Developmental Psychology*, *23*(1), 105–113.

Jay, S. (1989). Preparing for the pain. *Behavior Today*, *20*(17), 3–5.

Jeans, M. E. (1983). Pain in children — A neglected area. In P. Firestone, P. McGrath, & W. Feldman (Eds.), *Advances in behavioral medicine for children and adolescents* (pp. 23–37). Hillsdale, NJ: Erlbaum.

Johnston, C. C., & Strada, M. E. (1986). Acute pain response in infants: A multidimensional description. *Pain*, *24*, 373–382.

Kane, N. E., Lehman, M. E., Dugger, R., Hansen, L., & Jackson, D. (1988). Use of patient-controlled analgesia in surgical oncology patients. *Oncology Nursing Forum*, *15*(1), 29–32.

Lazarus, R. S., & Folkman, S. (1984). *Stress, appraisal, and coping.* New York: Springer.

Leventhal, H., & Everhart, D. (1979). Emotion, pain and physical illness. In C. E. Izard (Ed.), *Emotions in personality and psychopathology* (pp. 263–299). New York: Plenum.

Levy, D. M. (1960). The infant's earliest memory of inoculation: A contribution to public health procedures. *Journal of Genetic Psychology*, *96*, 3–46.

Lewis, N. (1978). The needle is like an animal. *Children Today*, *7*, 18–21.

Lollar, D. J., Smits, S. J., & Patterson, D. L. (1982). Assessment of pediatric pain: An empirical perspective. *Journal of Pediatric Psychology*, *7*(3), 267–277.

MacKinnon, P. C. B. (1954). Variations with age in the number of active palmar digital sweat glands. *Journal of Neurology and Neurosurgical Psychiatry*, *17*, 124–126.

Maier, H. W. (1978). *Three theories of child development* (3rd ed.). New York: Harper & Row.

Margolis, R. B., Tait, R. C., & Krause, S. J. (1986). A rating system for use with patient pain drawings. *Pain*, *24*(1), 57–65.

McCaffery, M. (1969). Brief episodes of pain in children. In B. S. Bergenson, E. H.

Anderson, M. Duffey, M. Lohr, & M. H. Rose (Eds.), *Current concepts in clinical nursing* (Vol. 3, pp. 178–191). St. Louis: C. V. Mosby.

McCaffery, M. (1977). Pain relief for the child: Problem areas and selected nonpharmacological methods. *Pediatric Nursing, 3,* 11–16.

McCaffery, M. (1979). *Nursing management of the patient with pain.* Philadelphia: J. B. Lippincott.

McGrath, P. A., deVeber, L. L., & Hearn, M. T. (1985). Multidimensional pain assessment in children. *Advances in Pain Research and Therapy, 9,* 387–393.

McGraw, M. B. (1941). Neural maturation as exemplified in the changing reactions of the infant to pin prick. *Child Development, 12*(1), 31–42.

Melzack, R. (1975). The McGill Pain Questionnaire: Major properties and scoring methods. *Pain, 1,* 277–299.

Melzack, R., & Torgerson, W. S. (1971). On the language of pain. *Anesthesiology, 34,* 50–59.

Melzack, R., & Wall, P. D. (1965). Pain mechanisms: A new theory. *Science, 150,* 971–979.

Mills, N. (1989). Acute pain behaviors in infants and toddlers. In S. Funk, E. Tornquist, M. T. Champagne, L. A. Copp, & R. A. Wiese (Eds.), *Key aspects of comfort: Management of pain, fatigue, and nausea* (pp. 52–59). New York: Springer.

Molsberry, D. (1979). *Young children's subjective quantification of pain following surgery.* Unpublished master's thesis, University of Iowa, Iowa City, IA.

Murphy, L. B., & Moriarty, A. D. (1976). *Vulnerability, coping, and growth.* New Haven: Yale University Press.

Norbeck, J. (1981). Young children's ability to conserve facial identity when facial emotion varies. *Nursing Research, 30*(6), 329–333.

Owens, M. E., & Todt, E. H. (1984). Pain in infancy: Neonatal reaction to a heel lance. *Pain, 20,* 77–86.

Piaget, J. (1971). *The child's conception of time.* New York: Ballantine Books.

Piaget, J. (1972). *Psychology of intelligence.* Totowa, NJ: Littlefield, Adams.

Piaget, J., & Inhelder, B. (1969). *The psychology of the child.* New York: Basic Books.

Porter, F. L., Miller, R. H., & Marshall, R. E. (1986). Neonatal pain cries: Effect of circumcision on acoustic features and perceived urgency. *Child Development, 57,* 790–802.

Price, D. D. (1988). *Psychological and neural mechanisms of pain* (pp. 1–18). New York: Raven Press.

Prugh, D., Staub, E., Sands, H., Kirschbaum, R., & Lenihan, E. (1953). A study of emotional reactions of children and families to hospitalization and illness. *American Journal of Orthopsychiatry, 23,* 70–106.

Rich, E. C., Marshall, R. E., & Volpe, J. J. (1974). The normal neonatal response to pin-prick. *Developmental Medicine and Child Neurology, 16,* 432–434.

Rosch, E., Mervis, C. B., Gray, W. D., Johnson, D. M., & Boyes-Braem, P. (1976). Basic objects in natural categories. *Cognitive Psychology, 8,* 382–439.

Ross, D. M. (1984). Thought-stopping: A coping strategy for impending feared events. *Issues in Comprehensive Pediatric Nursing, 7,* 83–89.

Ross, D. M., & Ross, S. A. (1984a). Childhood pain: The school-aged child's viewpoint. *Pain, 20,* 179–191.

Ross, D. M., & Ross, S. A. (1984b). The importance of type of question, psychological climate and subject set in interviewing children about pain. *Pain, 19*, 71–79.

Ross, D. M., & Ross, S. A. (1988). *Childhood pain: Current issues, research, and management*. Baltimore: Urban & Schwarzenberg.

Savedra, M., Gibbons, P., Tesler, M., Ward, J., & Wegner, C. (1982). How do children describe pain? A tentative assessment. *Pain, 14*, 95–104.

Savedra, M., Tesler, M., Holzemer, W., Wilkie, D., & Ward, J. A. (1989). Pain location: Validity and reliability of body outline markings by hospitalized children and adolescents. *Research in Nursing & Health, 12*, 307–314.

Savedra, M., Tesler, M., Ward, J. A., Wegner, C., & Gibbons, P. (1981). Description of the pain experience: A study of school-age children. *Issues in Comprehensive Pediatric Nursing, 5*, 373–380.

Schultz, N. (1971). How children perceive pain. *Nursing Outlook, 19*, 670–673.

Scott, P. J., Ansell, B. M., & Huskisson, E. C. (1977). Measurement of pain in juvenile chronic polyarthritis. *Annals of the Rheumatic Diseases, 36*, 186–187.

Scott, R. (1978). "It hurts red": A preliminary study of children's perception of pain. *Perceptual and Motor Skills, 47*, 787–791.

Shapiro, B., & Cohen, D. (1989). *Progress report to the Pediatric Pain Management Program Oversight Committee*. Philadelphia: Children's Hospital of Philadelphia, University of Pennsylvania.

Simmel, M. L. (1962). Phantom experiences following amputation in children. *Journal of Neurology, Neurosurgery and Psychiatry, 25*, 69–78.

Smith, E. C. (1977). Communicating with young children: Are you really communicating? *American Journal of Nursing, 77*, 1966–1968.

Steward, M. S., & Steward, D. S. (1981). Children's conceptions of medical procedures. In R. Bibace & M. Walsh (Eds.), *New directions for child development: Children's conceptions of health, illness, and bodily functions* (no. 14, pp. 67–83). San Francisco: Jossey-Bass.

Taylor, P. (1983). Post-operative pain in toddler and pre-school age children. *Maternal Child Nursing Journal, 12*(1), 35–50.

Tesler, M. D., Savedra, M. C., Ward, J. A., Holzemer, W. L., & Wilkie, D. J. (1989). Children's words for pain. In S. Funk, E. Tornquist, M. Champagne, L. A. Copp, & R. Wiese (Eds.), *Key aspects of comfort: Management of pain, fatigue, and nausea* (pp. 60–65). New York: Springer.

Tesler, M., Ward, J., Savedra, M., Wegner, C. B., & Gibbons, P. (1983). Developing an instrument for eliciting children's description of pain. *Perceptual and Motor Skills, 56*, 315–321.

Tesler, M., Wegner, C. B., Savedra, M., Gibbons, P., & Ward, J. (1981). Coping strategies of children in pain. *Issues in Comprehensive Pediatrics, 5-6*, 351–359.

Unruh, A., McGrath, P. J., Cunningham, S. J., & Humphreys, P. (1983). Children's drawings of their pain. *Pain, 17*, 385–392.

Varni, J. W., Thompson, K., & Hanson, V. (1987). The Varni-Thompson Pediatric Pain Questionnaire. I. Chronic musculoskeletal pain in juvenile rheumatoid arthritis. *Pain, 28*, 27–38.

Wall, P. D. (1979). On the relation of injury to pain: The John J. Bonica lecture. *Pain, 6*, 253–264.

Wallace, M. R. (1989). Temperament: A variable in children's pain management. *Pediatric Nursing, 15*(2), 118–121.

Webb, C. J., Stergios, D. A., & Rodgers, B. M. (1989). Use of patient-controlled analgesia by children. In S. Funk, E. Tornquist, M. Champagne, L. A. Copp, & R. Wiese (Eds.), *Key aspects of comfort: Management of pain, fatigue, and nausea* (pp. 80–86). New York: Springer.

Whaley, L., & Wong, D. L. (1991). *Nursing care of infants and children* (4th ed.). St. Louis: C. V. Mosby.

Wong, D. L., & Baker, C. M. (1988). Pain in children: Comparison of assessment scales. *Pediatric Nursing, 14*(1), 9–17.

9
Developmental Issues: Adolescent Pain

PATRICK J. MCGRATH AND SUSAN PISTERMAN

In this chapter we focus on the interface between the developmental stage of adolescence and the experience of pain. Detailed discussion of specific syndromes are not included in this chapter. Rather, we will examine more general issues that may be applied to any pain problem. Although adolescence marks major increases in the prevalence of a wide range of pain problems, pain in adolescents has been specifically addressed in only a few articles (e.g. Smith, Tyler, Womack, & Chen, 1989).

Adolescence is a time of transition between childhood and adulthood. It is often divided into three phases: early (10 to 13 years), middle (14 to 16 years), and late (17 to 21 years) (Felice, 1983). This time is marked by the maturation of cognitive functioning, changes in social and family interaction and by major physiological and physical changes.

Theories of Adolescence

Specific theories of adolescent cognitive (Piaget, 1970), moral (Kohlberg, 1976), emotional and biological (Tanner, 1962) development have been formulated but no comprehensive theory has gained widespread acceptance. Consequently, adolescence has been an underconceptualized area of research, and findings in one area or aspect of adolescence frequently are not theoretically integrated into other areas.

Cognitive Development

Traditionally, cognitive development has been seen as progressing through distinct, ordered stages (Piaget, 1970) culminating in the formal operations stage attained in adolescence. Although this simplistic stage view has been challenged (Asington, Harris, & Olson, 1988), the Piagetian model is the only one that has been applied to the adolescent's understanding of pain. According to the Piagetian view, between ages 7 years and approximately 11 years the child's thinking becomes more flexible and abstract. This level of abstraction is still, however, largely restricted to concrete objects and situations; hence, the term *concrete operational thought*. By about age 11 or 12 years the adolescent enters the stage of formal operational thinking, which is characterized by the ability to think about thoughts. This allows the adolescent to manipulate ideas and symbols in abstract ways. Thinking becomes more flexible and systematic. The attainment of formal operational thinking is, however, not universal.

Cognitive development has important effects on the experience of pain because understanding of pain changes with age. Moreover the ability to engage in different coping strategies for dealing with pain is also dependent on cognitive development.

Developmental changes in children's understanding and description of pain were found in work by Gaffney and Dunne (Gaffney & Dunne, 1986; Gaffney & Dunne, 1987; Gaffney, 1988), who studied 680 schoolchildren in Ireland between 5 and 14 years of age. They examined changes in the definitions, descriptions, and understanding of causality of pain. The adolescents in the study were divided into two groups according to Piagetian stages, up to age 10 years (concrete operations) and 11 to 14 years (formal operations). Younger adolescents used physical analogies to describe pain and demonstrated a developing awareness of the psychological concomitants of pain, such as the ability of pain to affect mood. Adolescents in the older age group gave definitions of pain that included both a physical and a psychological component. They viewed pain more actively and tended to define pain as something that has to be handled stoically.

Social Development

Major potentially stressful phenomena of adolescence include increasing independence from parental and family influences and increasing reliance on peers for social support and values. Within the family, issues of emancipation are important for many adolescents. An epidemiologic study of over 2,000 Finnish youths (Aro, 1987) found that girls were more likely to perceive increasing conflict with mother (18.1%) or father (14.6%) than were boys (11.2% and 9.2%, respectively).

As well, adolescence is the typical start of dating relationships. Adolescents will experience both the desire to engage in these relationships and peer pressure to participate even if they do not feel ready to do so.

Pressure to have sexual intercourse can be very strong and can come from peers or from abuse situations. Consultation for pain (especially, but not exclusively, gynecologic pain) may be an acceptable way for a nervous teenager to obtain help in dealing with sexual pressures or abuse.

During adolescence the pressure to make a vocational choice and the subsequent increasing academic demands may coincide with demands of part-time employment and social activity.

The role of emancipation issues in pain problems has not been elucidated. The principal mechanism may be the stress that these conflicts cause.

Although the relationship between stress in the adolescent and pain syndromes has not been well conceptualized there are several mechanisms likely to be acting. Stress might trigger ischemic pain such as muscle contraction headache by way of increased muscular tension. Stressful events can launch a cascade of biochemical or neural processes that may result in pain (e.g., migraine). Stress might contribute to changes in sleep, physical activity, or diet (especially alcohol, salt, or caffeine consumption), causing or exacerbating pain. In susceptible individuals, stress can lead to heightened awareness of bodily sensation and increase the tendency to label such sensations as pain. Finally, stress could contribute to a breakdown in the ability to cope adequately with pain and cause the onset of pain-related disability or handicap. Moreover, stress may have idiosyncratic mechanisms in the individual adolescent. For example, an adolescent under stress may become less compliant to a medical regimen and cause a flare-up in pain due to uncontrolled medical problems.

In summary, although the mechanisms are not well understood, for some individuals stress can play an important role in the etiology or maintenance of a pain problem.

Physical Development

Hormonal changes form the bases of many important physical and physiological changes in adolescence. However, these changes may be asynchronous. That is, changes occur at different times within the individual. Individual differences across adolescents also are common.

Puberty is a gradual process and often signals the first obvious transformation in the adolescent period. Usually girls experience puberty about 2 years earlier than most boys. In girls the initial signs of puberty (development of breast buds or pubic hair) begin at about age 9. For boys, physical changes (darkening of the scrotal skin and lengthening of the penis) begin at about age 11 years (Tanner, 1962).

The growth spurt associated with puberty typically manifests at pubertal onset in girls reaching peak growth early in the pubertal process. In contrast, boys reach their peak growth toward the end of puberty when girls of the same age are typically experiencing menarche. Menarche typically occurs in the middle of the fat/weight spurt in girls. On average, the pubertal process takes about 4 years but the timing and sequence of these changes show great individual variation.

The changes in physical development that occur in adolescence can impact on pain problems in at least four different ways. First, there can be hormonal alterations that directly influence the onset of pains such as migraine or dysmenorrhea.

Second, aspects of physical development may cause stress. For example, the timing of maturation can impact adolescents' self-perceptions of attractiveness. In particular, early-maturing girls and late-maturing boys may experience lowered self-esteem because of comparisons with peers.

Third, because of the obvious physical changes occurring in adolescence there may be a heightened self-awareness of somatic functioning and physical characteristics. Some evidence to support this comes from Hibbs, Kobos, and Gonzalea (1979), who found an age effect on the Minnesota Multiphasic Personality Inventory (MMPI) hypochondriasis subscale in which adolescents and young adults (ages 13 to 24 years) showed elevated scores compared to adults (aged 25 to 34 years). Whether this is a psychological phenomenon related to developmental biological changes or represents reporting of actual increases in physical problems is difficult to discern. The hypochondriasis subscale of the MMPI is actually a symptom-reporting checklist rather than a measure of overreporting or hypochondriasis per se.

Fourth, biological aspects can be mediated by individual, social, or situational factors that enhance or limit direct biological influences (Richards & Petersen, 1987). For example, a biological predisposition to constipation might have not resulted in pain during childhood because of maternal regulation of diet and a high activity level. However, if in adolescence the diet became lower in fiber because of decreasing parental control and increasing independence and if activity level decreased, recurrent abdominal pain might result. Likewise, skipping breakfast and lack of sleep might trigger migraine in a susceptible adolescent.

Similarly, the increasing social and academic demands that occur during adolescence might combine with occurrence of dysmenorrhea in a young adolescent who is ill-equipped to cope, producing a serious pain problem.

In addition, biological factors can be influenced by cultural beliefs or stereotypes. A classic example is the expectation in some subcultures that menstrual pain is disabling. These expectations may or may not change perception of pain but do have an impact on disability from pain.

Given the dramatic biological changes that occur during adolescence it is no wonder that many developmental theorists have posited these changes as underlying the psychosocial, psychological, and developmental tasks of this period (Elkind, 1970).

Prevalence of Pains

The importance of physical and physiological changes of adolescence are highlighted by the dramatic changes in prevalence and distribution of pain in the adolescent years. Sex differences in prevalence of recurrent pains emerge early in adolescence and vary with different types of pain. These differences in pain report could be due to actual differences in the occurrence of pain, reporting bias, or the maturational lag that males experience. There is little evidence of a reporting bias in which females are more ready to interpret sensations as pain. If a reporting bias were important, sex differences should occur in all pains, and this is not the case. For example, heartburn is more commonly reported in boys (Aro, 1987), and among adolescents attending an emergency room there was an overrepresentation of girls with abdominal pain but not chest pain (Pantell & Goodman, 1983). If a simple developmental lag were the cause boys should catch up 2 to 3 years later, but the prevalence data cannot be fitted to such a lag model.

Prevalence rates vary from study to study, perhaps because of differences in definition of the pain syndrome, differences in method of ascertainment, or because of actual differences in occurrence.

Naish and Apley (1951) found that in boys there was a steady incidence of abdominal pain of between 10% and 12% between 5 and 10 years of age, a steady fall in incidence after 10 years, with a subsequent rise to about 10% at age 14. In girls the incidence was similar to boys until age 8. At 9 there was a dramatic rise, with about one quarter affected. The incidence then showed a steady decrease. Oster (1972) also found a sex difference in recurrent abdominal pain and a peak incidence in girls of about 30% and boys of 21% at 9 years with a drop to approximately 5% in both sexes at the age of 16 to 17.

Dysmenorrhea occurs in approximately one third of female adolescents (Feldman, Hodgson, Corber, & Quinn, 1986). Disability from this pain is extremely variable and may be related to family factors. Ross and Ross (1988) have described how the high familial concordance of this problem could be the result of an interaction between biological factors and the tone and content of information given to the adolescent by her mother.

The prevalence of migraine headache in children and adolescents has been well examined in several studies (e.g., Bille, 1962; Sillanpaa, 1976, 1983a, 1983b). The picture is consistent, with increases for both boys and girls occurring at about age 10 years but a consistently higher prevalence for females compared to males once puberty begins. There appears to be a secular trend with prevalence increasing over time. Using the same instruments, Sillanpaa (1983a, 1983b) found the expected increase attributable to age as he followed children from 7 years to 13 years and a 200 to 250% increase in prevalence in 13-year-olds surveyed in 1980 compared to children in a different city surveyed in 1955 by Bille (1962). Similarly, increases over time in prevalence of migraine were found in children entering school in the same towns.

Although the prevalence of migraine increases with puberty, there is no indication that timing of puberty (late or early, for example) has any effect on headache or other symptoms (Aro, 1987).

Benign limb pains, especially "growing pains," are common in childhood but usually resolve by adolescence. An exception to this is the phenomenon of peripatellar knee pain, which occurs in up to 31% of adolescents (Fairbank, Pynsent, Van Poortvliet, & Philips, 1984).

Chest pain appears to be common in adolescents but most studies are very poorly designed and, as a result, the exact prevalence is not known (McGrath & Unruh, 1987). Most commonly, the major concern of the adolescent is that he/she has cancer or heart disease. Fortunately this is almost never the case. Back pain is rare in children (King, 1984) but the adult pattern of back pain begins in late adolescence.

Stress, Pain, and Adolescence

Stress is commonly associated with change at any stage of development and many somatic complaints are frequently assumed to be stress-related. Moreover, adolescence is usually seen as a period of great storm and stress. The classic notion of adolescence as a time of turmoil is not borne out by empirical research (Offer & Offer, 1975; Rutter, Graham, Chadwick, & Yule, 1976; Yankelovitch, 1974). For example, Offer and Offer (1975), in their longitudinal study of middle-class adolescent boys found that only about 20% had a tumultuous growth pattern marked by conflict and stress. Although the direction of the influence is not entirely clear, the families of these youths were more distressed and disorganized. Although stress may not be endemic in adolescence, there may be a relationship between stress and pain.

The evidence that adolescents under stress are more likely to have pain is mixed. Studies that focus on clinical samples have tended to find few differences between children and adolescents who suffer from pain and children and adolescents who do not. For example, in our own case-control studies of headache sufferers (Cunningham et al., 1987) and recurrent abdominal pain sufferers (McGrath, Goodman, Firestone, Shipman, & Peters, 1983) we found little evidence of the role of stress in the etiology of these pain problems. Similarly, Cooper, Bawden, Camfield, and Camfield (1987) found that a group of young adolescents with headache were not different from controls on measures of anxiety and stress. However, among the migraineurs, more anxious children had more frequent and severe headaches. Other case-control studies have been contradictory. Raymer, Weininger, and Hamilton (1984) found no relationship between stress and pain, whereas others have found a relationship (Crossley 1982; Greene, Walker, Hickson, & Thompson, 1985). Studies based on community samples, however, have consistently found that stress is related to pain problems (Aro, 1987; Larsson, 1988). For example, in a series of papers, Aro and her colleagues (Aro, 1987, 1988; Aro, Paronen, & Aro, 1987; Aro & Rantanen, in review; Aro & Taipale, 1987) described a longitudinal study of over 2,000 adolescents whose mean age at the beginning of the study was 14.5 years. Three assessments were conducted over 17 months from December, 1981 to May, 1983. Aro (1987) found a complex interaction between stress, gender, and symptoms. Stress was measured in terms of a 25-item life events scale and an interpersonal problems scale. The "psychosomatic" symptoms included headache, abdominal pain, sleep disturbance, loss of appetite, nausea or vomiting, dizziness, tremor, bowel problems, breathlessness, palpitations, and excessive perspiration. The level of symptoms was higher among girls at all three testings. As well, increases in symptoms occurred for both sexes over the three testings. For both sexes, life events and interpersonal problems were significantly correlated with symptoms. However these correlations were low (range .09 to .34; mean = .20). This suggests that interpersonal problems were more predictive of symptoms (range .17 to .34; mean = .26) than were life events (range .09 to .24; mean = .15). Predictions were equally good for boys and for girls, but increases in symptoms were more related to life events and interpersonal problems in boys than in girls. Although boys, in general, had fewer symptoms than girls, at the third testing, boys with many life events had the same number of symptoms as girls with many life events. In summary, this large, well-conducted study suggests that there may well be a significant but small relationship between stress and pain. The implications for the individual adolescent are not clear. It may be that a small proportion of adolescents are very sensitive to stress, or it may mean that there is a very small effect on a large proportion of adolescents.

Parental discord and divorce can be serious stressors for adolescents. Their relationship to symptoms such as pain has also been explored by Aro (1988). She found that 15- to 16-year-old adolescents who were in families experiencing discord or divorce were more likely to experience somatic and psychic symptoms. Unfortunately no breakdown is given for specific pain symptoms such as headache and abdominal pain.

Sexual abuse in childhood or adolescence is a stressor that has been linked to pain problems (Caldirola, Gemperle, Guzinski, Gross, & Doerr, 1984; Haber & Roos, 1985). The mechanism is not understood but is thought to follow the pattern of a posttraumatic stress disorder.

How Adolescents Learn to Cope

Although it is widely believed that children and adolescents learn to cope from their families, surprisingly little is known about the transmission of pain behavior and coping in families. The social learning processes of modeling, reinforcement, and punishment have been well documented in the experimental pain literature with adults (Craig, 1986) but well-controlled data with clinical pain in children are extremely scarce. It does appear that people who have pain problems are more likely to report having had parents that had pain problems as well (Harris and Associates, 1985; Sternbach, 1986). However, the specific roles of biological predisposition and learning have not been disentangled. In a recent study of adolescents following surgery we (Branson, McGrath, Craig, Rubin, & Vair, 1990) could not demonstrate any familial aggregation of coping strategies.

Families may contribute to pain problems in several other ways. For example, older adolescent girls and young women who report not having been prepared for menarche also report more severe menstrual symptoms and more negative feelings about menstruation (Brooks-Gunn & Ruble, 1983).

Family therapists have long described families in which parents are inappropriately overinvolved with their children (Minuchin et al., 1975). These "enmeshed" families are marked by poor coping with chronic illness. This pattern of interaction is associated with adolescents who are missing school because of chronic nonmalignant pain. In one study, (Dunn-Geier, McGrath, Rourke, Latter, & D'Astous, 1986) mothers of adolescents missing school because of pain were much more intrusive than mothers of adolescents who had similar pains but were not missing school. In this study, mothers supervised their adolescent children on a simple exercise task, which was videotaped and coded. Interestingly, the mothers of noncopers both encouraged and discouraged coping more than the mothers of adolescents who were coping well with similar pain. Because of the nature of the study we do not know how much of the parental overinvolvement is the cause of the adolescent's poor coping and how much is the result of it.

The Outcome of Coping

We have argued strongly for the need to separate pain conceptually and clinically from the resulting change in function or role that may result (Dunn-Geier et al., 1986; McGrath & Unruh, 1987; McGrath, Unruh, & Branson, 1990). Amount or severity of pain is often not directly related to the extent of disability. For example, two adolescents may have similar levels of pain from migraine but one will miss no school and have a rich and extensive social life, whereas the other will withdraw from social activities and school.

The World Health Organization's (WHO) International Classification of Impairments, Disabilities, and Handicaps (World Health Organization, 1980) provides a framework for making this distinction clear. According to this model, the effects of disease can be conceptualized as occurring in four planes of experience. The first plane is that of the occurrence of an abnormality (disease). The second plane of experience occurs when someone (usually the affected individual) becomes aware of the abnormality or develops a symptom. This is termed an impairment. Impairments are concerned with "abnormalities of body structures and . . . organ or system function resulting from any cause (World Health Organization, 1980, p. 14). The third plane of experience, disability, occurs when there is "any restriction or lack (resulting from an impairment) of ability to perform an activity in the manner or within the range considered normal" (p. 28). The fourth plane of experience, handicap, occurs when the experience is socialized. Handicaps are concerned with the social disadvantages experienced by the individual as a result of impairments and disabilities.

In summary, impairments are at the organ level, disabilities are at the level of the person, and handicaps are at the level of the social role. In terms of pain problems, pain would be an impairment, disruption of specific activities because of pain is a disability, and interruption of social roles is a handicap.

The WHO model should not be seen as competing with diagnostic nomenclatures such as the American Psychiatric Association's Diagnostic and Statistical Manual (DSM-III-R) (American Psychiatric Association, 1987), the International Classification of Diseases (ICD-9) (Commission on Professional and Hospital Activities, 1979), or the International Association for the Study of Pain's classification system (Merskey, 1986). Each of these is a system for identifying diseases or disorders. The WHO model focuses on the results of disease or disorder.

Appropriate interventions are likely to be very different for individuals who experience the same pain but whose levels of disability or handicap differ. For example, analgesics are the likely treatment of choice for the pain of simple migraine (an impairment). Encouragement and availability of short rest periods and analgesics at school might be appropriate for adolescents who are having difficulty staying at school when a headache is beginning (a disability). Intensive involvement by a mental health professional would be appropriate for an adolescent who has begun to fail school and who has become socially isolated because she is housebound with headaches (a handicap).

Clinical experience with adolescents who are seriously handicapped by pain is limited because such handicap is relatively rare. We have prepared some guidelines for parents and for clinicians, illustrated in Tables 9.1 and 9.2, that may assist in helping these patients.

Individual Differences

There are individual differences in response to painful stimuli. These differences may be due to differences in physiological reactivity, personality, prior experience with pain, coping skills, and expectations in the particular situation.

The stability of individual differences in reactivity to painful stimuli in adolescents has not been investigated. For example, we do not know if an adolescent who reacts strongly to menstrual pain will be a strong reactor to other pain such as from an injury. One area in which there has been some research is the tendency to be aware of and report symptoms. The personality construct of symptom reporting (Pennebaker, 1982) has been used to

TABLE 9.1. General guidelines for parents to help their adolescents who are having a difficult time coping with recurrent pain.

Never dispute that the adolescent has pain or argue about the severity of the pain. Do not accuse the adolescent of malingering. This will only encourage more pain behavior.

Encourage a calm, matter-of-fact approach to pain. Pain is no big deal.

Encourage the maintenance of normal activity (except during a severe pain attack).

Model coping behavior by parental maintenance of activities and calm approach to your own pain problems.

Discourage excessive complaining, pain behavior, and requests for special consideration by generally paying minimal attention to such behavior.

Empathize with the suffering by having preset times when complaints are carefully listened to and sympathy and understanding are given.

If adolescent is sick enough to miss school, he should be at home in bed with no television or special privileges.

If school absence of 1 or more days most weeks persists for more than 2 months, seek help from a mental health professional.

Note. From "Recurrent headaches in children and adolescents: Diagnosis and management" by P. J. McGrath and P. Humphreys, 1989, *Pediatrician, 16*, pp. 71–77. Copyright 1989 by S. Karger AG, Basel. Adapted by permission.

explain individual differences. Symptom reporting refers to the tendency to be aware of and report internal physiological states. Although pain is only one symptom that can be reported, it is believed that symptom reporting is a general predisposition rather than being limited to a given symptom such as pain. High levels of symptom reporting have been linked to family problems, parents' levels of symptom reporting, psychological abuse and maternal depression (Mechanic, 1980). Low levels of symptom reporting have been associated with the Type A behavior personality construct in children

TABLE 9.2. Guidelines for helping adolescents who are handicapped by pain.

Begin psychosocial assessment as soon as the adolescent becomes handicapped (e.g., starts missing school or withdrawing from social activities).

Unless the cause of pain is clearly evident, avoid the organic/psychogenic dichotomy.

Emphasize coping rather than curing.

Focus on family strengths rather than weaknesses; do not blame the family.

Investigate possible problems at school.

Teach coping skills such as relaxation and cognitive restructuring.

Listen to the adolescent; do not accuse patient of malingering or fabrication.

Educate the family and the adolescent about pain and the role of analgesics, rest, and maintenance of activities.

Understand without pitying.

Note. From "Recurrent headaches in children and adolescents: Diagnosis and management" by P. J. McGrath and P. Humphreys, 1989, *Pediatrician, 16*, pp. 71–77. Copyright 1989 by S. Karger AG, Basel. Adapted by permission.

(Leikin, Firestone, & McGrath, 1988). Symptom reporting may tend to aggregate in families and appears to be a trait that endures over many years from late childhood to adolescence (Mechanic, 1980). Unfortunately, little research has examined the developmental course of symptom reporting.

The Adolescent and the Health Care System

The health care system is usually considered the primary source of assessment and treatment for more-than-trivial pain problems. However, surprisingly little is known about adolescents' attitudes toward and use of the health care system.

A recent survey of 730 adolescents between 12 and 20 years of age in the Canadian national capital region, reported that 84.7% had consulted a physician in the previous year (Hodgson, Feldman, Corber, & Quinn, 1986). Most (78.9%) said they usually received care from a private physician. Females reported that they consulted more than males but there were no age or social class differences in rates of consultation. The rates of consultation in this study of Canadian adolescents were substantially higher than rates reported in American studies (e.g., Kovar, 1982), probably because there is universal free access to health care in Canada. The different health care system in the United States may limit generalization of these findings to that country. It is likely that the cost of health care would be a barrier to many adolescents in the United States.

Adolescents in this sample did not consult as much as they would like to, though. For example, although 31.5% of the female respondents worried about menstrual problems, only 43.3% of those who were concerned consulted a doctor. An additonal 40.0% of those suffering would like to have consulted. Similarly, 19.0% worried about stomachaches; 35.6% of these consulted and 25% more would have liked to consult.

Adolescents identified factors that were important to their patronizing a health care facility. They cited the following factors as very important: confidentiality (73.5%), friendliness of staff (70.7%), getting the doctor you like (52.9%), being able to get lab tests done at the same place (51.7%), and short waiting time (39.7%). The factors that were cited as "not very important" or "not important at all" included the age and sex of the staff (56.0%), proximity of the facility (42.7%), and availability of transportation to the clinic (41.0%).

Adolescents in this study recognized that their physician was an appropriate person to consult for pain but did not access the health care system as much as they would like. Adolescents, like other potential patients, may limit their access to health care because of misconceptions or anxieties about utilization of care.

Confidentiality

Physicians (and other health professionals) who see adolescents should establish early on in the relationship that information is confidential. Explicit discussion of confidentiality, outlining the ethical and legal rights of the adolescent patient and the limits of confidentiality, is appropriate. Children over 9 or 10 years of age should be routinely seen by their doctor, without their parents present, to discuss any private matters.

By adolescence, in order to obtain independent sampling of opinion, it is necessary to discuss issues separately from parents even if a parent is accompanying the adolescent. For example, queries about sexual activity in an adolescent female with abdominal pain are appropriate and answers are likely to be muted in the presence of parents.

Compliance

Adolescents are not necessarily less compliant than other patients. Treatment of pain may be plagued less by noncompliance than other problems, because of the inherent motivation to reduce pain. However, problems are likely to arise with complex treatment regimens that require considerable effort before there is any reduction in pain. A good example of such a regimen is the cognitive behavioral programs for recurrent headache (McGrath & Humphreys, 1989).

Life-Style and Pain

Specific aspects of adolescent life-style may impact on pain problems. A low fiber diet may lead to recurrent abdominal pain (Feldman, McGrath, Hodgson, Ritter, & Shipman, 1985). Skipping meals, lack of sleep, or wide variations in sleep patterns may trigger migraine (McGrath & Humphreys, 1989). High levels of athletic activity may lead to overuse injuries and pain. Risk taking may lead to athletic or accidental injuries and resulting pain. Unfortunately we have no data on the extent to which these factors impact on adolescent pain.

The modification of life-style is extraordinarily difficult. The wise health care professional will draw attention to the possible link between factors such as headache and sleep patterns but will not expect adolescents (or anyone else for that matter) easily to accomplish life-style changes. When life-style changes are required, systematic intervention with adequate follow-up is more likely to be successful than simple exhortations.

Development and Specific Treatments

Various forms of therapy, especially psychological treatment, are dependent on the adolescent's cognitive and social development. Cognitive therapy, in which the patient is taught to examine and modify his/her beliefs, attitudes, and self-statements and then to apply these skills in the natural environment, is unlikely to be effective in the preadolescent years. Although such cognitive strategies are within the capabilities of many preadolescents, they usually are unable to grasp the underlying principles and apply them to new situations.

In the areas of postoperative pain and in managing sickle-cell disease pain, patient-controlled analgesia, in which the patient controls the amount of intravenous analgesic by means of a small computer-pump can be understood by late childhood or early adolescence (Schechter, Berrien, & Katz, 1988). However, as these authors have found, inappropriate stereotypes of adolescent behavior in terms of drug-seeking behavior and medical personnel's misconceptions about adolescents' ability to self-regulate their behavior may be a barrier to implementation of adequate pain relief.

Group approaches can have the advantage of being less costly and exploiting the emerging importance of the peer group to enhance therapeutic efficacy. Few studies have been done to evaluate group treatments for pain in adolescents. In a study in our laboratory, Davies (1987) found that individual and group stress management therapy were superior to a placebo control group and quite similar in effectiveness to each other. However, adolescents with more severe headache were better served in the individual format than in the group format. Treatment was a combination of cognitive and behavioral therapy using a standardized treatment manual. Muscle relaxation, use of relaxing, pleasant images, cognitive restructuring, and problem solving were among the skills taught.

Family therapy, no matter what the orientation, presents a paradoxical situation. On one hand, adolescents are struggling for independence and autonomy, and treating pain in the family context may be perceived as opposing these trends. On the other hand, adolescents are embedded in the matrix of the family and their greatest strengths and resources as well as the source of the greatest stress are often in the family. Clinically we have resolved this matter by using family therapy only for adolescents who have become handicapped in their academic and social life by pain. For the rest, the vast majority of adolescent pain sufferers, we keep the family informed and may occasionally meet with them, but do not engage in family therapy.

Self-directed treatments based on a coping model in which the patient works largely on his/her own to learn stress management skills hold great promise for adolescent pain disorders such as migraine. Stress management approaches are the treatment of choice in severe pediatric and adolescent migraine because the most widely used prophylactic medication, propranolol, is not effective (Forsythe, Gillies, & Sills, 1984). Moreover, adolescents seem to be particularly averse to the use of drugs to control pain and will frequently refuse to take adequate medication. We have had to return grant money because adolescents declined participation in prophylactic drug studies! They have been convinced by the antidrug campaigns not to use medications to solve their pain problems and fear addiction from long term drug use.

We have recently completed randomized trials evaluating self-directed treatments for adolescent (McGrath, Humphreys, Goodman, Keene, Firestone, Lascelles, Capelli, & Cunningham, 1989) and adult migraine (Richardson & McGrath, 1989). In both trials, the self-directed treatment was as successful as the clinic-based treatment but much more cost-effective. The program is now available as a package with instructions for nurses, doctors, social workers, occupational therapists, or psychologists on how to deliver this treatment (McGrath, Cunningham, Lascelles, & Humphreys, 1990). A similar self-directed program using muscle relaxation has been described by Larsson (Larsson, Daleflod, Hakansson, & Melin, 1987).

Medical treatments for pain must also be evaluated on the basis of the age of the sufferer. Unfortunately, there has been little work documenting the safety and effectiveness with adolescents of treatments that are widely used with adults. Although in many cases the assumption that adolescents are similar to adults will be true, it is impossible to know when this will not be the case. For example, propranolol is probably not effective in prophylactic treatment of migraine in adolescents (Forsythe et al., 1984) and aspirin, a common and safe treatment for adult headache, has been linked to Reye's syndrome in adolescents.

Conclusions

Adolescence is a particularly important time period in the development of pain problems and the ability to cope successfully with such problems. However, surprisingly little attention has been focused on these issues. Much more careful research and conceptual work is needed to understand the interface between the biological, psychological, and social aspects of adolescence that may impact on prevalence, maintenance, and coping with pain. Better understanding of pain in adolescence is likely to improve clinical management in this population and may provide clues to understanding and perhaps preventing the serious burden of pain in adulthood.

Acknowledgments. The authors wish to thank J. T. Goodman, R. Pilon, A. Unruh, and J. Bush for assistance. R. Flynn first drew our attention to the utility of applying the WHO classification system to pain problems.

References

American Psychiatric Association. (1987). *Diagnostic and statistical manual of mental disorders* (3rd ed., rev.). Washington, DC: American Psychiatric Association.

Aro, H. (1987). Life stress and psychosomatic symptoms among 14 to 16 year old Finnish adolescents. *Psychological Medicine, 17,* 191-201.

Aro, H. (1988). Parental discord, divorce and adolescent development. *European Archives of Psychiatric and Neurological Sciences, 237,* 106-111.

Aro, H., Paronen, O., & Aro, S. (1987). Psychosomatic symptoms among 14-16 year old Finnish adolescents. *Social Psychiatry, 22,* 171-176.

Aro, H., & Rantanen, P. (in review). Parental loss and adolescent development. In C. Chiland & J. G. Young (Eds.), *The child and his family, Vol. 9: Yearbook of the International Association for Child and Adolescent Psychiatry and Allied Professions.* New Haven, CT: Yale University Press.

Aro, H., & Taipale, V. (1987). The impact of timing of puberty on psychosomatic symptoms among fourteen to sixteen year old Finnish girls. *Child Development, 58,* 261-268.

Asington, J., Harris, P. L., & Olson, D. R. (Eds.). (1988). *Developing theories of mind.* New York: Cambridge University Press.

Bille, B. (1962). Migraine in schoolchildren. *Acta Paediatrica Scandinavica, 51*(Suppl. 136), 1-151.

Branson, S., McGrath, P. J., Craig, K. D., Rubin, S. Z., & Vair, C. (1990). Spontaneous coping strategies for coping with pain and their origins in adolescents who undergo surgery. In D. Tyler & E. Krane (Eds.), *Pediatric pain, vol. 15, Pain research and therapy* (pp. 237-245). New York: Raven Press.

Brooks-Gunn, J., & Ruble, D. N. (1983). The experience of menarche from a developmental perspective. In J. Brooks-Gunn & A. C. Petersen (Eds.), *Girls at puberty: Biological and psychosocial perspectives* (pp. 155-177). New York: Plenum Press.

Caldirola, D., Gemperle, M., Guzinski, G., Gross, R., & Doerr, H. (1984). Chronic pelvic pain as related to abdominal pain in childhood and to psychosocial disturbance in the family. In R. Rizzi & M. Visentin (Eds.), *Pain: Proceedings of the joint meeting of the European chapters of the International Association for the Study of Pain* (pp. 291-297). Padua: Piccin and Butterworths.

Commission on Professional and Hospital Activities. (1979). *The international classification of diseases, clinical modification* (9th rev.). Ann Arbor, MI: Edwards Bros.

Cooper, P. J., Bawden, H. N., Camfield, P. R., & Camfield, C. J. (1987). Anxiety and life events in childhood migraine. *Pediatrics, 79,* 999-1004.

Craig, K. D. (1986). Pain in context: Social modeling influences. In R. A. Sternbach (Ed.), *The psychology of pain* (2nd ed., pp. 67-96). New York: Raven Press.

Crossley, R. B. (1982). Hospital admissions for abdominal pain in childhood. *Journal of the Royal Society of Medicine, 75,* 772-776.

Cunningham, S. J., McGrath, P. J., Ferguson, R. E., Humphreys, P., D'Astous, J., Latter, J., Goodman, J. T., & Firestone, P. (1987). Personality and behavioral characteristics in pediatric migraine. *Headache, 27,* 16-20.

Davies, K. E. (1987). *A comparison of group versus individually administered behavioral treatment for adolescent migraine.* Unpublished doctoral dissertation, University of Manitoba.

Dunn-Geier, J., McGrath, P. J., Rourke, B. P., Latter, J., & D'Astous, J. (1986). Adolescent chronic pain: The ability to cope. *Pain, 26*, 23–32.

Elkind, D. (1970). Egocentrism in adolescence. In E. D. Evans (Ed.), *Adolescents: Readings in behavior and development* (pp. 79–92). Hinsdale, IL: Dryden Press.

Fairbank, J. C. T., Pynsent, P. B., Van Poortvliet, J. A., & Philips, H. (1984). Mechanical factors in the incidence of knee pain in adolescents and young adults. *Journal of Bone and Joint Surgery, B, 66*, 685–693.

Feldman, W., Hodgson, C., Corber, S., & Quinn, A. (1986). Health concerns and health related behavior of adolescents. *Canadian Medical Association Journal, 134*, 489–493.

Feldman, W., McGrath, P. J., Hodgson, C., Ritter, H., & Shipman, R. T. (1985). The use of dietary fiber in the management of simple idiopathic recurrent abdominal pain: Results in a prospective double-blind randomized controlled trial. *American Journal of Diseases of Children, 139*, 1216–1218.

Felice, M. E. (1983). Adolescence: General considerations. In M. D. Levine, W. B. Carey, A. C. Crocker, & R. T. Gross (Eds.), *Developmental-behavioral pediatrics* (pp. 133–149). Philadelphia: W. B. Saunders.

Forsythe, W. I., Gillies, D., & Sills, M. A. (1984). Propranolol (Inderal) in the treatment of childhood migraine. *Developmental Medicine and Child Neurology, 26*, 737–741.

Gaffney, A. (1988). How children describe pain: A study of words and analogies used by 5–14 year olds. In R. Dubner, G. F. Gebhart, & M. R. Bond (Eds.), *Proceedings of the Vth World Congress on Pain. Vol. 3, Pain research and clinical management* (pp. 341–347). Amsterdam: Elsevier.

Gaffney, A., & Dunne, E. A. (1986). Developmental aspects of children's definition of pain. *Pain, 26*, 105–117.

Gaffney, A., & Dunne, E. A. (1987). Children's understanding of the causality of pain. *Pain, 29*, 91–104.

Greene, J. W., Walker, L. S., Hickson, G., & Thompson, J. (1985). Stressful life events and somatic complaints in adolescents. *Pediatrics, 75*, 19–22.

Haber, J. D., & Roos, C. (1985). Effects of spouse abuse and/or sexual abuse in the development and maintenance of chronic pain in women. In H. L. Fields, R. Dubner, & F. Cervero (Eds.), *Advances in pain research and therapy* (vol. 9, pp. 889–895). New York: Raven Press.

Harris, L. & Associates, Inc. (1985). *The Nuprin Pain Report. Study #851017*. New York: Author.

Hibbs, B. J., Kobos, J. C., & Gonzalea, J. (1979). Effects of ethnicity, sex, and age on MMPI profiles. *Psychological Reports, 45*, 591–597.

Hodgson, C., Feldman, W., Corber, S., & Quinn, A. (1986). Adolescent health needs. II. Utilization of health care by adolescents. *Adolescence, 21*, 383–390.

King, H. A. (1984). Back pain in children. *Pediatric Clinics of North America, 31*, 1083–1095.

Kohlberg, L. (1976). Moral stages and moralization: The cognitive developmental approach. In T. Lickona (Ed.), *Moral development and behavior: Theory, research and social issues* (pp. 31–58). New York: Holt, Rinehart and Winston.

Kovar, M. G. (1982). Health status of U.S. children and use of medical care. *Public Health Reports, 97*, 3.

Larsson, B. (1988). The role of psychological, health, behavioral and medical factors in adolescent headache. *Journal of Developmental Medicine and Child Neurology*, *30*, 616–625.

Larsson, B., Daleflod, B., Hakansson, L., & Melin, L. (1987). Therapist-assisted versus self-help relaxation treatment of chronic headaches in adolescents: A school based intervention. *Journal of Child Psychology and Psychiatry*, *28*, 127–136.

Leikin, L., Firestone, P., & McGrath, P. J. (1988). Physical symptom reporting in Type A and B children. *Journal of Consulting and Clinical Psychology*, *56*, 721–726.

McGrath, P. J., Cunningham, S. J., Lascelles, M., & Humphreys, P. (1990). *Help yourself: A program for treating migraine headaches*. Ottawa: University of Ottawa Press.

McGrath, P. J., Goodman, J. T., Firestone, P., Shipman, R., & Peters, S. (1983). Recurrent abdominal pain: A psychogenic disorder? *Archives of Disease of Childhood*, *58*, 888–890.

McGrath, P. J., & Humphreys, P. (1989). Recurrent headaches in children and adolescents: Diagnosis and management. *Pediatrician*, *16*, 71–77.

McGrath, P. J., Humphreys, P., Goodman, J. T., Keene, D., Firestone, P., Lascelles, M., Capelli, M., & Cunningham, S. J. (1989). Evaluation of a self-administered treatment for adolescent migraine. *Journal of Pain and Symptom Management*, 4, S2.

McGrath, P. J., & Unruh, A. (1987). *Pain in children and adolescents: Pain research and clinical management* (Vol. 1). Elsevier: Amsterdam.

McGrath, P. J., Unruh, A. M., & Branson, S. (1990). Chronic non-malignant pain with disability. In D. Tyler & E. Krane (Eds.), *Pediatric pain, Vol. 15, Pain research and therapy* (pp. 255–271). New York: Raven Press.

Mechanic, D. (1980). The experience and reporting of common physical complaints. *Journal of Health and Social Behavior*, *21*, 146–155.

Merskey, H. (1986). Classification of chronic pain: Description of chronic pain syndromes and definition of pain terms. *Pain*, (Suppl. 3, pp. S1-S225).

Minuchin, S., Baker, L., Rosman, B., Liebman, R., Milman, L., & Todd, T. (1975). A conceptual model of psychosomatic illness in children: Family organization and family therapy. *Archives of General Psychiatry*, *32*, 1031–1038.

Naish, J. M., & Apley J. (1951). "Growing pains": A clinical study of non-arthritic limb pains in children. *Archives of Disease of Childhood*, *26*, 134–140.

Offer, D., & Offer, J. B. (1975). *From teenage to young manhood*. New York: Basic Books.

Oster, J. (1972). Recurrent abdominal pain, headache and limb pains in children and adolescents. *Pediatrics*, *50*, 429–436.

Pantell, R. H., & Goodman, B. W. (1983). Adolescent chest pain: A prospective study. *Pediatrics*, *71*, 881–887.

Pennebaker, J. W. (1982). *The psychology of physical symptoms*. New York: Springer-Verlag.

Piaget J. (1970). Piaget's theory. In P. H. Mussen (Ed.), *Carmichael's manual of child psychology* (Vol. 1, pp. 703–732). New York: Wiley.

Raymer, D., Weininger, O., & Hamilton, J. R. (1984). Psychological problems in children with abdominal pain. *Lancet*, *1*, 439–440.

Richards, M., & Petersen, A. C. (1987). Biological theoretical models of adolescent development. In V. B. Van Hasselt & M. Hersen (Eds.), *Handbook of adolescent psychology* (pp. 34–52). New York: Pergamon Press.

Richardson, G. M., & McGrath, P. J. (1989). Cognitive-behavioral therapy for migraine headaches: A minimal-therapist-contact approach versus a clinic-based approach. *Headache, 29,* 352–357.

Ross, D. M., & Ross, S. A. (1988). *Childhood pain: Current issues, research and management*. Baltimore: Urban & Schwarzenberg.

Rutter, M., Graham, P., Chadwick, O. F. D., & Yule, W. (1976). Adolescent turmoil: Fact or fiction. *Journal of Child Psychology and Psychiatry, 17,* 35–36.

Schechter, N. L., Berrien, F. B., & Katz, S. (1988). The use of patient controlled analgesia in adolescents with sickle cell pain crisis: A preliminary report. *Journal of Pain and Symptom Management, 3,* 109–113.

Sillanpaa, M. (1976). Prevalence of migraine and other headache in Finnish children starting school. *Headache, 15,* 288–290.

Sillanpaa, M. (1983a). Prevalence of headache in prepuberty. *Headache, 23,* 10–14.

Sillanpaa, M. (1983b). Changes in the prevalence of migraine and other headaches during the first seven school years. *Headache, 23,* 15–19.

Smith, M. S., Tyler, D. C., Womack, W. M., & Chen, A. C. N. (1989). Assessment and management of recurrent pain in adolescence. *Pediatrician, 16,* 85–93.

Sternbach, R. A. (1986). Survey of pain in the United States: The Nuprin Pain Report. *Clinical Journal of Pain, 2,* 49–53.

Tanner, J. M. (1962). *Growth at adolescence*. Oxford: Blackwell Scientific Publications.

World Health Organization. (1980). *International classification of impairments, disabilities and handicaps*. Geneva: World Health Organization.

Yankelovitch, D. (1974). *The new morality: A profile of American youth in the 1970's*. New York: McGraw-Hill.

Part II
Specific Pain Populations

10
Recurrent Abdominal Pain

KAY HODGES AND DANIEL J. BURBACH

Recurrent abdominal pain (RAP), as described in Apley's (1975) seminal work, refers to a constellation of symptoms characterized by at least three episodes of abdominal pain, severe enough to interfere with psychosocial functioning, over a period of at least 3 months. In addition to the patient's own distress, RAP in children and adolescents often engenders feelings of frustration among family members and treating practitioners. In fact, the difficulties of assessing, diagnosing, and treating this ailment are considerable.

Although approximately 10 to 15% of children and adolescents have RAP, less than 10% are found to have an organic illness (Apley, 1975; Oster, 1972). As many as 100 different organic diseases can cause abdominal pain, requiring considerable vigilance on the part of the primary care physician (Levine & Rappaport, 1984). The pain is episodic, with symptoms often being vague, variable in location, and often accompanied by multiple extra-gastrointestinal complaints (Liebman, 1978; Stone & Barbero, 1970). Mental health professionals often view these families as lacking psychological-mindedness and consider them difficult to treat. In fact, the word *alexithymic* has been coined to describe the marked difficulty psychosomatic patients tend to experience in their attempts to express feelings in words (Nemiah, 1977).

The parents of these children are typically very worried about the health of their child, and reassurances from treating professionals do not appear to abate their concerns. For example, Faull and Nicol (1986) found that although 58% of the surveyed mothers had taken their child with RAP to the family doctor, most reported the physician unhelpful. Patients and their families have indicated that they feel rejected when referred to mental health professionals and that they feel treated in a pejorative way, if not dismissed, when the pain is attributed to "nerves."

Despite the lack of proven treatment strategies, the literature is replete with treatment advice from experienced clinicians, easily summarized as follows: Establish a therapeutic alliance with the family, assure them of the absence of organic illness, consider a trial of increased fiber in the diet, and be sensitive to the possibility of the following intrafamilial dynamics: a somatic orientation, anxiety and stress, and enmeshed relations between mother and child.

In this chapter, we restrict our focus to functional RAP, with the intention of excluding organically based RAP (i.e., caused by a known disease). We assume that for the most part, children with RAP do in fact experience the pain they report (with the possible exception of some malingerers) and that any conceptual model of RAP must attend to somatic as well as psychosocial factors. In contrast to some authors, we do not believe that functional RAP is equivalent to somatization disorder, a psychiatric diagnosis present in the Diagnostic and Statistical Manual of Mental Disorders (DSM-III-R) (American Psychiatric Association, 1987). Empirical data appear too scant to make such an assumption, and most likely, children with RAP constitute a heterogeneous group whose symptoms change in complex ways over the course of development. In the discussion that follows, we review the literature pertinent to RAP, including developmental issues, theoretical models, relevant empirical findings, assessment strategies, and treatment considerations. After reviewing the extant literature, suggestions for future research are provided.

Developmental Issues

An understanding of pediatric RAP requires, among other things, a familiarity with normal child development and an ability to distinguish between adaptive and aberrant patterns of physical, cognitive, and psychosocial maturation. Emphasized here will be those developmental issues that not only relate to the conceptualization of this disorder, but have assessment, diagnostic, and treatment implications as well.

Epidemiologic Considerations

At the most basic level, epidemiologic data reveal important developmental trends in the incidence and prevalence of RAP over the life span. For example, in a classic study by Apley and Naish (1958), which involved the assessment of 1,000 school-aged children between the ages of 4 and 16 years, it was found that RAP occurred at a rate of approximately 10 to 12% in boys ages 5 to 10 years and generally declined thereafter. In contrast, although RAP occurred in approximately 8 to 10% of girls ages 5 to 8 years, estimates dramatically increased to a rate of approximately 30% at age 9 years, and finally dropped to a rate of approximately 12 to 15% in 11- and 12-year-olds. Few cases were observed in girls older than 12 years. In an even larger sample of 6- to 19-year-old youngsters, Oster (1972) found that although RAP occurred somewhat more frequently in girls than boys, developmental trends in the prevalence of the disorder did not occur as a function of gender. The highest prevalence of RAP was observed in children between the ages of 8 and 10 years. On the basis of these and other epidemiologic studies, it is generally thought that (a) RAP occurs in approximately 10 to 15% of all school-age children; (b) the incidence of this disorder peaks between the ages of 9 and 12 years, with substantially fewer cases occurring in children less than 5 and older than 15 years; and (c) girls are affected somewhat more frequently than boys, at a ratio of approximately 5 : 3.

Course and Prognosis

Natural history studies suggest that there are also important developmental trends in the course and prognosis of this disorder. More specifically, current data indicate that although RAP may spontaneously remit in many affected children, approximately 25 to 50% of these youngsters continue to exhibit similar symptoms in adulthood (Apley & Hale, 1973; Christensen & Mortensen, 1975; Stickler & Murphy, 1979).

In addition to its apparent persistence, RAP may also signal the emergence of a more chronic, polysymptomatic hysterical or somatization disorder. Ernst, Routh, and Harper (1984) found that children with RAP reported an increasing number and duration of somatic complaints, both of which tended to reflect more diffuse involvement of bodily systems, than youngsters with known medical illness. An earlier study by Dahl and Haahr (1969, cited by Olson, 1987) also found this pattern. They followed 116 youngsters with RAP for 1 to 10 years and discovered that in addition to the 30% who exhibited persistent abdominal pain, another 16% had developed headaches and dizziness.

RAP and Developmental Tasks

Inasmuch as the peak incidence of RAP occurs between the ages of 9 and 12 years, it has been proposed that this disorder may be related to an inability to master important developmental tasks encountered during this phase of the life span (Coleman & Levine, 1986; Ulshen & Stabler, 1984). During this age range, youngsters are expected to develop considerable physical, cognitive, and social competence, the results of which often have important consequences for identity formation (Sarnoff, 1976). Examples of relevant tasks include increasing independence from parents, developing peer relations, meeting academic challenges at school, becoming more aware of the world at large, and adopting appropriate sex roles (Senn & Solnit, 1968). In general, children who are unable to successfully master these and other challenges are considered at risk for developing feelings of inferiority and shame, poor peer relations, and psychosocial symptoms or dysfunction. Thus, for many youngsters, a developmental stage that has sometimes been characterized as a rather calm period of childhood can be a complex, uneasy, and stressful phase of the life span (Sarnoff, 1976).

Additionally, children with RAP may have tempermental characteristics that complicate attaining mastery of some developmental tasks. For example, research by Faull and Nicol (1986) revealed an unusually high prevalence of RAP (approximately 25%) in a British sample of 5- and 6-year-olds, most of whom were experiencing difficulties settling into school. A majority of affected children exhibited difficult temperaments, characterized by behavioral irregularity in girls and a tendency to withdraw from new situations in boys. At 6- to 8-month follow-up (Davison, Faull, & Nicol, 1986), most of the children's RAP symptoms had abated but their temperamental characteristics had remained stable. These results raise the question of whether these same children may be at risk for similar symptoms when confronted by future developmental stressors, especially given the stability of temperament and the persistence of RAP.

Assessment and Treatment

There is also mounting evidence that developmental issues are important in the assessment and treatment of pain-related disorders in children (Bush, 1987; Lavigne, Schulein, & Hahn, 1986a). Children's concepts of physical illness (Burbach & Peterson, 1986), and to some extent pain (Bush, 1987; Lavigne et al., 1986a), tend to develop in a manner consistent with the Piagetian theory of general cognitive development. For example, during the age span when the prevalence of RAP peaks (i.e., 7 to 9 years old), youngsters' conceptualizations of illness tend to be quite global and nonspecific, with little appreciation for specific symptoms and the ways in which psychological factors such as stress can relate to illness. At this age children also tend to rely more on internal than external cues to determine when they are sick, with more anxious children also tending to believe that sickness is a consequence of misbehavior. To some extent, this latter tendency may also contribute to denial of illness and the stoic facades that are often seen in sick children at this age, particularly boys.

Learning more about the ways in which these youngsters conceptualize, experience, and cope with RAP may assist in efforts to communicate more effectively, reduce fears and anxieties, and educate them about this disorder and specific therapeutic interventions (e.g., Brown, O'Keefe, Sanders, & Baker, 1986; Siegel & Smith, 1989). Determination of this type of information is also necessary if children are to be maximally involved in their treatment and other health-care decisions that affect them, a strategy that may help increase adherence to recommended therapeutic regimens (Bush & Davidson, 1982). In light of recent survey data suggesting that health care professionals have a limited understanding of children's illness concepts (Perrin & Perrin, 1983), increased attention to the ways in which children conceptualize illness and related issues over the course of their development appears warranted.

Toward a Theoretical Model

Theoretical models serve an important role in guiding both research and clinical endeavors. Until relatively recently, however, a theoretical model has been absent for RAP, with the exception of several unidimensional models based upon an overly simplistic dichotomy between organic and functional illness (i.e., psychosomatic, psychogenic). Given current knowledge, it would seem that any model of RAP should, at minimum (a) recognize the interplay between "body" (i.e., somatic) and "mind" (i.e., psychological); (b) include family and other environmental influences (e.g., school, peers) that mutually influence the child; (c) account for individual differences in degree of pain, according to the role that various factors play for the individual child; (d) recognize that pain behaviors (i.e., verbal and nonverbal indicators that pain is being experienced) can be shaped by behavioral conditioning; (e) account for why health services are sought by some families, but not by others; (f) include variables that have been identified by clinicians as important, but have not yet been empirically tested (i.e., the hypotheses present in the literature); and (g) account for the influence of development on the child's symptomatology and vice versa.

Perhaps the most comprehensive model to date for conceptualizing RAP was developed by Levine and Rappaport (1984), who postulated that "multiple predisposing factors" (p. 971) interact to create the symptoms of pain and modulate its severity and impact. These factors include (a) somatic predisposition, dysfunction, or disorder; (b) life-style and habit; (c) milieu and critical events; and (d) temperament and learned response patterns.

Somatic Factors

A review of the many organic diseases that cause abdominal pain is beyond the scope of this chapter; however, excellent reviews can be obtained elsewhere (Galler, Neustein, & Walker, 1980; Levine & Rappaport, 1984). We will restrict our discussion to the somatic predispositions and dysfunctional states that have been most empirically studied, apparently because they are thought potentially to play a role in the development of this disorder. They include lactase deficiency, constipation and bowel motility, irritable bowel syndrome (IBS), and autonomic dysfunction.

Lactase Deficiency

Lactase deficiency has been the most extensively researched somatic factor in RAP. In brief, lactase deficiency occurs when there are insufficient levels of lactase, an intestinal enzyme needed for the complete metabolism of lactose (milk sugar), in the gastrointestinal tract. The ingestion of lactose by lactase deficient individuals (i.e., lactose malabsorbers) produces lactose intolerance, a condition characterized by bloating, cramping, gas, constipation, loose stools, diarrhea, and at times abdominal pain. These symptoms, which differ greatly in terms of frequency, duration, and severity, usually occur within 2 hours after the ingestion of lactose.

The diagnosis of lactase deficiency is usually made on the basis of the breath hydrogen test (Galler et al., 1980). On this test, lactase deficient individuals will produce increased levels of bacterial fermentation upon ingestion of lactose due to its incomplete metabolism in the small intestine (Barr, Watkins, & Perman, 1981). Suggested treatments include reduction of milk products in the diet and commercially available enzyme products such as Lactaid. The use of milk substitutes such as yogurt and soy preparations have also been advocated. In addition, it has been suggested that a 6- to 12-month abstinence from lactose may be sufficient to allow for the occasional intake of milk without symptomatic response (Coleman & Levine, 1986).

Despite initial enthusiasm, which stemmed from findings suggesting that lactase deficiency might be of etiologic significance in as many as 30 to 40% of all cases of childhood RAP (Barr, Levine, & Watkins, 1979; Bayless & Huang, 1971; Liebman, 1979), subsequent research has been much less supportive (Christensen, 1980; Lebenthal, Rossi, Nord, & Branski, 1981; McGrath, Goodman, Firestone, Shipman, & Peters, 1983; Wald, Chandra, Fisher, Gartner, & Zitelli, 1982). In brief, these latter studies have indicated that neither the onset nor sensation of RAP is significantly associated with the presence of lactase deficiency or ingestion of lactose and consequently, that lactase deficiency probably explains only a limited number of cases of this disorder.

Constipation and Bowel Motility

According to Levine and Rappaport (1984), constipation and other less common dysfunctions of bowel motility (e.g., irritable colon) are among the most frequent somatic predispositions to RAP. Constipation can produce intermittent pain secondary to colonic distention, gas formation, and difficult passage of fecal material. The pain itself ranges from dull to cramping and tends to localize in the lower abdominal region, especially in the left lower quadrant and periumbilical area. At present, suspected etiologies include colonic spasms, often secondary to emotional stress; inefficient defecation; significantly delayed transit time; and inattention or insensitivity to the gastrocolic reflex (i.e., bodily cues indicating a need to defecate) (Coleman & Levine, 1986).

Diagnosis of constipation is usually complicated by several factors, including the often misleading nature of child and parent report, the variable symptom picture, and the fact that routine physical exams are often negative in the presence of stool retention (Barr et al., 1979; Levine & Rappaport, 1984). Consequently, it has been recommended that plain supine (postvoiding) X-rays of the abdomen be utilized in the diagnosis of constipation, especially when it is a suspected cause of RAP. Once identified, constipated children are usually treated with the use of stool softeners, laxatives, enemas, behaviorally based bowel training programs, and dietary fiber (Levine & Rappaport, 1984).

Although constipation may indeed play a causal role in RAP, less than 25% of affected youngsters experience constipation (Dimson, 1971). In addition, in their clinical work, Galler et al. (1980), have identified few children whose constipation caused their RAP. Thus, existing data suggest that constipation probably plays only a small role in the occurrence of RAP.

Irritable Bowel Syndrome

IBS usually occurs during the preschool years and early adolescence (Levine & Rapport, 1984), and is thought to be of etiologic significance in RAP approximately 10% of the time (Apley, 1975). IBS presents with a history characterized by alternating patterns of diarrhea, constipation, normal bowel movements, and abdominal pain. IBS-related pain, while usually more severe during diarrheal episodes, is similar in nature and location to constipation-related pain. Although pain is usually relieved upon passage of gas and stools, feelings of incomplete evacuation are apparently quite common (Coleman & Levine, 1986).

Despite the lack of precise etiologies, it has been proposed that the colonic functions of children with IBS may be hypersensitive to stress (Davidson, 1987). Given the multifactorial nature of IBS, recommended treatment strategies usually include reducing environmental stress, teaching affected children more effective coping and problem solving skills, stabilizing bowel habits, and a variety of dietary manipulations (e.g., increasing dietary fiber, decreasing fat intake, reducing the quantity of milk consumed). Results are often positive (Wooley, Blackwell, & Winget, 1978).

Autonomic Dysfunction

Several forms of autonomic nervous system dysfunction, including autonomic imbalance, instability, and hypersensitivity, have also been implicated in the etiology of RAP. Despite minor differences, all are based on the thesis that a constitutional sensitivity to stress can compromise the functioning of the autonomic nervous system in ways that can interfere with bowel motility and other gastrointestinal functions, which, in turn, leads to the occurrence of RAP, constipation, IBS, and other difficulties potentially mediated by the autonomic nervous system (e.g., migraine headache).

At present, experimental data relevant to the existence of autonomic dysfunction in RAP are regarded as intriguing but equivocal and difficult to interpret (Lavigne, Schulein, & Hahn, 1986b; McGrath & Feldman, 1986). For example, in an early study, Kopel, Kim, and Barbero (1967) found that when compared to controls (i.e., healthy children and children with ulcerative colitis), youngsters with RAP exhibited increased rectosigmoid motility in response to Prostigmin. This finding was thought to support the notion of autonomic hypersensitivity or a more diffuse autonomic imbalance in

RAP. Two studies have used pupillary response to cold pressor stress as a measure of autonomic reactivity. In the first (Rubin, Barbero, & Sibinga, 1967), it was found that when compared to normal controls, children with RAP exhibited increased recovery time in pupillary response. In the second (Apley, Haslam, & Tulloh, 1971), although investigators failed to replicate the findings of Rubin et al. (1967), children with RAP appeared to experience a more "unstable" recovery in pupillary response than healthy controls. Although "unstable" was insufficiently defined, this latter finding was thought to support a more general autonomic instability in RAP. In a more recent and methodologically rigorous study by Feuerstein, Barr, Francoeur, Houle, and Rafman (1982) that also involved the use of cold pressor stress, the autonomic, somatic, subjective, and behavioral responses of youngsters with RAP were compared to those of children in carefully matched hospital and normal control groups. Although cold pressor stimulation resulted in significant arousal in all domains assessed, significant group differences were not observed. Given the equivocal nature of current data, clinical reliance on autonomic measures in the diagnosis of RAP is probably premature.

Psychological Factors and Personality

Based on the clinical literature, the major hypothesis regarding children with RAP is that they are "high strung" or anxiety prone (Apley, 1975; Stone & Barbero, 1970), an observation that has been supported by the empirical literature (Hodges, Kline, Barbero, & Woodruff, 1985; Walker & Greene, 1989a). However, these children do not appear more anxious than children with organic gastrointestinal (GI) illness (Walker & Greene, 1991) or frank psychiatric disturbance (Hodges, Kline, Barbero, & Woodruff, 1985). Together, these findings indicate that although children with RAP seeking health care are more anxious than healthy children, they are no more anxious than other youngsters seeking medical and/or psychiatric care for their respective difficulties.

The presence of depression has also been examined in four studies (Hodges, Kline, Barbero, & Flanery, 1985; McGrath et al., 1983; Raymer, Weininger, & Hamilton, 1984; Walker & Greene, 1989). Only in Walker and Greene (1989) did the children with RAP report more depressive symptoms than healthy controls. However, their overall level of depression was not different than that of the comparison organic group.

In addition to the above, the prevalence of concomitant DSM-III diagnoses among children with RAP has been investigated by Wasserman, Whitington, and Rivara (1988) and by Astrada, Licamele, Walsh, and Kessler (1981). Unfortunately, neither had a control group for the diagnostic interviews, and the sample for Astrada et al. (1981) was a select group of children referred for psychiatric evaluation. In both studies, far more children were given anxiety diagnoses (i.e., 30% and 32%) than diagnoses of depression (i.e., 11% and 9%). Thus, based on both a self-report questionnaire and clinical interview data, the majority of the RAP patients appear to have some type of underlying anxiety, whereas perhaps a smaller portion are found to have heightened depressive symptoms. Longitudinal studies are now needed to determine whether the symptomatology of these children change with development and whether other variables, such as gender, shape the course of RAP.

In both of the above diagnostic studies, it is also noteworthy that RAP patients met DSM-III criteria for one of the somatoform disorders (i.e., conversion disorder, hypochondriasis, somatization disorder, or psychogenic pain disorder [the latter changed to somatoform pain disorder in DSM-III-R]). Other data, based on symptom checklist (Walker & Greene, 1989) and on retrospective review of medical charts (Ernst et al., 1984), also suggest that RAP children may be more likely to develop somatization disorder. Although this may be borne out by longitudinal studies, making the diagnosis of somatization disorder in RAP patients is somewhat complex.

In fact, there are no criteria for somatization disorder for children and adolescents in DSM-III-R (Shapiro & Rosenfeld, 1987). Furthermore, many of the RAP children would meet formal diagnostic criteria for this disorder by the very nature of their RAP-related symptomatology. However, they would not necessarily have the associated features included in the informal description of the disorder, and the disorder is considered rare in children and adolescents (Regan & Regan, 1989). Also, careful differential diagnosis is obviously important as physical symptoms are commonly associated with other psychiatric diagnoses, and, in fact, serve as criteria for several other psychiatric disorders (i.e., overanxious disorder, separation anxiety).

Stress and Life-Style Factors

In the clinical literature, an association between RAP and life stress has been frequently noted (e.g., MacKeith & O'Neill, 1951). Several studies have used the Coddington (1972) life events measure to compare RAP and various control groups, including healthy children, psychiatric outpatients, children with Crohn's disease, and children with ulcer-related disorders (Hodges, Kline, Barbero, & Flanery, 1984; McGrath et al., 1983; Raymer et al., 1984; Walker & Greene, 1991; Wasserman et al., 1988).

Only one study (Hodges et al., 1984) found a significant difference, with the RAP group reporting more events as well as more stress compared to healthy controls, but not significantly more than psychiatric outpatients. When type of event was examined, illness, death, and hospitalization primarily distinguished the RAP group from the control group, as well as the psychiatric group. Wasserman et al. (1988) also found significant effects for specific events (i.e., hospitalization of the child, hospitalization of the parent, and death of a grandparent), even though there was no main effect for diagnostic group. Walker and Greene (1991) found that over a 3-month period, level of life stress was significantly related to symptom resolution for RAP patients, but not organic controls. Higher levels of stress predicted poorer outcomes for the RAP group. The above studies offer some support for the clinical observation that children with RAP report stress from life events, especially illness and death-related events. However, a stronger relationship might be expected given the data suggesting that utilization of health services is usually associated with stress (Beautrais, Fergusson, & Shannon, 1982; Gortmaker, Eckenrode, & Gore, 1982; Tessler, Mechanic, & Dimond, 1976). In this regard, Gortmaker et al. (1982) have found that information on daily stresses as well as life events independently affected service utilization, with each tapping qualitatively different types of stresses. Daily stresses associated with school and peer relationships may be good predictors for RAP children, in light of the clinical data indicating frequent school absences and poor social skills (Apley, 1975; Faull & Nicol, 1986; Hughes & Zimin, 1978). Moreover, the ratio of stress to personal resources or coping skills may be more important, to a certain point, than the absolute amount of life stress.

Almost no attention has been focused on life-style and habit variables as described by Levine and Rappaport (1984). These authors have proposed that (a) an enjoyable life probably contributes to building a higher pain threshold, whereas the opposite may be true for children living more empty lives; (b) poor bowel habits, which can lead to painful constipation, may result from a frantic life-style or poor teaching; and (c) patients are inattentive to their diet, consuming foods that obviously exacerbate painful episodes (e.g., fatty foods in IBS). Levine and Rappaport (1984) appear to be referring in part to preventative efforts that can be undertaken by the patient. This is consistent with the recent emphasis in our culture on educating the public about life-style variables that can have a powerful effect on long-term health. In any case, this area is one that appears ripe for further research, especially regarding a psychoeducational model of treatment that helps patients and their families understand the nature and course of chronic abdominal pain and provides them with insight into how painful episodes may be minimized.

Family-Related Factors

In this section, we present clinical hypotheses and empirical findings regarding the association between family variables and RAP. We will emphasize several areas of research, including (a) psychological functioning of the parents, (b) learning of a somatic orientation through modeling and/or operant reinforcement, and (c) interpersonal dynamics within the family.

Psychological Functioning of the Parents

Two studies have assessed maternal depressive and anxiety symptomatology (Hodges, Kline, Barbero, & Flanery, 1985; Hodges, Kline, Barbero, & Woodruff, 1985; Walker & Greene, 1989), and a third examined depression only (Zuckerman, Stevenson, & Bailey, 1987). There were positive findings in all three studies, although elevated symptomatology was not unique to the RAP group. Mothers of the RAP group reported more symptoms of depression and anxiety than control mothers. However, they did not differ from mothers of behaviorally disordered children (Hodges, Kline, Barbero, & Flanery, 1985; Hodges, Kline, Barbero, & Woodruff, 1985) or an organic group (Walker & Greene, 1989). In the Zuckerman et al. (1987) study of mothers of preschoolers, recurrent stomachaches were associated with maternal depression, serious health problems, and marital problems. These authors suggested that preschool children may more readily obtain attention from a depressed mother if they present with somatic complaints, which further reinforces the symptoms. In any case, this research suggests that RAP may be related to an interaction among variables related to maternal well-being (i.e., depressive feelings, preoccupation with one's own health, and/or marital problems).

In addition to the maternal variables, Hodges, Kline, Barbero, and Woodruff (1985) found that the fathers of RAP children reported more anxiety than the fathers of psychiatric outpatients and the fathers of control children. However, they did not report more depression (Hodges, Kline, Barbero, & Flanery, 1985). There were no significant findings for the fathers in Walker and Greene's (1989) study.

Learning of Chronic Illness Behavior

Social learning refers to the modeling of behaviors relative to pain, either the modeling of pain complaints or the modeling of coping with pain (McGrath & Feldman, 1986). Violon and Giurgea (1984) conceptualized this as unwittingly teaching the child to respond to life stresses in a somatic way, resulting in aggravation or exaggeration of pain. In contrast, operant conditioning of pain results from direct or indirect positive reinforcement and failure to reinforce nonpain responses.

Modeling of a somatizing orientation could take the form of modeling of pain perception (i.e., threshold at which attention is given to pain), reporting of pain, and/or nonverbal or verbal behaviors displayed when experiencing pain (Lavigne et al., 1986b). There are considerable data indicating that the parents and relatives of children with RAP tend to have somatic symptomatology, which could be indicative of biological and/or environmental transmission (Apley & Naish, 1958; Oster, 1972; Routh & Ernst, 1984). Furthermore, Apley and Hale (1973) found that having parents with somatic complaints is an indicator of a poor prognosis in RAP. Studies of parent behavior or parent-child interactions around pain management could be conducted, examining a variety of dimensions such as (a) parents with and without maladaptive pain behavior (e.g., adult back pain patients), (b) parents of children who are high versus low health care utilizers, and (c) parents of children who have high versus low levels of symptomatology or functional disability.

Very little attention has been given to the potential role of operant reinforcement in modifying the consequences of abdominal pain. This reinforcement of chronic illness behavior may involve reinforcement of actual behaviors (verbal and nonverbal), reinforcement for attending to health issues, or reinforcement of cognitive processes that "catastrophize" the experience of pain (Lavigne et al., 1986b). Two studies have demonstrated that operant techniques can reduce complaints of RAP (Miller & Kratochwill, 1979; Sank & Biglan, 1974).

In the adult literature, it has been shown that people with IBS, compared to those with peptic ulcer and the population in general, are characterized by more chronic illness behavior (defined as having multiple somatic complaints, frequent utilization of health services, and avoidance of work or social obligations because of illness) (Whitehead, Winget, Fedoravicius, Wooley, & Blackwell, 1982). In a study of adolescents with chronic nonabdominal pain, Dunn-Geier, McGrath, Rourke, Latter, and D'Astous (1986) found that the mothers of children who missed school, compared to mothers of children who missed very little school, often made comments discouraging coping. Studies similar to Dunn-Geier et al. (1986), as well as studies assessing children's self-statements during pain experiences, would also generate information about the role of operant pain in RAP.

Family Dynamics

With the exception of a study by Wasserman et al. (1988), which indicated no significant differences between a RAP group and matched controls on the Family Environment Scale (FES: Moos & Moos, 1981), there are no empirical studies assessing the family dynamics of children with RAP. However, the clinical literature suggests that these families are characterized by maternal overprotectiveness, interpersonal tensions between parents, and excessively anxious parents who are preoccupied with the child's state of health (Apley, 1975; Hughes & Zimin, 1978; Liebman, 1978; Stone & Barbero, 1970; Zuckerman et al., 1987). These characteristics are similar to those identified by Minuchin et al. (1975) in the families of children with psychosomatic illness (i.e., enmeshment, overprotectiveness, lack of conflict resolution, and rigidity). In the chronic illness literature, maternal behavior similar to overprotectiveness was observed in recently diagnosed diabetic children (Hauser et al., 1986) and in families in which the child coped poorly with his pain (Dunn-Geier et al., 1986). Longitudinal studies that follow families after their first diagnostic workup and observe family interaction patterns of good and poor copers would help identify family prognostic indicators.

Assessment and Measurement Issues

Pain

Most experts agree that the assessment of RAP, like any pain syndrome, must begin with a complete medical evaluation both to rule out the presence of unlikely organic disease and to identify somatic factors that may be of etiologic significance (Coleman & Levine, 1986; Galler et al., 1980; Levine & Rappaport, 1984). The evaluation typically includes a careful history, a thorough physical exam, and limited laboratory studies, including an analysis of blood and urine and the testing of stools for parasites and ova. Although most organic causes of RAP can be identified at this initial phase of the evaluation, additional workup is necessary if questions of organic involvement remain.

A thorough behavioral assessment of the child's pain is also recommended, as pain is a subjective experience that is frequently unrelated to the nature, extent, and severity of organic involvement (Katz, Varni, & Jay, 1984). This is especially true in RAP where organic disease and dysfunction are rarely identified (Masek, Russo, & Varni, 1984). As a result, it is important to identify nonorganic factors that might contribute to, maintain, or exacerbate RAP, either in isolation or in concert with important somatic factors. The existing literature suggests that the behavioral assessment of RAP should include at minimum an evaluation of observable responses as well as internal experiences. Unfortunately, as our earlier summary indicated, data generated using psychophysiologic procedures are often equivocal and difficult to interpret and consequently, their clinical value remains unclear at this point (Lavigne et al., 1986a).

Observable Responses

Observable pain responses in RAP have been assessed with indirect measures and behavioral observation scales. Several indirect measures of RAP have been reported in the literature including days absent from school, requests to attend the school sick room, and presence in the school sick room (Sanders et al., 1989; Sank & Biglan, 1974), all of which seem to be sensitive to changes in symptomatology.

Behavioral observation scales, which are generally thought to yield the most valid and reliable data regarding pain behavior in children (Katz et al., 1984), are used to document the occurrence of operationally defined pain-related behaviors in specific situations during specified time intervals. The pain observation record used by Sanders and his colleagues (Sanders et al., 1989) provides an excellent example of how behavioral observation methods can be utilized in the assessment of RAP. The mothers were instructed to record the presence or absence of specified behaviors using time-sampling procedures (i.e., observations occurred in 1-hour time blocks both before and after the child attended school) over a 12-week period. Specific behaviors identified included pain complaints, requests for assistance, crying, and various nonverbal pain behaviors (e.g., rubbing, grimacing, sighing). In another study (Feuerstein et al., 1982), facial expressions were used to measure the intensity of pain in RAP and non-RAP children. In both studies, these measures were found to be quite reliable.

Internal Experiences

Although a variety of methods have been developed to assess the subjective experience of pain in children (Bush, 1987; Katz et al., 1984; Lavigne et al., 1986a; Masek et al., 1984), few have been employed in the assessment of RAP. However, measures that have been successfully used include Likert-type scales (Feuerstein et al., 1982; Sank & Biglan, 1974), visual analogue scales (Sanders et al., 1989), and diaries (McGrath, 1983). These have yielded valuable information relevant to the most important dimensions of RAP, including location, quality, frequency, and duration of pain as well as associated symptoms, alleviating factors, and exacerbating variables (McGrath, 1983). As such, these measures hold much promise for investigators in their attempts to delineate more homogeneous subgroups of RAP patients and assess progress.

Psychosocial Functioning

Similar to the medical evaluation, it seems appropriate to proceed in a graduated fashion with the psychosocial assessment, using progressively deeper probes as needed to answer pertinent questions. Early in this process, it seems wise to explain to patients and their families that (a) it is known that there is an interactive relationship between the body and mind, and (b) sometimes psychological interventions can help reduce symptoms, even when the pain is not caused by psychological factors.

In the first level of assessment, it is our persuasion that the focus should be on factors that may contribute to preoccupation with RAP. Such factors include the child's personality, the child and parents' beliefs about the child's abdominal pain and about health maintenance in general, potential secondary gains, and exogenous stress.

The assessment of personality disposition, especially the child's tendency to be a "worrier," appears important given research that shows that children with RAP tend to be anxious. This can be accomplished by using one of the anxiety symptom questionnaires (e.g., the State Trait Anxiety Inventory for Children; Spielberger, 1973). Informal questioning or structured interviews, such as the worry and fears sections of the Child Assessment Schedule (CAS: Hodges, Kline, Stern, Cytryn, & McKnew, 1982) can also be used. The CAS has been used successfully in research with psychosomatic and anxiety-disordered children (Hodges, Kline, Barbero, & Woodruff, 1985; Turner, Beidel, & Costello, 1987). In fact, it was originally developed for use with pediatric RAP patients because more traditional psychiatric measures did not inquire about many of the worries and concerns of these children.

It is also important to inquire into the child's and parents' beliefs about the current illness, their general expectations about their ability to influence the quality of their health (i.e., health locus of control), and their strategies for coping with pain. Additionally, interviewing the parents about the child's pain behaviors and their responses to these nonverbal and verbal behaviors may have implications for treatment and prevention. Inquiry can be made about the child's pain behaviors, what seems to increase or decrease the pain, others' responses to the child's expressions of pain, and child or family activities that are interrupted as a result of illness episodes (Fordyce, 1976).

Life events and associated stresses can be evaluated by informal interview or by one of the available life events inventories (e.g., Coddington, 1972). Understanding the subjective impact of the event (i.e., intensity and valence) and whether it represents a recent change for the child appear to be important. Within this domain, the practitioner should be alert to the possibility that two factors may be of particular importance, school avoidance and sexual abuse, neither of which is likely to be spontaneously reported. Given that children who have been sexually abused often report abdominal pain as well as other somatic symptoms (Rimsza, Berg, & Locke, 1988), it is important to keep this in mind in the evaluation of both males and females. Also, maintaining school attendance is an important part of treatment.

Further assessment focusing on the child's psychological functioning may be indicated if the family continues to seek services because previous treatment has been unsuccessful, or if the clinician is concerned about the child's adjustment. A typical assessment battery might include a diagnostic interview, a self-esteem measure, and an evaluation of the child's cognitive abilities. The goal would be to determine the extent and type of psychological and intellectual deficits (and assets) and to identify treatment needs.

In both clinical and research settings, there is considerable advantage to using one of the structured diagnostic interviews, particularly for the assessment of psychiatric disorders (for a review of these interviews, see Edelbrock & Costello, 1988; Hodges & Cools, 1990). Given the poor parent-child concordance found for internalizing disorders (i.e., anxiety and depression), it is important to interview the child directly even when the parent is interviewed (see Achenbach, McConaughy, & Howell, 1987; Hodges, Gordon, & Lennon, 1990).

Obtaining a measure of the child's self-esteem or perceived competence across various spheres of functioning (e.g., school, social) can also help the practitioner evaluate the child's strengths and weaknesses as well as the degree to which the child is realistic about him/herself. In a study using the measure developed by Harter (1985), anxiety-disordered children were found to have expectations of themselves that far exceeded their own self-reported competence level (Hodges, 1989). Additionally, intellectual and academic testing may be indicated if the child is avoidant of school, has frequent absences, or appears to have learning difficulties. A questionnaire completed by the teacher about the child's behavior is also desirable.

A third and final level of psychosocial assessment should involve a more in-depth evaluation of the family context. This would be indicated if the child appears poorly adjusted or if the dynamics observed in the family appear dysfunctional enough to render the child vulnerable to other anomalies. Inquiry about the family might include an interview with the parents about their own and extended family members' psychiatric history; screening measures to assess depression and anxiety in the parents; inquiry about life stresses, including marital discord; and assessment of the family dynamics via informal or formal observation.

Treatment Studies

The treatment of RAP is currently based upon the experiences and biases of individual practitioners because there have been few methodologically sound empirical studies. Three single case studies involving behaviorally based interventions utilizing operant strategies (Sank & Biglan, 1974), time-out procedures (Miller & Kratochwill, 1979), and covert positive reinforcement (Wasserman, 1978) have all reported positive results. In another case study (Linton, 1986), treatment emphasizing the use of relaxation and coping skills was successful in reducing the RAP of an adolescent female. In our review, we found only two well-controlled treatment studies. Sanders' et al. (1989) cognitive-behavioral treatment package, consisting of differential reinforcement of well behavior, coping skills training, and generalization/relapse prevention techniques, resulted in significant improvements in a sample of pediatric RAP patients relative to nontreatment controls. With respect to somatic factors, Feldman, McGrath, Hodgson, Ritter, and Shipman (1985) conducted a prospective, randomized, double-blind, placebo-controlled study of 52 youngsters with RAP. Approximately twice as many children given 10 mg/day of dietary fiber experienced 50% fewer painful episodes than those given dietary placebo. As such, this study suggests that although the etiology of RAP may indeed be multifactorial in nature, a treatment approach based solely on somatic factors may be useful and bring relief to many patients. However, it is important to emphasize that although a somatic approach may be efficacious for a patient this does not necessarily imply that the etiology itself is totally somatic in nature.

Although there is little research data on treatment efficacy, the empirical data base that has been accumulated on RAP provides sufficient guidance for the development of treatment protocols. Some of the various treatments that could be compared include (a) a psychoeducational approach, which could be developed from Apley and Hale (1973) and Apley and MacKeith (1968); (b) a pain management program, similar to that described by McGrath (1987) for headaches; (c) cognitive-behavioral intervention for managing anxiety, with particular attention to anxiety related to health and death issues; (d) family therapy, along the lines presented in Haggerty (1983); and (e) somatic remedies, such as increased dietary fiber.

Suggestions for Future Research

Current research in the area of pediatric RAP has the methodological flaws typically found in the preliminary stages of investigation, including failure to (a) use comparison groups, (b) match groups on important variables, (c) operationalize the diagnostic criteria for RAP beyond the general guidelines provided by Apley (1975), (d) establish reliability of diagnostic procedures and of inquiry into the child's physical symptomatology, and (e) use blind procedures or other procedures (e.g., standardized formats) that help minimize observer bias and expectancy effects. In particular, operationalization of diagnostic criteria for RAP and development of psychometrically sound measures to assess the criteria will result in better opportunities for collaborative studies and more systematic growth of accumulative knowledge about RAP. An example is the Walker-Greene Functional Disability Inventory (Walker & Greene, 1988), which has been successfully used with RAP patients to assess disruption of normal physical and social activity.

With these methodological improvements, we can proceed to study important, remaining questions about children with RAP and their families. Several of the more salient questions are:

How do children for whom help services are sought differ from those who are not taken to the doctor?   Research with adult IBS patients has found that only a minority of IBS sufferers seek health care services at all, and those who do differ from those who do not (Sandler, Drossman, Nathan, & McKee, 1984; Thompson & Heaton, 1980).

What are the important predictors of outcome?   Outcome can be assessed by numerous variables such as chronicity and severity of abdominal pain as well as non-GI symptoms, psychological functioning, functional disability (e.g., school attendance), health care services utilization, and impact of the illness on the other family members. Given the empirical findings, predictors might include degree of trait anxiety in the child, history of family life events related to illness and death, mono- versus polysymptomatic presentation, extent of parental somatic symptomatology, and parental stress and psychological functioning. Based on the untested hypotheses that have been generated from the clinical literature on RAP, other predictors might include (a) stressfulness associated with expectations placed on the child relative to academic and social developmental tasks (i.e., competence relative to expectations), (b) general coping skills as well as specific coping skills for managing pain, and (c) parental behavior relevant to pain management. It is important to determine if these findings are unique to children with RAP and their families. Do they also apply to children who are organically ill, who have pain-free conditions, who have other "functional" symptom presentations (e.g., headaches), or who experience high levels of stress (e.g., psychiatrically disordered)?

What are the mediating variables involved in the impact of parental responses on the child's ability to manage pain? The relative role of operant reinforcement and modeling of pain management behavior needs to be addressed. Furthermore, family therapists would question whether changes in parental responses would remain stable unless other changes in the family system are made (e.g., mother can only give up her preoccupation with the child by reinvesting her psychic energy some place else, such as her husband or other activities).

Does the course of the illness vary as a function of age (or developmental stage), gender, or age of onset of symptomatology? Are the predictors differentially related to outcome as a function of these variables? Based on their long-term follow-up review of treated and untreated patients, Apley and Hale (1973) observed that there was a better prognosis for females and for children with an onset after 6 years of age. Walker and Greene (1991) found that being female was associated with higher symptomatology at 3-month follow-up.

What is the treatment efficacy of various approaches and is treatment efficacy improved by matching patient/family characteristics with type of treatment? Are combinations of treatment approaches more effective than single modality approaches? Does the length of time between onset of symptoms and the initiation of treatment affect treatment efficacy?

Conclusions

Although pediatric RAP has not received as much systematic attention as many of the other pain-related syndromes discussed in this volume, it is clear that this disorder is a significant and common malady affecting the lives of many children and families and the work of practitioners. Given its multifactorial nature, RAP offers a multitude of challenges to both clinicians and researchers, many of which were identified here. To meet these challenges, it is necessary to consider not only the individual and interactive effects of somatic, psychological, and environmental factors in RAP but also the ways in which these phenomena relate to developmental variables over the life span. With such a knowledge base, it will be possible to delineate more useful models for assessment and treatment of this disorder, with the ultimate goal of improving the quality of life for these children and their families.

References

Achenbach, T., McConaughy, S., & Howell, C. (1987). Child/adolescent behavioral and emotional problems: Implications of cross informant correlations for situational specificity. *Psychological Bulletin, 10*, 213–237.

American Psychiatric Association. (1987). *Diagnostic and statistical manual of mental disorders* (rev. 3rd ed.). Washington, DC: American Psychiatric Association.

Apley, J. (1975). *The child with abdominal pains* (2nd ed.). Oxford: Blackwell Scientific Publications.

Apley, J., & Hale, B. (1973). Children with recurrent abdominal pain: How do they grow up? *British Medical Journal, 3*, 7–9.

Apley, J., Haslam, D., & Tulloh, C. (1971). Pupillary reaction in children with recurrent abdominal pain. *Archives of Diseases of Childhood, 46*, 337–340.

Apley, J., & MacKeith, R. (1968). *The child and his symptoms: A comprehensive approach* (2nd ed.). Oxford: Blackwell Scientific Publications.

Apley, J., & Naish, N. (1958). Recurrent abdominal pains: A field survey of 1,000 school children. *Archives of Diseases of Childhood, 33*, 165–170.

Astrada, C., Licamele, W., Walsh, T., & Kessler, E. (1981). Recurrent abdominal pain in children and associated DSM-III diagnoses. *American Journal of Psychiatry, 138*, 687–688.

Barr, R., Levine, M., & Watkins, J. (1979). Recurrent abdominal pain of childhood due to lactose intolerance. *New England Journal of Medicine, 300*, 1449–1459.

Barr, R., Watkins, J., & Perman, J. (1981). Mucosal function and breath hydrogen excretion: Comparative studies in the clinical evaluation of children with nonspecific abdominal complaints. *Pediatrics, 68*, 526.

Bayless, T., & Huang, S. S. (1971). Recurrent abdominal pain due to milk and lactose intolerance in school-age children. *Pediatrics, 47*, 1029–1032.

Beautrais, A., Fergusson, D., & Shannon, F. (1982). Life events and childhood morbidity: A prospective study. *Pediatrics, 70*, 935–940.

Brown, J., O'Keefe, J., Sanders, S., & Baker, B. (1986). Developmental change in children's cognition to stressful and painful situations. *Journal of Pediatric Psychology, 11*, 343–357.

Burbach, D., & Peterson, L. (1986). Children's concepts of physical illness: A review and critique of the cognitive developmental literature. *Health Psychology, 5*, 307–325.

Bush, J. (1987). Pain in children: A review of the literature from a developmental perspective. *Psychology and Health, 1*, 215–236.

Bush, P., & Davidson, F. (1982). Medicine and drugs: What do children think? *Health Education Quarterly, 2*, 209–223.

Christensen, M. (1980). Prevalence of lactose intolerance in children with recurrent abdominal pain. *Pediatrics, 65*, 681.

Christensen, M., & Mortensen, O. (1975). Long-term prognosis in children with recurrent abdominal pain. *Archives of Diseases of Childhood, 50*, 110–114.

Coddington, R. (1972). The significance of life events as etiologic factors in the diseases of children: II. A study of normal population. *Journal of Psychosomatic Research, 16*, 205–213.

Coleman, W., & Levine, M. (1986). Recurrent abdominal pain: The cost of the aches and the aches of the cost. *Pediatrics in Review, 8*, 143–151.

Davidson, M. (1987). Functional problems associated with colonic dysfunction. *Pediatric Annals, 16*, 776–795.

Davison, I. S., Faull, C., & Nicol, A. R. (1986). Research note: Temperament and behaviour in six-year-olds with recurrent abdominal pain: A follow up. *Journal of Child Psychology and Psychiatry, 27*, 539–544.

Dimson, S. (1971). Transit time related to clinical findings in children with recurrent abdominal pain. *Pediatrics, 47*, 666.

Dunn-Geier, B., McGrath, P. J., Rourke, B., Latter, J., & D'Astous, J. (1986). Adolescent chronic pain: The ability to cope. *Pain, 26*, 23–32.

Edelbrock, C., & Costello, A. (1988). Structured psychiatric interviews for children. In M. Rutter, A. Tuma, & I. Lann (Eds.), *Assessment and diagnosis in child psychopathology* (pp. 87–112). New York: Guilford.

Ernst, A., Routh, D., & Harper, D. (1984). Abdominal pain in children and symptoms of somatization disorder. *Journal of Pediatric Psychology, 9*, 77–86.

Faull, C., & Nicol, A. (1986). Abdominal pain in six-year-olds: An epidemiological study in a new town. *Journal of Child Psychology and Psychiatry, 27*, 251–260.

Feldman, W., McGrath, P. J., Hodgson, C., Ritter, H., & Shipman, R. (1985). The use of dietary fiber in the management of simple, childhood, idiopathic, recurrent, abdominal pain. *American Journal of Diseases in Childhood, 139*, 1216–1218.

Feuerstein, M., Barr, R., Francoeur, E., Houle, M., & Rafman, S. (1982). Potential biobehavioral mechanisms of recurrent abdominal pain in children. *Pain, 13*, 287–298.

Fordyce, W. (1976). Behavioral concepts in chronic pain and illness. In P. Davidson (Ed.), *The behavioral management of anxiety, depression, and pain* (pp. 147–188). New York: Brunner/Mazel.

Galler, J., Neustein, S., & Walker, W. (1980). Clinical aspects of recurrent abdominal pain in children. *Advances in Pediatrics, 27*, 31–53.

Gortmaker, S., Eckenrode, J., & Gore, S. (1982). Stress and the utilization of health services: A time series and cross-sectional analysis. *Journal of Health and Social Behavior, 23*, 25–38.

Haggerty, J. (1983). The psychosomatic family: An overview. *Psychosomatics, 24*, 615–623.

Harter, S. (1985). *The Self-Perception Profile for Children: Revision of the Perceived Competence Scale for Children Manual*. Denver: University of Denver.

Hauser, S., Jacobson, A., Wertlieb, D., Weiss-Perry, B., Follansbee, D., Wolfsdorf, J., Herskowitz, R., Houlihan, J., & Rajapark, D. (1986). Children with recently diagnosed diabetes: Interactions with their families. *Health Psychology, 5*, 273–296.

Hodges, K. (1989). *Self-perceived competence in anxiety, affective and conduct disordered children*. Unpublished manuscript.

Hodges, K., & Cools, J. (1990). Structured diagnostic interviews. In A. M. LaGreca (Ed.), *Through the eyes of the child: Obtaining self-reports from children and adolescents* (pp. 109–149). Boston: Allyn and Bacon.

Hodges, K., Gordon, Y., & Lennon, M. (1990). Parent-child agreement on symptoms assessed via a clinical research interview for children: The Child Assessment Schedule (CAS). *Journal of Child Psychology and Psychiatry, 31*, 427–436.

Hodges, K., Kline, J., Barbero, G., & Flanery, R. (1984). Life events occurring in families of children with recurrent abdominal pain. *Journal of Psychosomatic Research, 28,* 185–188.

Hodges, K., Kline, J., Barbero, G., & Flanery, R. (1985). Depressive symptoms in children with recurrent abdominal pain and in their families. *Journal of Pediatrics, 107,* 622–626.

Hodges, K., Kline, J., Barbero, G., & Woodruff, C. (1985). Anxiety in children with recurrent abdominal pain and their parents. *Psychosomatics, 26,* 859–866.

Hodges, K., Kline, J., Stern, L., Cytryn, L., & McKnew, D. (1982). The development of a child assessment interview for research and clinical use. *Journal of Abnormal Child Psychology, 10,* 173–189.

Hughes, M., & Zimin, R. (1978). Children with psychogenic abdominal pain and their families. *Clinical Pediatrics, 17,* 569–573.

Katz, E. R., Varni, J. W., & Jay, S. M. (1984). Behavioral assessment and management of pediatric pain. *Progress in Behavior Modification, 18,* 163–193.

Kopel, F., Kim, I., & Barbero, G. (1967). Comparison of rectosigmoid motility in normal children, children with recurrent abdominal pain, and children with ulcerative colitis. *Pediatrics, 39,* 539–545.

Lavigne, J., Schulein, M., & Hahn, Y. (1986a). Psychological aspects of painful medical conditions in children. I. Developmental aspects and assessment. *Pain, 27,* 133–146.

Lavigne, J., Schulein, M., & Hahn, Y. (1986b). Psychological aspects of painful medical conditions in children: II. Personality factors, family characteristics and treatment. *Pain, 27,* 147–169.

Lebenthal, E., Rossi, R., Nord, K., & Branski, D. (1981). Recurrent abdominal pain and lactose absorption in children. *Pediatrics, 67,* 828–832.

Levine, M., & Rappaport, L. (1984). Recurrent abdominal pain in school children: The loneliness of the long-distance physician. *Pediatric Clinics of North America, 31,* 969–991.

Liebman, W. (1978). Recurrent abdominal pain in children: A retrospective survey of 119 patients. *Clinical Pediatrics, 17,* 149–153.

Liebman, W. (1979). Recurrent abdominal pain in children: Lactose and sucrose intolerance, a prospective study. *Pediatrics, 64,* 43–45.

Linton, S. J. (1986). A case study of the behavioral treatment of chronic stomach pain in a child. *Behavior Change, 3,* 70–73.

MacKeith, R., & O'Neill, D. (1951). Recurrent abdominal pain in children. *Lancet, ii,* 278–282.

Masek, B., Russo, D., & Varni, J. (1984). Behavioral approaches to the management of chronic pain in children. *Pediatric Clinics of North America, 31,* 1113–1131.

McGrath, P. A. (1987). The multidimensional assessment and management of recurrent pain syndromes in children. *Behaviour Research and Therapy, 25,* 251–262.

McGrath, P. J. (1983). Psychological aspects of recurrent abdominal pain. *Canadian Family Physician, 29,* 1655–1659.

McGrath, P. J., & Feldman, W. (1986). Clinical approach to recurrent abdominal pain in children. *Developmental and Behavioral Pediatrics, 7,* 56–61.

McGrath, P. J., Goodman, J., Firestone, P., Shipman, R., & Peters, S. (1983). Recurrent abdominal pain: A psychogenic disorder? *Archives of Diseases of Childhood, 58,* 888–890.

Miller, A., & Kratochwill, T. (1979). Reduction of frequent stomach complaints by time out. *Behavior Therapy, 10,* 211–218.

Minuchin, S., Baker, L., Rosman, B., Liebman, R., Milman, L., & Todd, T. (1975). A conceptual model of psychosomatic illness in children. *Archives of General Psychiatry, 32*, 1031–1038.

Moos, R., & Moos, B. (1981). *Family Environment Scale manual*. Palo Alto, CA: Consulting Psychologists Press.

Nemiah, J. (1977). Alexithymia: Theoretical considerations. *Psychotherapy and Psychosomatics, 28*, 199–206.

Olson, A. (1987). Recurrent abdominal pain: An approach to diagnosis and management. *Pediatric Annals, 16*, 834–842.

Oster, J. (1972). Recurrent abdominal pain, headache and limb pains in children and adolescents. *Pediatrics, 50*, 429–436.

Perrin, E. C., & Perrin, J. M. (1983). Clinicians' assessments of children's understanding of illness. *American Journal of Diseases in Children, 137*, 874–878.

Raymer, D., Weininger, O., & Hamilton, J. (1984). Psychological problems in children with abdominal pain. *Lancet, 1*(8374), 439–440.

Regan, J., & Regan, W. (1989). Somatoform disorders. In C. Last & M. Hersen (Eds.), *Handbook of child psychiatric diagnosis* (pp. 343–355). New York: John Wiley.

Rimsza, M., Berg, R., & Locke, C. (1988). Sexual abuse: Somatic and emotional reactions. *Child Abuse and Neglect, 12*, 201–208.

Routh, D., & Ernst, A. (1984). Somatization disorder in relatives of children and adolescents with functional abdominal pain. *Journal of Pediatric Psychology, 9*, 427–437.

Rubin, L., Barbero, G., & Sibinga, M. (1967). Pupillary reactivity in children with recurrent abdominal pain. *Psychosomatic Medicine, 29*, 111–120.

Sanders, M., Rebgetz, M., Morrison, M., Bor, W., Gordon, A., Dadds, M., & Shepherd, R. (1989). Cognitive-behavioral treatment of recurrent nonspecific abdominal pain in children: An analysis of generalization, maintenance, and side effects. *Journal of Consulting and Clinical Psychology, 57*, 294–300.

Sandler, R., Drossman, D., Nathan, H., & McKee, D. (1984). Symptom complaints and health care seeking behavior in subjects with bowel dysfunction. *Gastroenterology, 87*, 314–318.

Sank, L., & Biglan, A. (1974). Operant treatment of a case of recurrent abdominal pain in a 10 year old boy. *Behavior Therapy, 5*, 677–681.

Sarnoff, C. (1976). *Latency*. New York: Jason Aronson.

Senn, M., & Solnit, A. (1968). *Problems in child behavior and development*. Philadelphia: Lea and Febiger.

Shapiro, E., & Rosenfeld, A. (1987). *The somatizing child: Diagnosis and treatment of conversion and somatization disorders*. New York: Springer-Verlag.

Siegel, L., & Smith, K. (1989). Children's strategies for coping with pain. *Pediatrician: International Journal of Child and Adolescent Health, 16*, 110–118.

Spielberger, C. (1973). *Preliminary test manual for the State Trait Anxiety Inventory for Children*. Palo Alto, CA: Consulting Psychologist Press.

Stickler, G., & Murphy, D. (1979). Recurrent abdominal pain. *American Journal of Diseases in Childhood, 133*, 486–489.

Stone, R., & Barbero, G. (1970). Recurrent abdominal pain in childhood. *Pediatrics, 45*, 732–738.

Tessler, R., Mechanic, D., & Dimond, M. (1976). The effect of psychological distress on physician utilization: A prospective study. *Journal of Health and Social Behavior, 17*, 353–364.

Thompson, W., & Heaton, K. (1980). Functional bowel disorders in apparently healthy people. *Gastroenterology*, *79*, 283–288.

Turner, S., Beidel, D., & Costello, A. (1987). Psychopathology in the offspring of anxiety disorder patients. *Journal of Consulting and Clinical Psychology*, *55*, 229–235.

Ulshen, M., & Stabler, B. (1984). Recurrent abdominal pain. In V. C. Kelley (Ed.), *Practice of pediatrics* (Vol. 5, pp. 1–17). Philadelphia: Lippincott.

Violon, A., & Giurgea, D. (1984). Familial models for chronic pain. *Pain*, *18*, 199–203.

Wald, A., Chandra, R., Fisher, S. E., Gartner, J. C., & Zitelli, B. (1982). Lactose malabsorption in recurrent abdominal pain of childhood. *Journal of Pediatrics*, *100*, 65–68.

Walker, L., & Greene, J. (1988). *Development and validation of a measure of functional disability for children and adolescents.* Paper presented at the Florida Conference on Child Health Psychology, Gainesville, FL.

Walker, L., & Greene, J. (1989). Children with recurrent abdominal pain and their parents: More somatic complaints, anxiety, and depression than other patient families? *Journal of Pediatric Psychology*, *14*, 231–293.

Walker, L., & Greene, J. (1991). Negative life events and symptom resolution in pediatric abdominal pain patients. *Journal of Pediatric Psychology*, *16*, 39–57.

Wasserman, A., Whitington, P., & Rivara, F. (1988). Psychogenic basis for abdominal pain in children and adolescents. *Journal of American Academy of Child and Adolescent Psychiatry*, *27*, 179–184.

Wasserman, T. (1978). The elimination of complaints of stomach cramps in a 12 year old child by covert positive reinforcement. *Behavior Therapy*, *1*, 13–14.

Whitehead, W., Winget, C., Fedoravicius, A., Wooley, S., & Blackwell, B. (1982). Learned illness behavior in patients with irritable bowel syndrome and peptic ulcer. *Digestive Diseases and Sciences*, *27*, 202–208.

Wooley, S., Blackwell, B., & Winget, C. (1978). A learning theory model of chronic illness behavior: Theory, treatment, and research. *Psychosomatic Medicine*, *40*, 379–401.

Zuckerman, B., Stevenson, J., & Bailey, V. (1987). Stomachaches and headaches in a community sample of preschool children. *Pediatrics*, *79*, 677–682.

Johnson, R., Kerr, G.D. (1980): Functional bowel disorders are an anxiety
feeling (expp. Theorypublishng): 39 281-285.

Magni, G., Salmi, A., De Cristo, G. (1987): Psychopathology in the origin of
and of severe chronic Annual Journal of Gastritits and Clinical Psychology 39
51-55.

Olness, K.J., Stiehm, S. (1984): Recurrent abdominal pain in V.C. Strubb, J.C.
Crombie (ed) Pain (Vol 2, pp. 1-10). Wessschmidt: Longmann.

Walker, A., Zeltzer, L.T. (1986): Painful interactions for chronic pain. Clin. Lin. 1986
201.

Walker, A.C., Garber, G., Greene, B.R., Cutting, J.D., Kettels, H. (1992): Recurrent
and abdominal: is it just your abdominal pain of childhood. Journal of Pediatrics
200 85-92.

Walker, L.A., Cutting, J. (1991): Parent reinforcement of well behaviors a resource of
pain complaints in children and adolescents. Paper presented at the Society for Pediatrics in children. Ann Arbor. Chicago. Ill.

Walker, L.A., Garber, J. (1991): Children with recurrent abdominal pain and their
parents. More somatic symptoms and depression than other pain patients?
Implications in pediatric Psychology 15 231-244.

Walker, L.A., Greene, J.W. (1991): Negative life events and symptom resolution in
pediatric abdominal pain patients. Journal of Pediatric psychology 15 341-360.

Weigert, G.A., Cottrell, R.A., Hofeld, J., Lesnik, R. (1991): Risk factors for abdominal
pain and other functional gastrointestinal disorders: a study of Rochester New and
controls. Gastroenterology 1 102 232.

Wiltrauten, H.J. (1988): The elimination of abdominal sickness attacks in a 17 year
old boy through contingency management. Behaviour Therapy. 1 12.

White, John K., Wortz, G., Liebskind, J.C., Whaler, T.A., Bancroft, W. (1987):
Chronic illness theory in the pediatric abdominal bowel symptoms and symptom behavior. In Ann Annual Review, 79. 766 3898.

Woolfolk, G., Miller, J., & Wahler (1979): A family cycles in children through the
street families. Journal of Community and Clinical Psychology of Childhood. 266,
141-155.

Zeltzer, L.K., Schwab-Stone, D., Hein, J. & Ghahremani, E., Kronenberger, N.J.,
Stressors, Children Sommation in adult life. In J. Pediatr. 80, 512-520.

11
Burn Injury and Treatment Pain

MARLENE MARON AND JOSEPH P. BUSH

Pediatric burn injuries pose tremendous physical and psychological challenges to victims and their families. Burns are among the most excruciatingly painful of injuries, and treatment procedures can be extremely aversive as well. Unfortunately, the signal function of acute pain, that of motivating adaptive avoidance behavior, may interfere with adaptation to debridement and other therapies aimed at facilitating skin healing and minimizing difficulties such as contractures and scarring. In addition to pain, children with severe burns are confronted with the possibility of life-altering disability and disfigurement. Discharge from the hospital may be followed by further disruption of life activities with the burn victim continuing to participate in aggressive physical and occupational therapies. Limitations in activities of daily living and on return to school are common. The intensity and duration of the stresses of treatment and recovery for the patient and family may well exceed their expectations. For the burned child, the physical pain of the injuries and treatment are often coupled with considerable psychological distress, blurring any distinction between physical pain and emotional distress. Assessment and intervention should therefore address both physical and emotional concomitants of injury-related and procedural pain as well as the psychological consequences of disfigurement and altered body image for the child and family.

In recent years, increasing attention has been devoted to factors that influence the child's experience and expression of pain. McGrath and Vair (1984) identified five physical and seven psychological factors affecting pediatric pain. Physical factors included (a) amount, type, and location of tissue damage; (b) integrity of the peripheral and central nervous systems; (c) individual differences in pain threshold and tolerance; (d) adequacy of analgesia; and (e) physical stimulation (e.g., application of heat, cold, and debridement). Psychological factors included (a) the child's understanding of the meaning and causes of pain and hospitalization; (b) previous painful experiences; (c) gender; (d) age; (e) current and previous reactions of others to the child's pain; (f) levels of anxiety and depression; and (g) cultural and familial strategies and models for dealing with pain.

The developmental level of the burned child affects his/her experience of pain and has implications for provision of clinical services. The child's cognitive skills play a fundamental role in determining his/her understanding of treatment procedures in ways that will affect both emotional distress and coping responses. Communication between child and care provider is also influenced by developmental variables; this in turn affects interpersonal support and the conveying of information. Evidence suggests substantial gaps between children's pain expressions and adults' interpretations of these expressions (Perrin & Perrin, 1983). These and other developmental considerations have implications for both the focus and the techniques of pain assessment and intervention across disciplines.

Epidemiology

In previous years, mortality rates due to severe burns in children were considerably higher than they are today (Carvajal & Parks, 1982). Therefore, treatment and long-term care for burned children have become increasingly important. Fires and burns still claim the lives of more children between the ages of 1 and 14 years than any other type of unintentional injury occurring in the home (East, Jones, Feller, Saxon, & Wolfe, 1988). According to the National Burn Information Exchange, as of 1985 nearly 30,000 of 92,034 cases on file from 133 burn centers in the United States involved children under 18 years of age (East et al., 1988). Infants and toddlers account for 52% of all childhood burns; children from birth through 23 months comprise 28% and 2- to 4-year-olds 24%. Children between the ages of 5 and 12 account for 27% and 13- to 18-year-olds make up 21% of the pediatric burn population. Very young children are more likely to die due to their injuries than are older children and young adults (Carvajal & Parks, 1982). More boys sustain burn injuries than girls, particularly later in childhood. At 0 to 23 months the ratio of boys to girls is 1.5:1, whereas in the 13 to 18 year range the ratio of boys to girls is 3.5:1 (East et al., 1988).

Infants and toddlers are most frequently burned by scalds, whereas burns caused by flame or contact with hot solids comprise the second most frequent source of these children's injuries. The majority of these burns are incurred as a result of pulling on objects (e.g., pots on the stove) (Feller, Tholen, & Cornell, 1980). In 2- to 4-year-olds, flame burns become more common and scalds less so than in younger children. In this age group, play activities and experimentation with matches are frequently implicated. Flame burns are most common in children between the ages of 5 and 12 and are usually due to playing with or standing near fire. Finally, 13- to 18-year-olds are most frequently burned by flames. Their injuries are associated with a wider range of activities, such as lighting fires, automobile accidents, and working with corrosive or flammable materials (East et al., 1988).

An alarming number of children are burned due to the intentional abusive actions of others. Documented child abuse accounts for 10 to 25% of pediatric burn admissions (Deitch & Staats, 1982), and burn injuries have been estimated to account for approximately 10% of all child abuse incidents (Purdue, Hunt, & Prescott, 1988). In one sample, 61% of children with inflicted burns and 71% of those whose burns were attributed to accidents associated with neglect had parents who had been previously identified to child protective services agencies (Ayoub & Pfeifer, 1979).

Burn Injury and Treatment Characteristics

During the first few days of hospitalization, medical efforts are aimed at survival. Clearing airways, restoring and maintaining body fluids, and preventing sepsis (infection) are of primary concern. Immediate psychological reactions to severe burns may often include anxiety, withdrawal, disorientation, recent memory loss, restlessness and delirium, hallucinations and delusions (Schubert Walker & Healy, 1980). Parents' initial reactions are varied, often including shock, fear, denial, guilt, and distrust and hostility toward medical caregivers.

As the child becomes medically stable, treatment of the wounded areas begins. For many children, burn treatment procedures are the most aversive aspect of hospitalization. Researchers have not yet been able to discriminate the traumatizing role of this procedural pain from other sources, such as disfigurement, in contributing to psychological problems in survivors. Most patients, typically those with extensive second-degree burns, undergo "open treatment" twice daily. Such treatment consists of removal of bandages, exposure of wounds, removal of devitalized tissue and adhesions (debridement), hydrotherapy, and application of topical antibacterial cream. Each of these elements of wound care can be extremely difficult to endure. Bandages can stick to burned skin and may therefore be painful to remove. Exposure of affected areas to air can cause discomfort, and debridement is usually very painful due to the abrasion needed to remove wound adhesions. Hypersensitivity to temperature changes can lead to discomfort, pain, and suffering during hydrotherapy (Kelley, Jarvie, Middlebrook, McNeer, & Drabman, 1984). Finally, while awaiting application of new bandages, the burned child has the opportunity to see his/her wounds without any covering to minimize the visual impact of the insult to body integrity.

Understandably, many children experience considerable anxiety and distress in connection with these procedures. Some actively resist by kicking, screaming, attempting to escape or delay treatment. Others may respond catatonically. This may represent stress-induced analgesia or (more likely) lethargic indifference associated with learned helplessness (Kavanaugh, 1983). Some children urinate or defecate in the hydrotherapy tub, causing infection risks. Some refuse to eat, which presents a threat to skin healing at a time when adequate nutrition is crucial. Insertion of a nasogastric feeding tube is sometimes necessary to ensure adequate caloric intake.

Skin grafting is usually required for children with third-degree burns. A thin layer of healthy skin from an unaffected site on the child's body (or from a donor) is patched over the burned area(s). Children often complain of itchiness and discomfort around the graft and donor sites. After grafting, a period of rest is usually required to promote healing; this period of relative immobility can be difficult for a normally active child.

Along with wound care and grafting procedures, children on burn units participate in physical and occupational therapies, both of which are often resisted. It is difficult for children to comply with treatments that require that they exercise wounded areas. Yet, working to improve range of motion, prevent contractures, and promote circulation are critical to healing.

As skin healing progresses, the focus of treatment shifts to include resocialization and psychological concerns for patients and their families. Although psychological issues previously revolved around pain and anxiety management during wound care and therapies, the effects of disfigurement, altered body image, and fears of peer rejection now move into the foreground. Children and parents often require assistance as they negotiate changing roles, expectations, and reintegration.

Child Characteristics Influencing Burn Injury and Treatment Pain

Developmental Issues

Each developmental phase carries particular challenges for coping with pain and hospitalization. Infants must contend with separation, and preschoolers with conceptual distortions and communication deficits. School-age children are vulnerable to other sorts of distorted perceptions regarding their wounds and treatment procedures; adolescents face the threat of peer rejection and loss of control. The likelihood that stage-specific difficulties will arise and persist to the point of disrupting attainment of developmental milestones or subsequent adjustment may depend upon pretraumatic or hospital treatment factors.

One developmentally specific vulnerability affecting pain management in burned children involves prolonged hospitalization. Separation and stranger anxiety are, in fact, thought to be the most frightening aspects of hospitalization for many young children (Steward & Steward, 1981). According to Sroufe (1979), the quality of infant-caregiver attachment is an important predictor of later coping competencies and capacity to tolerate stress. Sroufe noted that infants, normally dependent on primary caretakers, rely on these adults to be psychologically available. Psychological availability implies that the parent is physically present, sensitive and responsive to the child's needs. Such a parent provides a secure base from which the child can explore and deal with fear-arousing stimuli. Securely attached infants are likely to develop into competent preschoolers, in whom competence is, however, manifested differently than in the infant. Preschoolers seek instrumental assistance when ill, injured, or otherwise in need, but behave in a generally autonomous fashion. Sroufe sees the quality of the child's adaptation as continuous; given initial secure attachment, healthy development is likely to ensue. The child learns to maintain support-seeking contact with others while functioning increasingly independently.

Extended hospitalization may deprive the infant of adequate stimulation and relationship experiences (King & Ziegler, 1981), potentially depriving the child of coping resources as well as risking interference with the ongoing development of competence. Since the infant is prelinguistic, discerning his/her needs and distress is difficult. The staff must infer the nature of the baby's distress from his/her cry. In addition, the usual methods of soothing a baby such as holding or gentle stroking might be difficult or impossible due to the location of the burns. Thus, the infant's need for and expectation of parental comfort and protection are frequently frustrated. The baby must tolerate separation and painful experiences with many different hospital personnel. Consistent care may not be available from either parents or hospital staff. Fortunately, several hospitals have become increasingly responsive to the needs of child patients and have extended parental visiting hours, provisions for parental rooming-in, and assign primary care nurses to pediatric patients. It cannot be overemphasized, however, that the presence of a parental figure will be most helpful if the parent is well prepared and capable of being emotionally available and instrumentally supportive to the child, and if her/his participation is well accepted by unit staff. Parents often need help dealing with their anxiety and revulsion due to the child's disfigurement, as well as in playing a consensually validated role in the child's inpatient care.

Perhaps the experience of hospitalization limits the child's ability to master separation and reunion or exploratory behavior, hampering the establishment or maintenance of secure attachment. On the other hand, perhaps those very young children who show extreme manifestations of regression are those for whom attachment is already insecure. These possibilities merit further investigation.

Another central developmental issue for very young children relates to the cognitive characteristics of their comprehension of causality and the nature of their injuries. It has been argued, based on interview data, that preschoolers commonly interpret their pain and hospitalization as punishment for real or imagined wrongdoing (Bibace & Walsh, 1980; Brewster, 1982; Eiser, 1985; Perrin & Gerrity, 1981). This notion of "imminent justice" is consistent with other phenomenistic and magical beliefs typical of the preoperational child (Piaget, 1965). Some children hold themselves responsible for burn injuries even though their culpability is clearly nonexistent from an adult perspective. This issue is, however, particularly complicated when the child was injured as a result of misbehavior (e.g., playing with matches). Another potential problem inheres in the preschooler's inability to understand the rationale for painful treatment and tendency to focus upon proximal perceptual cues in constructing his/her own explanation. Beales (1982) noted that the young child might equate wound visibility with damage, and therefore believe that it should be covered up and left alone. Likewise, this child might believe that, because treatment hurts, (s)he is being damaged (pain equals injury) or attacked (pain equals punishment).

Beales (1982) observed and interviewed 60 4-week to 15-year-old children hospitalized for burn injuries and found that beliefs about treatment and recovery were strongly associated with anxiety and expectations of pain. These children were reported to perceive wound care and physical therapy as painful and therefore harmful. It was found that these treatment procedures conflicted with most children's concrete beliefs about healing and about self-care. In general, these children appeared to be perceptually centered on pain and obvious breaches of bodily integrity as signals indicating damage. Thus, painful procedures would be seen as harmful, whereas bandaging and rest of affected areas would be seen as therapeutic. The young child might have difficulty understanding that wounds must be exposed, rubbed, and exercised to promote healing. The ability to rationalize such painful treatment procedures as benign is rendered even more difficult by the fact that wound manipulation may become more painful as healing progresses, due to regeneration and functional recovery of peripheral nerve endings (Mumford & Bowsher, 1976). Beales also found that hearing other patients talk about or cry during treatment and the staff discussing a child's wound care often elevated children's anxiety levels, as did seeing a loaded instrument trolley. Feelings of helplessness and powerlessness were noted in children who were restrained for wound care; such feelings often led to escalated anxiety and anticipation of pain.

Language development is also an important variable in the hospital experience of young children. To the extent that children lack adult-like verbal skills, their caretakers are likely to have difficulty understanding their pain, distress, and other needs. Children communicate to elicit support and information from adult caretakers; without sophisticated verbal skills, young children are left to resort to behaviors that may be perceived as maladaptive, aggressive, or otherwise unacceptable rather than as nonverbal coping attempts. This can inhibit the child's attempts to achieve mastery. Brewster (1982), for example, examined comprehension of the intent of medical procedures in 50 5- to 12-year-olds hospitalized for chronic illness. She reported that the 7- to 10-year-olds typically did understand that treatment was intended to help them recover, but believed that caregivers would not recognize that they were in pain unless they screamed and cried. Thus, cognitive factors are difficult to separate from developmental characteristics in children's manner of communicating about pain.

Although school-age children have greater cognitive sophistication than younger children, they too have developmentally specific vulnerabilities. Beales, Keen, and Lennox Holt (1983) reported that 7- to 11-year-olds showed little appreciation for the beneficial aspects of painful procedures and tended to perceive such procedures as damaging. Similar to the preschooler, the school-age child may display noncompliance due to developmentally predictable cognitive distortions. For example, children at the concrete operational stage of development might become anxious in response to beliefs that their injuries are contagious (Bibace & Walsh, 1980). These children, however, are able to recognize multiple external causes for their injuries, which could serve to offset guilt or other cognitive distortions. Adolescent cognitive development allows for more accurate understanding of the injury and treatment. However, it also makes possible reflection upon more remote, possibly negative consequences. Some concerns of youngsters in this age group relate to surgical procedures and anesthesia, physical appearance and peer acceptance, and autonomy. Pride in their burgeoning independence and the belief that they are becoming increasingly in control of their lives can make hospital rules and procedures difficult for teenagers. In the hospital, autonomy is severely curtailed; inpatients cannot choose what they wear, how they structure their time, or whether they will have to endure skin grafting. Upon discharge, they don't usually get to decide when to return to school or work and often find themselves tired and physically less able to participate in normal activities. Understandably, adolescents may resist aspects of their nursing care and physical therapy. Perhaps the most obvious difficulties for burned teenagers, however, involve their altered appearance and body image. This may be especially problematic for youngsters who have yet to undergo plastic surgery and may try to hold on to fantasies of recovering preburn appearance (Giljohann, 1980).

The normal course of adjustment to hospitalization for burned children includes more extreme disruptions of behavioral and cognitive functioning than are typically observed in the general pediatric population (Knudson-Cooper & Thomas, 1988). Regression is common (e.g., loss of previously acquired abilities such as walking, talking, toilet training), as are psychological symptoms such as anxiety, hyperactivity, and depression. Although some authors consider regression in the burn patient to be necessary and adaptive (e.g., Solnit & Priel, 1975), others hold the view that although regression should be tolerated and understood, attempts to facilitate developmentally appropriate coping are important. For example, Stoddard (1982) recommends consistent nurturing relationships for very young children, distraction techniques for preschoolers, adaptive fantasy, hypnosis, and biofeedback for school-age children, and medication, self-hypnosis, and relaxation for adolescents as ways to mitigate the effects of severe regression and to facilitate coping. Whether regression will represent transient reactions or the beginnings of long-term dysfunctional sequelae may, like developmental challenges, relate to premorbid individual and family functioning and to hospital practices. Further study of the relationships among these variables is warranted.

Pretraumatic Functioning

A child who has previously undergone painful medical procedures or experienced extended hospitalization may bring to the burn event residual behavioral or emotional issues, e.g., difficulty trusting hospital staff and feelings of helplessness or powerlessness in anticipation of inadequately managed pain. In addition, the child's family may have experienced a drain of financial and social support resources in the course of previous medical treatment and find themselves overwhelmed and less emotionally available to their burned child. Pretraumatic psychopathology in the child may also exacerbate maladjustment and intolerance of painful procedures, requiring skilled adaptation of intervention techniques.

Environmental Systems' Influences on Child Burn Injury and Treatment Pain

The characteristics and circumstances of the burn injury can be expected to bear upon the child's pain experience. The depth and extent of burns will directly influence the child's pain experience, as will the number and extensiveness of required surgeries, duration of treatment, and degree of disfigurement. The manner in which the family mobilizes its resources and responds to the challenge of facilitating the child's recovery is also likely to affect the child's pain experience and overall adjustment. Pretraumatic familial factors, family functioning throughout the child's hospitalization, and postdischarge interaction patterns may affect the child's long- and short-term adjustment. Family functioning has been linked to patient compliance and adjustment in the general pediatric population (Jay, Ozolins, Elliott, & Caldwell, 1983; Johnson, 1985; Pless, Roghmann, & Haggerty, 1972). The precise nature of the relationship between family functioning, patient compliance, and posthospitalization adjustment merits further investigation.

The Hospital Environment

Support for the view that hospital factors might mediate developmental risks is provided by research that suggests that although particular developmental tasks may be affected by treatment for burns, some of these effects can be minimized or prevented. For example, in commenting on a report on the effects of allowing mothers to room-in and visit frequently with their preschool children (Woodward, 1959), Jackson (1974) noted that the incidence of psychological disturbance was drastically reduced after liberalizing visiting policies. On the other hand, the presence of a parent who, due to either situational anxiety or inhibition or to deficient parenting skills, may exacerbate distress and disruptive behavior in the child (Bush & Cockrell, 1987; Gross, Stern, Levin, Dale, & Wojnilower, 1983) might not be warranted. There has been little research to date, however, specifically investigating parental participation in children's burn treatment.

The clinical sensitivity and pain management policies of burn unit personnel have a direct and massive effect on the burned child's pain and suffering. Overly routinized analgesic prescribing and administration practices coupled with a lack of sophistication in recognizing developmental influences on the variety of ways in which young children express pain (see chapter 7), can lead to inadequate care. For example, one 6-year-old boy was observed to demonstrate severe withdrawal and regressive behavior for several days following admission to a pediatric burn unit. It was not until his dosage of morphine was doubled and administered on a regular basis that he began to disengage from a fetal position and interact with others on the unit. This child apparently required unusually large doses of analgesics, and was able to tolerate the increased dosage without untoward effects. It is noteworthy that there had been considerable staff resistance to interpreting his withdrawal as a response to pain and to considering augmenting his analgesia; his behavior had been seen as deliberate manipulative noncompliance. The widespread tendency to undermedicate children in pain has been noted by a number of researchers (Bush, Holmbeck, & Cockrell, 1989; see chapter 3, this volume).

The Family Environment

The ways in which family members characteristically cope with pain is likely to be important with regard to the burned child's experience. If a child is taught to "keep a stiff upper lip" and be stoic, (s)he might feel compelled to show little visible distress in response to burn or procedural pain. Similarly, if the family climate is one in which dramatic expression of even mild pain is encouraged, the child might be inclined to be more vocal and expressive. For such a child, freedom to express pain vocally, even if presenting a management challenge to the staff, should be encouraged. On the other hand, if the burned child has learned that pain expression is a means toward a desired end, inappropriate pain behavior is likely to persist. Modes of pain expression also reflect cultural and ethnic norms in ways that are as yet poorly understood (Reid & Bush, 1990).

In a discussion of the impact of children's illnesses on families, Johnson (1985) noted that marital disharmony, financial problems, sibling conflicts, and diminished attention to nonpatient siblings have been documented as common problems. The impact of these problems on parental availability to burned children remains to be clarified. Identification of factors that facilitate or hamper utilization of resources that are related positively to postburn adjustment is also incomplete. To date, research has shown that social support (for parents and children), marital integrity, an atmosphere of open discussion, family participation in community activities, communication of a sense of hopefulness, and the opportunity for parents to mourn along with their children can contribute to a positive outcome for children (Browne et al., 1985; Clarke, 1980; Davidson, Bowden, & Feller, 1981; Giljohann, 1980; Love, Byrne, Roberts, Browne, & Brown, 1987; Seligman, MacMillan, & Carroll, 1971).

As noted previously, appropriate parental participation has been found to relate to adjustment in hospitalized children. Benians (1974) reported a statistically significant relationship between severe psychological disturbance and irregular parental visiting. In his study, children whose parents did not visit daily showed poorer physical and emotional in-hospital adjustment. Additionally, those children had greater incidences of both pre- and posthospitalization problems, including weak school performance. Benians, consistent with Jackson (1974), noted that reinstatement of daily visiting was associated with improved psychological functioning in the children. Another factor that could be expected to impact postburn adjustment in children is the occurrence of major family events coincident with injury and recovery. The presence of additional stressors (e.g., financial and emotional pressures attendant to a housefire) and how they are handled may affect parent emotional availability. Likewise, how parents marshall the resources to facilitate their own coping is likely to be important. Finally, parental cooperation with hospital procedures and participation in the child's treatment could play a role in the child's adjustment.

Previous psychiatric history in the parents might also affect the burned child's pain experience. A lack of available psychological resources and disturbed functioning can be problematic. A severely depressed parent, for example, might have difficulty helping the child with wound care and other aversive procedures. High rates of depressive and posttraumatic stress responses were identified in parents of even mildly burned children (Cella, Perry, Poag, Amand, & Goodwin, 1988) relative to parents of demographically similar children hospitalized for other (nonemergency) procedures. A highly anxious parent might transmit his/her anxiety to the child and escalate the child's anxiety level (Bush, 1987), which can in turn escalate the subjective experience of pain. The frequent implication of parental abuse in pediatric burns provides further evidence that psychological disturbance in the parent(s) and in the parent-child relationship may be prevalent in this population.

Psychological Sequelae

It is difficult to determine the precise nature of the long-term impact of burn and burn treatment–related pain. Much has been written about the psychological adjustment of burned children but systematic attempts to tease out the effects of the injuries themselves, the pain engendered, and the degree to which pain was adequately managed are extremely difficult and rare.

The psychological characteristics, coping skills, and environmental resources associated with better adjustment in the burned child have been described in several reviews and studies (e.g., Breslin, 1975; Giljohann, 1980; Holter & Friedman, 1969; Long & Cope, 1961; Martin, 1970; Seligman et al., 1971; Vigliano, Hart, & Singer, 1964; Wright & Fulwiler, 1974). Most of these investigators report that the majority of children showing adjustment problems subsequent to their injuries also had difficulties or came from families with difficulties that predated their burns. Pretraumatic problems were reported to be more common among burn victims than in the general population. Conversely, Woodward (1959) concluded that burn injuries in themselves are sufficient to produce significant emotional disturbances, even without a history of difficulty in the child. However, Woodward did not assess the pretraumatic mental health of the mothers and relied heavily on maternal verbal report, with comments such as "I've never been the same since" to indicate the pathognomic nature of childhood burns for patients and their parents. More recent empirical work (Tarnowski, Rasnake, Linscheid, & Mulick, 1989) suggests that previous estimates of the prevalence of long-term behavioral sequelae in burned children may have been substantially exaggerated, perhaps due to overreliance on subjective outcome measures.

Giljohann (1980) found that the children who adjust most favorably were those who tended to cope in an active, assertive fashion. Seligman et al. (1971) also discussed coping style as a pretraumatic factor in postburn adjustment. These authors noted that children may employ an adaptive form of denial. For example, if a child who might otherwise be devastated by his/her disfigurement denies the extent of physical alteration for a while, he/she may thereby be able to keep stress and anxiety at a manageable level, enabling him/her to cope with painful physical exercises. Later, when treatment involves fewer painful procedures, the child might begin to incorporate a new body image.

Browne et al. (1985) reported that maternal adjustment and coping style, as defined by scores on the Billings and Moos (1981) Coping Scale and the Psychological Adjustment to Illness Scale, distinguished adequate from poor adjusters to childhood burns. They stated that children who adjusted poorly had mothers whose adjustment was also rated as poor, who tended to cope using avoidance and emotional distance, engaged in few recreational activities, and came from families with minimal moral and religious emphasis. Interestingly, despite the use of the same data set as Byrne et al. (1986), Browne's team found maternal factors to be significant predictors of postburn adjustment in children, whereas Byrne's did not. This discrepancy may have been due to the fact that Browne addressed a variety of dimensions of postburn adjustment, whereas Byrne focused primarily on social competence. Other preburn family variables that have been associated with postburn adjustment in children include number of family moves (with a greater number being more problematic), adequacy of the family's living space, and number of children under the age of five needing supervision (Martin, 1980; Sawyer, Minde, & Zucker, 1982). Social support, particularly within the family, is considered to be the most important predictor of postburn adjustment by Knudson-Cooper (1984).

In an important, though methodologically flawed longitudinal study, Benians (1974) interviewed burned children and their families from time of admission until several months postdischarge from a children's burn unit in England. He began interviewing as soon after admission as possible in an attempt to ascertain the relationship between preburn psychological functioning and disturbance arising both in the hospital and after discharge. In some cases, intelligence testing and school records were obtained. Chi-square analyses were computed to determine relationships between preburn factors (e.g., psychological disturbance) and outcome. The author noted that he functioned both as therapist and investigator and that his methodology was thus compromised. No significant relationship was found between severe psychological disturbance arising while the child was in the hospital and symptoms after discharge. There also was no significant relationship between mothers' psychiatric symptoms and "severe" psychological disturbance in children on the burn unit. Benians also claimed that burned children showed high rates of preexisting psychological disturbance and were likely to come from disorganized families (wherein mothers showed increased incidence of depression and phobic symptoms), relative to cited rates in nonclinical community populations. Furthermore, he suggested that the trauma of injury and hospitalization may magnify existing problems in these children, since posttreatment psychological disturbance seemed to be associated with pretraumatic maladjustment.

To evaluate the predictive power of pretraumatic physical and mental health more definitively, preburn information must be gathered and multivariate analyses of preburn functioning along with other potential predictors are necessary. In much of the previous research, methodologically sound data pertaining to pretraumatic functioning were not collected and multivariate designs were not employed.

Developmentally Sensitive Intervention

Pain management in burned children is progressing from an intuitive to a more empirically based level of practice. Developmentally specific interventions must address needs and vulnerabilities that have been shown to differ with the child's age, and should utilize modalities suited to the child's cognitive and communication abilities and coping skills. Descriptive studies focusing on developmentally specific vulnerabilities and on the emergence of children's cognitive abilities and coping resources are strongly suggestive of interventions best suited to children of different ages. Thus, programs and policies that enhance parental availability and interventions to support optimal parental functioning can be made responsive to the problems arising from separation in infants and preschoolers. Use of developmentally appropriate language in providing information relating to misperceptions and cognitive distortions is indicated in preschool and school-aged children. With adolescents, opportunities should be provided to address cosmetic and peer group concerns, whereas school-aged as well as adolescent children should be helped to exercise their needs for autonomy and control in treatment procedures in ways that facilitate rather than impair therapeutic outcomes. A variety of distraction, relaxation, and other coping techniques have been shown to be effective during intensely painful procedures. Research to date, however, has not empirically addressed the developmental specificity of particular interventions. Rather, studies have supported the effectiveness of certain interventions with burned children of certain ages, but have neglected age as a variable that mediates treatment effects. Most of these studies deal specifically with pain and anxiety management during wound care.

Unfortunately, undermedication of pediatric patients' pain and beliefs that pain does not have a lasting effect on children are still common in pediatric medical centers (Bernstein, 1976; Beyer & Byers, 1985; Bush et al., 1989; Mather & Mackie, 1983; McCaffery, 1977; McGrath & Vair, 1984; Perry & Heidrich, 1982; Ross & Ross, 1984). Anxiolytic and analgesic medications are now often employed, but treatment facilities remain in which limited use of narcotics and inadequately scheduled medications (p.r.n. – as necessary – only or up to 1 hour before wound care) are typical. Also, nonpharmacological interventions for pain and anxiety management are not employed with sufficient regularity. Several nonpharmacological approaches to pediatric pain management have been described in the literature (reviewed in Ross & Ross, 1988). These include supportive psychotherapy, behavior modification, relaxation training (with hypnosis and stress management components), and cognitively oriented behavioral interventions.

One innovative behavioral approach to the management of pediatric burn pain was reported by Kelley et al. (1984). These authors evaluated the effects of contingent cartoon viewing and star chart reinforcement for two children (ages 4 and 6 years) undergoing hydrotherapy. Using a replicated single subject reversal design, the authors demonstrated that distraction (cartoons) along with star chart feedback resulted in a significant decrease in pain behavior. In addition, therapist and maternal ratings of child pain, anxiety, and cooperativeness were correlated significantly with observer ratings. Other behavioral interventions shown to be successful with children include contracting for treatment compliance, contingency management, and modeling. Simons et al. (1978) used behavioral contracting to improve dietary compliance in a severely burned 5- year-old, and to improve compliance with medication in a 13-year-old. Varni, Bessman, Russo, and Cataldo (1980) demonstrated reduced pain behaviors and enhanced coping in a 3-year-old girl, using a multiple baseline across settings with reversal design. More delayed reinforcement was found to be effective in improving on-unit behavior in a severely burned hyperactive 13-year-old, by using a point system in combination with peer modeling (Zide & Pardoe, 1976).

Relaxation training, stress management, and hypnosis have also been reported to be effective for reducing children's distress in response to painful burn treatment. Knudson-Cooper (1981) found significantly lower observed and self-reported anxiety and pain in 27 7- to 16-year-olds who received biofeedback or relaxation training, compared with children (matched on age, sex, and extent of burn) who received only pharmaceutical intervention. Similarly, LaBaw (1973) found "adjunctive trance therapy" useful for combating appetite and feeding problems and encopresis in 23 severely burned 6-month to 14-year-old children. Elliott and Olson (1983) assessed the efficacy of a stress-management package consisting of distraction, relaxation (breathing exercises), emotive imagery and/or reinterpretation of the context of pain, and reinforcement. The authors reported that the program produced substantial reductions in treatment-related distress in 4 5- to 12-year-olds, but that the reduction was only evident when the psychologist was present. The benefits of stress management interventions clearly need to be extended by means of more efficacious generalization training.

Kavanaugh (1983) noted that providing information and maximizing predictability and control may have powerful positive effects on burned children. This view is consistent with the observations reported by Beales (1982). Kavanaugh reasoned that burned children's negative emotional responses, including anxiety, depression, fear, and anger, are in large part caused by learned helplessness, including the expectation that painful events are unpredictable and uncontrollable and that coping behaviors are ineffective. Using a sample of nine severely burned 2- to 12-year-olds, her experimental design compared interventions to maximize predictability and control, to standard hospital procedures (emphasizing staff control and distraction of children). Intervention strategies included warning the children that a painful procedure was upcoming by means of nurses wearing red aprons, and encouraging the child to participate in treatment by asking him/her to remove splints, hold bandages, etc. Experimental group children, in comparison to controls, showed significantly less maladaptive behavior during the first 2 weeks of hospitalization, less nonresponsiveness to noxious stimuli, and less depression at discharge. Similar findings were reported by Tarnowski, McGrath, Calhoun, and Drabman (1987), using a single-subject reversal design with a severely burned 12-year-old. Observed behavioral distress was significantly less when this child was allowed to debride himself than during standard procedure (i.e., debridement by the physical therapist). In addition, the child reported greatly preferring self-mediated debridement, which was rated by the therapist as having been performed satisfactorily. Possible problems with this procedure included its taking a somewhat longer time, and an apparent reactivity effect in which heightened distress followed the child's relinquishing the debriding task to the therapist. Together with Kavanaugh's (1983) findings, these results suggest that substantially enhanced cooperation and satisfaction may be achieved by increasing children's perceptions of control over aversive stimuli through increased participation and information. In addition to studying generalizability, further research is needed regarding other techniques for enhancing perceived control, as well as for determining optimal interventions to enhance predictability and control in a manner that is consistent with the ways in which children at different developmental levels and with different coping repertoires operate on their environments (see Siegel & Smith, chapter 6).

In addition to pain management programs, psychological intervention with burned children can include crisis intervention, supportive therapy with patients and their families, group contact, and ongoing follow-up support. Assistance with discharge planning and school reentry are particularly important. Bernstein (1983) and Cahners (1978; Cahners & Bernstein, 1979) are among several writers who have stressed the importance of psychological support throughout the entire recovery process.

Several general recommendations for staff behavior aimed at minimizing adverse aspects of burn treatment have been presented in the literature. Most authors agree that assessment and treatment should be multifaceted and take into account the child's developmental level. Repeating age-appropriate explanations to children (e.g., with the help of puppets, dolls, drawings, etc.), and carefully assessing the meaning for the child of his/her pain, the circumstances surrounding injury and treatment, and ideas about the future are recommended. It is important, however, first to elicit the child's understanding, so that this may be used as a point of departure for provision of more accurate and corrective explanations. In addition, avoidance of p.r.n. prescriptions has been suggested in order to assure adequate provision of analgesics and to avoid reinforcing pain behaviors. Intervention attempts should incorporate anxiety and depression management, maximize predictability and control, utilize relaxation and distraction, and target the responses of family members and caregivers. For example, staff members can be encouraged to consider the likelihood that they offer inordinate sympathy to a physically attractive child or that they tend to avoid the badly disfigured child in considerable pain (McGrath & Vair, 1984).

Beales (1982) offered several treatment suggestions based on observations of the ways in which children's understanding of their burns and treatment-related pain impacted their ability to master wound care and therapies. Beales recommended against the following: the use of physical restraint, exposing the patient to discussion of the gruesome aspects of burn care, visual exposure to treatment instruments in advance of wound care or to exposed wounds during debridement or bandaging, and interruption of the child's attention to distracting media (e.g., stories, television, music) during the course of treatment. In addition, tailoring explanations about treatment to children's cognitive levels was strongly urged. For example, a preschooler can be told that the silver sulfadiazine, which is applied to the affected areas after debridement, will work like magic and make the wound shrink. A concrete operational child might benefit from factual information coupled with an analogy, (e.g., a skin graft will function on skin like a patch on clothing).

A recent positive trend in pediatric burn care involves the use of a multidisciplinary team approach (see Gillman & Mullins, chapter 5). In this model, physicians, nurses, psychologists, social workers, physical and occupational therapists, as well as parents, cooperate to develop comprehensive evaluation and treatment plans. Clinical observations suggest that such collaboration can be especially valuable. Unfortunately, multidisciplinary teams are not employed at all burn care facilities. Perhaps with empirical evidence of their effectiveness, more widespread acceptance of multidisciplinary treatment packages would ensue.

It is difficult to determine if any one intervention approach is superior to others for the treatment of the emotional and physical concomitants of burns in an individual child patient. This is largely because systematic comparative treatment outcome studies are unwieldy for many burn units. Selecting appropriate dependent variables, ethical constraints, and limited resources all contribute to difficulties in designing and carrying out quality studies. One promising avenue for evaluating treatment effectiveness lies in single case time series research. More work in this area is warranted.

Program evaluation studies that address the nature of the physical and psychological environments of hospital burn units should be encouraged. It would be useful to ask what services are available at different burn centers and to investigate relationships between service delivery variables and children's pain experiences. For example, does a particular hospital have a staff person available whose primary responsibility is to support patients and families? Does the unit provide adequate analgesia? Are nonpharmacological pain management approaches utilized extensively? Does the center encourage family participation in treatment? Are siblings and noninjured family members considered targets for intervention? Does the hospital encourage involvement in long-term follow up activities? Have staff members been adequately trained in pediatric pain management and are they aware of developmental differences in children's pain expression? Although efforts to develop and evaluate psychological interventions are underway, attention to investigating optimal hospital practices that might offset some of the potentially iatrogenic aspects of pediatric burn treatment is still needed.

Future Directions and Recommendations

One way to think about potential areas for change is to consider what is currently lacking in pediatric burn care. Use of inadequate assessment tools continues to be problematic. Efforts to develop, evaluate, and employ developmentally appropriate pain assessment devices should be encouraged. Another critical issue involves the level of staff awareness of developmental aspects of children's pain experiences and expression. Ongoing continuing education and in-service training to improve and maintain sensitivity to treatment aspects unique to pediatric burn patients are recommended. Similarly, psychological support for burn care professionals and assistance with their understanding of psychological factors that influence children's burn recovery would be valuable. Family involvement, wherever appropriate, has been demonstrated to be beneficial. Many hospital burn units discourage parental involvement in wound care or rooming-in, due to concerns about infection and interference with the smooth management of the unit. Many of these units are mixed, with adult and pediatric beds.

Current knowledge suggests that burned children should be admitted to pediatric burn units or burn care sections of pediatric wards, where the staff are trained pediatric health care workers. Peer interaction could facilitate children's coping with disfigurement and peer reactions. Parental involvement could mitigate the separation problems that are so salient for younger children. Mental health support for siblings and parents, throughout the child's hospitalization and continuing beyond discharge, might ease the family's coping. Since for some families the burn event is merely one crisis event in a series of dysfunctional or chaotic family experiences, support and guidance during admission can be an important step toward improved family functioning.

Further empirical attention to pediatric pain assessment and intervention as well as to psychological sequelae in burned children is warranted. Practical, effective, and empirically validated prevention and treatment approaches are necessary. Multidisciplinary treatment planning and execution are promising; collaborative work not only serves to encourage multifaceted treatment programs, it can also allow for provision of support for nurses and other professionals in their efforts to maintain sensitivity and responsiveness while conducting necessary painful procedures. Clinical experience has shown us that nursing and therapeutic staff are usually receptive to and actively pursue opportunities for learning to improve their effectiveness with child patients. Making ongoing training and support experiences available to staff can increase the likelihood that children's burn pain will be managed with optimal sensitivity and sophistication. Also recommended is the provision of training for surgery residents in the areas of child development and its relation to children's pain experiences and expression, pharmacological and alternative methods of analgesia and anxiety management, and psychological factors that have the potential to exacerbate pain and therefore require medical attention.

References

Ayoub, C., & Pfeifer, D. (1979). Burns as a manifestation of child abuse and neglect. *American Journal of Diseases in Childhood, 133*, 910–914.

Beales, J. (1982). Factors influencing the expectation of pain among patients in a children's burns unit. *Burns, 9*, 187–192.

Beales, J., Keen, J., & Lennox Holt, P. (1983). The child's perception of the disease and the experience of pain in juvenile chronic arthritis. *Journal of Rheumatology, 10*, 61–65.

Benians, R. (1974). A child psychiatrist looks at burned children and their families. *Guy's Hospital Reports, 123*, 149–154.

Bernstein, N. (1976). *Emotional care of the facially burned and disfigured*. Boston: Little, Brown.

Bernstein, N. (1983). Child psychiatry and burn care. *Journal of the American Academy of Child Psychiatry, 22*(2), 202–204.

Beyer, J., & Byers, M. (1985). Knowledge of pediatric pain: The state of the art. *Children's Health Care, 13*(4), 150–159.

Bibace, R., & Walsh, M. (1980). Development of children's concepts of illness. *Pediatrics, 66*(6), 912–917.

Billings, A., & Moos, R. (1981). The role of coping responses and social resources in attenuating the stress of life events. *Journal of Behavioral Medicine, 4*(2), 139–157.

Breslin, P. (1975). The psychological reactions of children to burn traumata: A review. *Illinois Medical Journal, 148*, 519–524 and 595–602.

Brewster, A. (1982). Chronically ill children's concepts of their illness. *Pediatrics, 69*, 355–362.

Browne, G., Byrne, C., Brown, B., Pennock, M., Streiner, D., Roberts, R., Eyles, P., Truscott, D., & Dabbs, R. (1985). Psychosocial adjustment of burn survivors. *Burns, 12*, 28–35.

Bush, J. (1987). Pain in children: A review of the literature from a developmental perspective. *Psychology and Health, 1*, 215–236.

Bush, J., & Cockrell, C. (1987). Maternal factors predicting parenting behaviors in the pediatric clinic. *Journal of Pediatric Psychology, 12*(4), 505–518.

Bush, J., Holmbeck, G., & Cockrell, J. (1989). Patterns of PRN analgesic drug administration in children following elective surgery. *Journal of Pediatric Psychology, 14*(3), 433–448.

Byrne, C., Love, B., Browne, G., Brown, B., Roberts, J., & Streiner, D. (1986). The social competence of children following injury: A study of resilience. *Journal of Burn Care and Rehabilitation, 7*(3), 247–252.

Cahners, S. (1978). Group meetings benefit families of burned children. *Scandinavian Journal of Plastic and Reconstructive Surgery, 13*, 169–171.

Cahners, S., & Bernstein, N. (1979). Rehabilitating families with burned children. *Scandinavian Journal of Plastic and Reconstructive Surgery, 13*, 173–175.

Carvajal, H., & Parks, D. (1982). Survival statistics in burned children. *Journal of Burn Care and Rehabilitation, 3*(2), 81–84.

Cella, D., Perry, S., Poag, M., Amand, R., & Goodwin, C. (1988). Depression and stress responses in parents of burned children. *Journal of Pediatric Psychology, 13*(1), 87–99.

Clarke, A. (1980). Thermal injuries: The care of the whole child. *Journal of Trauma, 20*, 823–829.

Davidson, T., Bowden, M., & Feller, I. (1981). Social support and postburn adjustment. *Archives of Physical Medicine and Rehabilitation, 62*, 274–278.

Deitch, E., & Staats, M. (1982). Child abuse through burning. *Journal of Burn Care and Rehabilitation, 3*(2), 89–92.

East, M., Jones, C. Feller, I., Saxon, M., & Wolfe, R. (1988). Epidemiology of burns in children. In H. Carvajal & D. Parks (Eds.), *Burns in children: Pediatric burn management* (pp. 3-10). Chicago: Year Book Medical Publishers.

Eiser, C. (1985). Children's understanding of medical procedures. *Practitioner, 229,* 371-373.

Elliott, C., & Olson, R. (1983). The management of children's distress in response to painful medical treatment for burn injuries. *Behaviour Research and Therapy, 21,* 675-683.

Feller, I., Tholen, D., & Cornell, R. (1980). Improvements in burn care, 1965 to 1979. *Journal of the American Medical Association, 244,* 2074-2090.

Giljohann, A. (1980). Adolescents burned as children. *Burns, 7,* 95-99.

Gross, A., Stern, R., Levin, R., Dale, J., & Wojnilower, D. (1983). The effect of mother-child separation on the behavior of children experiencing a diagnostic medical procedure. *Journal of Consulting and Clinical Psychology, 51*(5), 783-785.

Holter, J., & Friedman, S. (1969). Etiology and management of severely burned children, psychosocial considerations. *American Journal of Diseases of Children, 118,* 680-686.

Jackson, D. (1974). The psychological effects of burns. *Burns, 1,* 70-74.

Jay, S., Ozolins, M., Elliott, C., & Caldwell, S. (1983). Assessment of children's distress during painful medical procedures. *Journal of Health Psychology, 2*(2), 133-147.

Johnson, S. B. (1985). The family and the child with chronic illness. In D. Turk & R. Kerns (Eds.), *Health, illness and families: A lifespan perspective* (pp. 220-254). New York: Wiley.

Kavanaugh, C. (1983). Psychological intervention with the severely burned child: Report of an experimental comparison of two approaches and their effects on psychological sequelae. *Journal of Child Psychiatry, 22*(2), 145-156.

Kelley, M., Jarvie, G., Middlebrook, J., McNeer, M., & Drabman, R. (1984). Decreasing burned children's pain behavior: Impacting the trauma of hydrotherapy. *Journal of Applied Behavior Analysis, 17,* 147-158.

King, J., & Ziegler, S. (1981). The effects of hospitalization on children's behavior: A review of the literature. *Children's Health Care, 10*(1), 20-28.

Knudson-Cooper, M. (1981). Adjustment to visible stigma: The case of the severely burned child. *Social Science Medicine, 15B,* 31-44.

Knudson-Cooper, M. (1984). What are the research priorities in the behavioral areas for burn patients? *Journal of Trauma, 24*(9), 197-201.

Knudson-Cooper, M., & Thomas, C. (1988). Psychosocial care of the severely burned child. In H. Carvajal & D. Parks (Eds.), *Burns in children: Pediatric burn management* (pp. 345-362). Chicago: Year Book Medical Publishers.

LaBaw, W. (1973). Adjunctive trance therapy with severely burned children. *International Journal of Child Psychotherapy, 2*(1), 80-92.

Long, R., & Cope, O. (1961). Emotional problems of burned children. *New England Journal of Medicine, 264,* 1121-1127.

Love, B., Byrne, C., Roberts, J., Browne, G., & Brown, B. (1987). Adult psychosocial adjustment following childhood injury: The effect of disfigurement. *Journal of Burn Care and Rehabilitation, 8*(4), 280-285.

Martin, H. L. (1970). Antecedents of burns and scalds in children. *British Journal of Medical Psychology, 43,* 39-47.

Martin, H. L. (1980). Psychological effects of accidental injury in childhood with particular reference to burns and scalds. *Burns, 7*(2), 90-94.

Mather, L., & Mackie, J. (1983). The incidence of postoperative pain in children. *Pain*, *15*, 271–282.

McCaffery, M. (1977). Pain relief for the child. *Pediatric Nursing*, *3*(4), 11–16.

McGrath, P. J., & Vair, C. (1984). Psychological aspects of pain management of the burned child. *Children's Health Care*, *13*, 15–19.

Mumford, J., & Bowsher, D. (1976). Pain and protopathic sensibility. A review with particular reference to the teeth. *Pain*, *2*, 223–243.

Perrin, E., & Gerrity, P. (1981). There's a demon in your belly: Children's understanding of illness. *Pediatrics*, *67*, 841–849.

Perrin, E., & Perrin, J. (1983). Clinicians' assessments of children's understanding of illness. *American Journal of Diseases of Children*, *137*, 874–878.

Perry, S., & Heidrich, G. (1982). Management of pain during debridement: A survey of U.S. burn units. *Pain*, *13*, 267–280.

Piaget, J. (1965). *The moral judgement of the child*. New York: Free Press.

Pless, I., Roghmann, K., & Haggerty, R. (1972). Chronic illness, family functioning, and psychological adjustment: A model for the allocation of prevention mental health services. *International Journal of Epidemiology*, *1*, 271–277.

Purdue, G., Hunt, J., & Prescott, P. (1988). Child abuse by burning—An index of suspicion. *Journal of Trauma*, *28*(2), 221–224.

Reid, V., & Bush, J. (1990). Ethnic factors influencing pain expression: Implications for clinical assessment. In T. Miller (Ed.), *Chronic pain: Clinical issues in health care management* (pp. 117–145). Madison, CT: International Universities Press.

Ross, D., & Ross, S. (1984). Childhood pain: The school-aged child's viewpoint. *Pain*, *20*, 179–191.

Ross, D., & Ross, S. (1988). *Childhood pain: Current issues, research, and management*. Baltimore: Urban & Schwarzenberg.

Sawyer, M. G., Minde, K., & Zucker, R. (1982). The burned child: Scarred for life? *Burns*, *9*, 205–213.

Schubert Walker, L., & Healy, M. (1980). Psychological treatment of a burned child. *Journal of Pediatric Psychology*, *5*(4), 395–403.

Seligman, R., MacMillan, B., & Carroll, S. (1971). The burned child: A neglected area of psychiatry. *American Journal of Psychiatry*, *128*, 52–57.

Simons, R., McFadd, A., Frank, H., Green, L., Malin, R., & Morris, J. (1978). Behavioral contracting in a burn care facility: A strategy for patient participation. *Journal of Trauma*, *18*(4), 257–260.

Solnit, A., & Priel, B. (1975). Scared and scarred: Psychological aspects in the treatment of soldiers with burns. *Israeli Annals of Psychiatry*, *13*, 213–220.

Sroufe, L. (1979). The coherence of individual development: Early care, attachment, and subsequent developmental issues. *American Psychologist*, October, 834–841.

Steward, M., & Steward, D. (1981). Children's conceptions of medical procedures. In R. Bibace & M. Walsh (Eds.), *Children's conceptions of health, illness, and bodily functions* (pp. 67–84). San Francisco: Jossey-Bass.

Stoddard, F. (1982). Coping with pain: A developmental approach to treatment of burned children. *American Journal of Psychiatry*, *139*(6), 736–740.

Tarnowski, K., McGrath, M., Calhoun, B., & Drabman, R. (1987). Pediatric burn injury: Self- versus therapist-mediated debridement. *Journal of Pediatric Psychology*, *12*(4), 567–579.

Tarnowski, K., Rasnake, L., Linscheid, T., & Mulick, J. (1989). Behavioral adjustment of pediatric burn victims. *Journal of Pediatric Psychology, 14*(4), 607-615.

Varni, J., Bessman, C., Russo, D., & Cataldo, M. (1980). Behavioral management of chronic pain in children: A case study. *Archives of Physical and Medical Rehabilitation, 61*, 375-378.

Vigliano, A., Hart, L., & Singer, F. (1964). Psychiatric sequelae of old burns in children and their parents. *American Journal of Orthopsychiatry, 34*, 753-761.

Woodward, J. (1959). Emotional disturbances of burned children. *British Medical Journal, 1*, 1009-1013.

Wright, L., & Fulwiler, R. (1974). Long range emotional sequelae of burns: Effects on children and their mothers. *Pediatric Research, 8*, 931-934.

Zide, B., & Pardoe, R. (1976). The use of behavior modification therapy in a recalcitrant burned child. *Plastic and Reconstructive Surgery, 57*(3), 378-382.

12
Chronic and Recurrent Pain: Hemophilia, Juvenile Rheumatoid Arthritis, and Sickle Cell Disease

Gary A. Walco and James W. Varni

Pain in children represents a complex cognitive-developmental phenomenon, involving a number of biobehavioral components that synergistically interact to produce differential levels of pain perception and verbal and nonverbal manifestations (Varni, 1983). In marked contrast to the rather extensive literature on adult chronic pain assessment and management, the systematic investigation of pediatric chronic and recurrent pain from a cognitive-biobehavioral perspective represents a relatively new area of inquiry (Varni, Jay, Masek, & Thompson, 1986; Varni, Katz, & Dash, 1982). Given children's various cognitive developmental stages, conceptualizations of pain and discomfort must be taken into consideration (Thompson & Varni, 1986). Thus, an accurate understanding of pain perception in children cannot be gleaned from simply applying downward the knowledge of pain perception in adults; rather, research and clinical practice in pediatric pain assessment and management must develop a separate, if not parallel, data base from the adult field that is sensitive to the unique characteristics of children. In the past several years a growing number of investigators have begun generating a substantial data base from which the clinical potential of cognitive-biobehavioral techniques in managing pediatric chronic and recurrent pain has become clear (McGrath, 1987a; Varni, Walco, & Wilcox, 1990).

Varni (1983) has identified four primary categories of pediatric pain: (a) pain associated with a disease state (e.g., hemophilia, arthritis, sickle cell disease); (b) pain associated with an observable physical injury or trauma (e.g., burns, lacerations, fractures); (c) pain not associated with a well-defined or specific disease state or identifiable physical injury (e.g., migraine and tension headaches, recurrent abdominal pain); and (d) pain associated with medical and dental procedures (e.g., lumbar punctures, bone marrow aspirations, surgery, injections, venipuncture, tooth extractions). In this chapter, we focus exclusively on chronic and recurrent pain associated with the pediatric chronic diseases of hemophilia, juvenile rheumatoid arthritis (JRA), and sickle cell disease. The other three categories of pediatric pain are addressed in other chapters in this book. Furthermore, in discussing interventions for such pain syndromes, we will emphasize cognitive-biobehavioral techniques that have received considerable empirical attention over the last several years (Varni et al., 1990), and minimize descriptions of pharmacologic treatments (see Lovell & Walco, 1989; and Shapiro, 1989, for details of pharmacologic interventions in juvenile rheumatoid arthritis and sickle cell disease, respectively).

Pediatric Chronic and Recurrent Pain

In the cognitive-biobehavioral assessment and management of pediatric pain, it is essential to distinguish between acute, chronic, and recurrent pain (McGrath, 1987b; Varni, 1983; Varni et al., 1990). Acute pain serves an adaptive biological warning signal, directing attention to an injured part or disease condition, functioning within an avoidance paradigm to encourage escape or avoidance of harmful stimuli and indicating the need for rest, immobilization, or treatment of the injured area. Although neurophysiological processes may distinguish acute from chronic pain (Bonica, 1977), it is often the intensity of acute pain and its associated anxiety reaction that most parsimoniously differentiate acute from chronic pain expression (Varni, 1983).

Pediatric chronic pain, on the other hand, is typically characterized by the absence of an anxious component, with a constellation of reactive features such as compensatory posturing, lack of developmentally appropriate behaviors, depressed mood, and inactivity or restriction in the normal activities of daily living. These chronic pain behaviors may eventually be maintained independently of the original nociceptive impulses and tissue damage, being reinforced by socioenvironmental influences (Crue, 1985; Fordyce, 1976; P. A. McGrath, 1986; Varni, Bessman, Russo, & Cataldo, 1980). Acute pain, in contrast, typically occurs in temporal proximity with a pathogenic agent or noxious stimulus.

In pediatric chronic diseases, the chronic musculoskeletal pain associated with JRA and hemophilic arthropathy correspond to the chronic pain model described above. In the recurrent, episodical pain of acute bleeding episodes in hemophilia and of vaso-occlusive crises in sickle cell disease, the clear distinction between acute and chronic pain is not evident. The following sections will describe further the differential assessment and management strategies inherent in chronic and recurrent pain comprehensive care.

Pediatric Chronic and Recurrent Pain Assessment

Central to the assessment of pediatric chronic or recurrent pain is children's conceptualizations of their illness. We know of no studies specifically addressing the relationship between cognitive development, concepts of illness, and pain experience in children with any of the chronic illnesses under discussion. In fact, in cases where these issues were ignored, pain assessment data may be quite misleading. For example, two early studies focused on pain intensity in subjects with arthritis using simple visual analogue scales or four-point descriptive scales (Laaksonen & Laine, 1961; Scott, Ansell, & Huskisson, 1977). Results showed relatively low levels of pain in children, and it was concluded that children with JRA experience less pain than adults with rheumatoid arthritis. However, these authors did not sufficiently attend to developmental factors (a number of children were unable to respond adequately to visual analogue scales, for example), and thus the reliability of these data are questionable.

Beales, Keen, and Lennox Holt (1983) took cognitive developmental issues into account to a greater degree and found that children with JRA were able to describe discomfort in their joints. These authors subsequently divided their sample based on chronologic age (6 to 11 years, 12 to 17 years) and performed midpoint splits on visual analogue scores for pain intensity, and found that older children tended to report higher levels of pain. Although it is not clear why the data were analyzed in this manner, it was concluded that with increasing age comes greater understanding of key concepts related to illness and disease, leading to increased significance of pain and discomfort and thus reports of greater pain intensity. This notion was not tested, however.

Thompson and Varni (1986) discussed the relationship between pain assessment and the stages of children's concepts of illness as described by Bibace and Walsh (1980) (for details, see chapter 8). Such concepts were also integrated into their development of a pain questionnaire for chronic and recurrent pain in children.

For adult chronic pain patients, the most widely used and respected assessment instrument has been the McGill Pain Questionnaire (MPQ; Melzack, 1975). Subsequent to its publication, other investigators have further shown the reliability, validity, and clinical utility of the MPQ across a diversity of adult pain syndromes (Reading, 1983). Modeled after the MPQ but designed to be sensitive to the cognitive-developmental conceptualizations of children, the Varni/Thompson Pediatric Pain Questionnaire (PPQ; see Appendix to this chapter) is a comprehensive, multidimensional assessment instrument specifically designed for the study of acute, chronic, and recurrent pain in children, with child, adolescent, and parent forms.

The PPQ-child form addresses the intensity of pain through visual analogue scales and colors (representing relative levels of pain) on a body outline (through which specific sites are also identified). Verbal descriptors are also used to help delineate the sensory, evaluative, and affective qualities of pain perception. The PPQ-adolescent form additionally addresses potential socioenvironmental influences on pain perception. The PPQ-parent form consists of similar components to the PPQ-child and PPQ-adolescent forms to allow for cross-validation. A comprehensive family history section addresses the child's pain history and the family's pain history with questions pertaining to symptomatology, past and present treatments for pain, and socioenvironmental situations that may influence pain perception.

Thus far, the published reliability and validity of components of the PPQ are available for chronic musculoskeletal pain in JRA (Thompson, Varni, & Hanson, 1987; Varni, Thompson, & Hanson, 1987; Varni, Wilcox, Hanson, & Brik, 1988). Data are emerging on the psychometric properties and clinical utility of the PPQ for children and adolescents with sickle cell disease (Walco & Dampier, 1990; Walco, Dampier, & Djordjevic, 1987) and there are ongoing studies by Varni and other investigators at different sites on its applicability to a range of pediatric acute, chronic, and recurrent pain syndromes. In the following sections, details of certain aspects of the PPQ will be described.

Visual Analogue Scale

Present pain and worst pain intensity for the previous week are assessed in the PPQ by a visual analogue scale (VAS). Each VAS is a 10-cm horizontal line with no numbers, marks, or descriptive vocabulary words along its length. The child VAS is anchored with developmentally appropriate pain descriptors (e.g., "not hurting," "hurting a whole lot") and happy and sad faces. The adolescent and parent VAS are anchored by the phrases "no pain" and "severe pain" in addition to the descriptors "hurting" and "discomfort." The instructions for the VAS ask the child/adolescent/parent to place a vertical mark through the horizontal VAS line that represents the intensity of pain along the continuum from no pain to severe pain.

The assessment of pediatric pain must fulfill the requirements for any measurement instrument, including reliability, validity, minimum inherent bias, and versatility (Beyer & Knapp, 1986; P. A. McGrath, 1986; P. J. McGrath, 1986; Varni et al., 1987). As reviewed by P. A. McGrath (1986), the VAS, although deceptively simple, has demonstrated the reliability, validity, minimum inherent bias, and versatility necessary for an objective pain measure in a variety of experimental and clinical pain studies. Historically, the VAS has been used extensively with adult pain subjects because of its sensitivity and reproducibility (Huskisson, 1983). As a continuous measurement scale, the VAS avoids the spurious clustering of pain reports that occur with stepwise or categorical pain scaling methods (Levine, Gordon, Smith, & Fields, 1981).

In both children and adults, the VAS has demonstrated excellent construct validity in postoperative medication studies, showing the expected reduction in pain subsequent to analgesia intake (Aradine, Beyer, & Tompkins, 1988; Levine et al., 1981; O'Hara, McGrath, D'Astous, & Vair, 1987; Taenzer, 1983), and in chronic musculoskeletal pain, demonstrating the expected increase in perceived pain intensity with greater rheumatic disease activity (Thompson et al., 1987; Varni et al., 1987). Finally, in a recent study it was found that in children and adolescents with sickle cell disease, VAS scores were related to physician estimates of disease severity, increased dramatically with the onset of severe vaso-occlusive episodes, and were sensitive to analgesic effects in patients hospitalized for uncomplicated vaso-occlusive crises (Walco & Dampier, 1990).

A 10-cm line length has been found to have the smallest measurement error in comparison to line lengths of 5 or 20 cm (Seymour, Simpson, Charlton, & Phillips, 1985). In adults, vertical and horizontal VASs exhibit extremely high correlations ($r = .99$; Scott & Huskisson, 1979). It has been suggested that especially for young children, a vertical line may be more easily conceptualized, and thus more psychometrically sound (Aradine et al., 1988), but these impressions have not been supported with data.

From a psychophysical measurement perspective, the VAS is considered a direct scaling method and a form of cross-modality matching in which the length of a line is adjusted to match the intensity of pain (Huskisson, 1983; P. A. McGrath, 1986). P. A. McGrath has investigated the measurement properties of the VAS in a series of psychophysical studies with both children and adults (McGrath & deVeber, 1986; McGrath, deVeber, & Hearn, 1985; Price, McGrath, Rafii, & Buckingham, 1983) and demonstrated that the VAS has ratio rather than interval scale properties. Interval scales reflect equal distances in the variables being quantitatively ordered where the zero point is arbitrarily determined and does not represent the complete absence of the variable being measured. Ratio scales are the same as interval scales except that there is a true zero point. Clearly, for the measurement of pain, the latter is highly desirable.

In a study of chronic musculoskeletal pain in juvenile rheumatoid arthritis by Varni et al. (1987) using the PPQ, the child's report of pain on the child VAS correlated highly with both parental ($r = .72, p < .001$) and physician ($r = .65, p < .001$) ratings of the child's pain independently recorded on the adult VAS. Parent and physician ratings also correlated highly ($r = .85, p < .001$). In a similar study of vaso-occlusive pain in sickle cell disease (Walco & Dampier, 1990), these respective correlation coefficients were $r = .21$ ($p > .05$), $r = .67$ ($p < .001$), and $r = .62$ ($p < .001$). Finally, focusing on pediatric postoperative pain, P. J. McGrath and colleagues (P. J. McGrath et al., 1985) found a correlation of $r = .91$ between observer and nurse ratings on the VAS. The nurse and observer ratings on the VAS also correlated highly with a pain behavior checklist, $r = .81$ and $r = .86$, respectively.

The high correlations between the observer and nurse VAS ratings and the pain behavior checklist suggest that the paths of decision making regarding pediatric pain perception by observers may be the same for the observer VAS and the pain behavior checklist; i.e., manifestation of overt verbal and nonverbal pain behaviors by the child are a necessary (but most likely not sufficient) condition for the ratings of pediatric pain perception by objective observers. However, it is clear that a child can experience pain without necessarily exhibiting overt pain behaviors, consequently resulting in considerable measurement error for adult observation techniques in accurately assessing pediatric pain perception.

This point was discussed by Walco and Dampier (1990) with respect to the correlations reported above for pediatric sickle cell pain. In assessing the intensity of children's pain, physicians and parents appear to rely heavily on observations of overt pain behaviors (and thus their estimates intercorrelate). Additionally, physicians possess knowledge of disease characteristics and severity, which also likely contributes to their estimates of pain. Neither, however, have access to the private subjective experience of the child, and thus correlations with the child's pain estimates may be rather low (as was the case for child/parent VAS scores for present pain). This effect may be especially so when pain is episodic (such as with sickle cell disease) in contrast with chronic and ongoing pain (as is often the case for the musculoskeletal pain of JRA).

It is important to note that Walco and Dampier (1990) did not therefore question the validity of the children's self-reported pain intensity on the VAS. Indeed, the child VAS has been shown to be a reliable and valid measure of children's pain perception with children as young as 5 years of age (McGrath & deVeber, 1986; P. A. McGrath et al., 1985; Varni et al., 1987). To question child pain self-report because of a lack of significant correlations with observer estimates of child pain is an erroneous concept. Pain is a subjective phenomenon and it cannot be expected that another individual can accurately and without measurement error assess another person's private experience of it. In a study of adult pain, for example, the correlation between patients' VAS scores and nurses' VAS scores was only $r = .38$ (Teske, Dart, & Cleeland, 1983). This finding did not lead these investigators to subsequently question the validity of these adults to assess their pain! We strongly feel that children should be accorded the same degree of consideration; i.e., they are the best judges of their pain experience. Throughout the rest of this chapter we hope to make this point further by providing both research and clinical findings that support the validity of children's self-reports of their pain experience.

Pain Threshold and Chronic Clinical Pain

In the history of the literature on the assessment of clinical pain in children, initial emphasis was placed on the accurate assessment of the subjective pain experience. More recently, greater attention has been paid to the various factors that may affect that experience. Details of a comprehensive predictive model of disease-related and socioenvironmental factors related to joint pain in JRA will be presented below. One recent study, however, has focused on a little studied aspect of pediatric pain—pain threshold.

In the adult literature, experimental pain measures include pain threshold (the lowest level of stimulation labeled as "pain"), pain tolerance (the maximal level of noxious stimulation that the subject can tolerate), and pain reactivity (an index of a specific response to painful stimuli). Pain threshold is generally thought to be a sensory event that is physiologically loaded, whereas pain tolerance and reactivity are the result of one's physiologic sensitivity (pain threshold) in tandem with psychologic variables (Merskey, 1973; Sternbach, 1975; Wolff, 1983). Although the latter two factors are probably most closely related to clinical pain experience, for ethical reasons research involving experimentally induced pain at tolerance or reactance levels in pediatric populations is limited.

Walco and his colleagues (Walco, Dampier, Hartstein, Djordjevic, & Miller, 1990) investigated the relationship between pain threshold levels and clinical pain experience in four groups of children between 5 and 16 years of age: children with JRA (a chronic illness in which chronic and recurrent pain is a feature), children with sickle cell disease (a chronic illness in which recurrent episodes of acute pain is a common feature), asthma (a chronic illness in which pain is typically not a feature), and healthy controls. Pain threshold was measured through direct pressure to a joint and through circumferential pressure stimulation, whereas present clinical pain was assessed through visual analogue scales. Although no direct relationship was observed between these two measures, it was found that children with JRA and sickle cell disease had significantly lower pain thresholds than did their healthy peers. Furthermore, pain threshold values were found to be internally consistent over repeated trials and across stimulus modes, and were not found to be significantly related to measures of psychological adaptation or perceived self-competence and did not predict behavioral indices such as school attendance. Thus, it was concluded that pain threshold is a factor worthy of further consideration and that it may not be principally physiologically determined. It is also possible that experience with recurrent pain sensitizes children to future pain stimulation. Clearly, chronic pain in children is not a unidimensional construct and thus requires the assessment of a number of intrapersonal and socioenvironmental factors, a conceptualization that will be described in more detail for each of the major chronic illnesses to be described below.

Cognitive-Biobehavioral Treatment

The primary cognitive-biobehavioral treatment techniques utilized in the management of pediatric chronic and recurrent pain have been categorized by Varni (1983) into (a) *pain perception regulation* modalities through such self-regulatory techniques as progressive muscle relaxation, meditative breathing, and guided imagery, and (b) *pain behavior regulation*, which identifies and modifies socioenvironmental factors that influence pain expression and rehabilitation. The following sections will describe the utilization and clinical research findings of cognitive-biobehavioral assessment and management techniques for three pediatric chronic diseases: hemophilia, juvenile rheumatoid arthritis, and sickle cell disease.

Hemophilia

Whereas recurrent acute pain in the hemophiliac is associated with a specific bleeding episode, chronic musculoskeletal pain as a result of hemophilic arthropathy (similar to osteoarthritis and caused by repeated hemorrhages into the joint areas) represents a sustained condition over an extended period of time. Thus, pain perception in the hemophiliac truly represents a complex psychophysiological event, complicated by the existence of both recurrent bleeding pain and chronic arthritic pain, requiring differential treatment strategies. More specifically, acute pain of hemorrhage provides a functional signal, indicating the necessity of intravenous infusion of factor replacement that temporarily replaces the missing clotting factor, converts the clotting status to normal, and allows a functional blood clot to form. Arthritic pain, on the other hand, represents a potentially debilitating chronic condition that may result in impaired life functioning and analgesic dependency (Varni & Gilbert, 1982). Consequently, the development of an effective alternative to analgesic dependency in the reduction of perceived chronic arthritic pain secondary to hemophilic arthropathy that does not interfere with the essential functional signal of acute recurrent bleeding pain has been the goal of the behavioral medicine approach to hemophilia pain management (Varni, 1981a).

Varni and his associates (Varni, 1981a; Varni, 1981b; Varni & Gilbert, 1982; Varni, Gilbert, & Dietrich, 1981) have reported on a series of studies investigating chronic arthritic pain management in both child and adult hemophiliacs. Instruction in the cognitive-biobehavioral self-regulation of arthritic pain perception consists of three sequential phases. The child is first taught a 25-step progressive muscle relaxation sequence involving the alternative tensing and relaxing of major muscle groups (see Varni, 1983 for more details). The child is then taught meditative breathing exercises, consisting of medium deep breaths inhaled through the nose and slowly exhaled through the mouth. While exhaling, the child is instructed to say the word "relax" silently to himself and to initially describe aloud and subsequently visualize the word "relax" in warm colors, as if written in colored chalk on a blackboard. Finally, the child is instructed in the use of guided imagery techniques, consisting of pleasant, distracting scenes selected by the child. Initially, the child is instructed to imagine himself actually in the scene, not simply to observe himself there. The scene is evoked by a detailed multisensory description by the therapist and subsequently described aloud by the child. Once the scene is clearly visualized by the child, the therapist instructs the child to experiment with other, different scenes to maintain interest and variety. The child is instructed to practice these techniques on a regular basis in the home, and to return for sessions with the therapist to maintain technique and for encouragement and problem solving. Data have demonstrated the successful utilization of these techniques with both child and adult patients in controlling chronic musculoskeletal pain secondary to hemophilic arthropathy.

Juvenile Rheumatoid Arthritis

In children with chronic musculoskeletal pain, the prototype for inflammatory chronic arthropathy is juvenile rheumatoid arthritis (Varni & Jay, 1984). The disease typically manifests itself before 16 years of age, with peak onset in the age groups 1 to 3 and 8 to 12 years. In general, girls are affected twice as often as boys. Although the precise mechanisms of joint pain in JRA are not fully understood, it is clear that the effects of this pain are substantial and, from a clinical standpoint, pain is seen as the major mediating factor in one's ability to cope with the disease (Lovell & Walco, 1989).

Varni and his colleagues (Thompson et al., 1987; Varni et al., 1987; Varni et al., 1988) have developed an empirical model using multiple regression analysis to statistically predict pain perception and functional status in children with JRA. The criterion variable (dependent measure) for pain was the child VAS, and the predictor variables included child psychological adjustment, family psychosocial environment, and disease parameters. This empirical model was able to statistically predict 72% of the variance in child perception and report of worst pain for the previous week (Thompson et al., 1987). Taking the model one step further, Varni entered into the multiple regression analysis worst pain for the previous week in addition to the other predictor variables, this time to predict the criterion variable of functional status. The model accounted for 57% of the variance in activities of daily living (Varni et al., 1988). The following case study illustrates this comprehensive approach to chronic pain assessment.

The child was an 11-year-old female with polyarticular JRA. At the time of assessment, she had morning stiffness for approximately 4 hours each day. Sixteen joints exhibited active disease. A pediatric rheumatologist rated the child's overall disease as moderate (4) on a 5-point scale. Naprosyn (a nonsteroidal anti-inflammatory drug) was reported as being used to control pain episodes.

The child's mother completed the PPQ-parent form (see Appendix). The PPQ documented the child's pain as adversely affecting her mobility, appetite, sleep, social activities, and school attendance. On the 10-cm VAS, the child's mother estimated her child's present pain intensity at 9 cm (quite severe pain). The words "burning," "aching," "tiring," and "sharp" were chosen from the PPQ's word list by the mother to describe her child's pain. On the PPQ body diagram, the mother localized her child's pain in the shoulder, elbows, wrists, knees, ankles, toes, and fingers.

On the PPQ's word list, the child chose words "sharp," "pinching," and "squeezing" to describe her pain. On the 10-cm child VAS, the child estimated her present pain at 5 cm. She estimated her worst pain for the previous week at 9.5 cm (a rating very close to her mother's rating of her present pain intensity). The attending rheumatologist estimated the child's present pain at 7 cm. When localizing the pain on the PPQ's body diagram, the child indicated pain in her shoulders, elbows, wrists, knees, ankles, toes, and fingers; the exact same locations chosen independently by her mother.

On the PPQ's color scale, the child chose red to represent no hurt, yellow to represent a little hurt, blue to represent more hurt, and green to represent a lot of hurt (no pain, mild pain, moderate pain, severe pain, respectively), which illustrates the importance of allowing the child to select the color-intensity match, because most children select red to represent severe pain (Thompson & Varni, 1986; Varni et al., 1987). Consistent with a diagnosis of polyarticular arthritis, she colored in with green (severe pain) both knees and her left temporomandibular joint. Both hands, wrists, and shoulders, and her right temporomandibular joint were colored in blue (moderate pain). Both elbows, feet, and ankles were colored with yellow (mild pain). The rest of her body was colored in red (no pain). Thus, although red was selected to represent severe pain by 52% of the children in the original study (Varni et al., 1987), individual children should be given the opportunity to make their own developmentally appropriate color-intensity match.

The child's psychological adjustment scores on the Child Behavior Checklist (Achenbach & Edelbrock, 1983), completed by the mother, were within normal limits on most subscales. However, there was a large elevation on the depressive symptomatology scale for this child. Although this score was not in the clinical depression range, it was elevated to the extent that it suggested increased risk for some psychological adjustment problems in the area of depressive symptomatology. The Family Environment Scale (Moos & Moos, 1981), also completed by the mother, was used to develop a profile of family psychosocial functioning. In general, for this family the scores were within the normal limits on all subscales.

This multidimensional assessment battery (see Thompson et al., 1987, for a complete description of all the instruments used) provides a comprehensive basis for developing pediatric chronic and recurrent pain management interventions. By using such a developmentally appropriate instrument as the PPQ, pain intensity, pain location, and the qualitative aspects of the pain experience can be obtained from the child, as well as potentially modifiable psychological and socioenvironmental factors.

Indeed, in an ongoing study of cognitive-biobehavioral interventions for pain associated with JRA (Walco, Varni, Hartstein, & Ilowite, 1988), the PPQ is used for initial assessment and components are being employed to assess both immediate as well as long-term effects of the intervention. Children between the ages of 5 and 16 years are seen for a total of eight sessions in which they are taught progressive muscle relaxation, meditative breathing, and guided imagery in an attempt to moderate joint pain and increase adaptive functioning. Preliminary data indicate that there is tremendous short-term benefit of these strategies as virtually all subjects have been able to dramatically reduce their level of subjective pain as measured by the 10-cm VAS. The mean pretreatment score was 4.89 cm (S.D. = 1.53, range of 2.0 to 7.0 cm) and the mean posttreatment score was 0.68 cm (S.D. = 0.75, range of 0 to 2.0 cm). This difference was highly significant, $t = 8.14$, $p < .0001$. In addition, preliminary descriptive analyses show a reasonable degree of generalization from clinic sessions to strategies employed at home. Follow-up data, being gathered at regular intervals, focus not only on pain experience, but also on daily activities, school attendance, psychological adjustment, and family psychosocial functioning.

Sickle Cell Disease

Reversible microvascular occlusion at the arteriolar or capillary level affecting bone or bone marrow circulation causes the characteristic painful "crisis" (painful episode) that is the hallmark of sickle cell disease. Although a variety of biochemical (Karayalcin, Lanzkowsky, & Kazi, 1981; Lawrence & Fabry, 1986) or hematologic (Warth & Rucknagel, 1984) variables are altered during acute painful episodes, most are nonspecific and thus are not diagnostic for this event.

Assessment of Sickle Cell Pain

The frequency and severity of pain due to vaso-occlusive episodes varies greatly both across and within individuals. Recent data indicate that the average pediatric sickle cell disease patient experiences one to two severe episodes per year (Dampier, Walco, & Zimo, in review). The variation is great, however, in that some patients may experience no pain in a year, whereas others experience pain more than once a week. Furthermore, within a given individual, there may be extended periods that are pain free followed by a number of vaso-occlusive episodes over a relatively short period of time.

Although some of the variance may be accounted for by type of hemoglobinopathy (for example, HbSS is generally more severe than HbSC), there are no specific factors that have been identified to account for the observed differences. Relatedly, there are few reliable hematologic parameters by which the severity of a vaso-occlusive episode may be gauged. Thus, unlike the pain associated with acute bleeds in hemophilia or joint flare-ups in arthritis in which there are objective indices of medical factors related to pain, in sickle cell disease one is limited to subjective reports of the patient and behavioral observations as a means of evaluating the intensity of pain due to vaso-occlusion.

The PPQ and Sickle Cell Disease

A study has been conducted utilizing the PPQ to assess sickle cell pain (Walco & Dampier, 1990). Thirty-five subjects between the ages of 5 and 15 years were evaluated in the outpatient clinic. Results indicated that the relative infrequency of vaso-occlusive episodes apparently limited the number of opportunities parents had to evaluate their child's pain, and thus retrospective accounts of pain intensity were poor. Significant relationships among physician estimates of disease severity, restrictions in activity, impact on daily functioning, and reported levels of present pain were consistently shown. Furthermore, it was clear that pain adjectives, colors (for younger children), and body outlines could be used meaningfully to describe pain.

As a second aspect of the study, the present pain VAS and pain adjective checklist were used on a daily basis with patients admitted to the hospital for uncomplicated painful episodes. Findings indicate that the VAS was quite useful in this situation as patients were able to express different levels of discomfort throughout the course of their hospitalization and VAS ratings correlated with dosage of analgesic (an independent criterion, as the house physician was not privy to VAS ratings). In addition, patients utilized the adjective checklist in a meaningful way throughout the hospitalization. It was noted that a large number of pain descriptors were selected at the beginning of the hospital stay, and steadily dropped as days passed. This trend was especially obvious for the affective and evaluative pain descriptors. Finally, body outlines proved to be worthwhile as patients labeled specific pain sites and to a large extent differentiated relative levels of pain intensity among the sites.

Treatment of Sickle Cell Pain

Vaso-Occlusion and Recurrent Acute Pain

By and large, sickle cell crises may be conceptualized as recurrent acute painful episodes. Thus, the average patient appears to maintain a relatively normal life-style that is interrupted periodically by vaso-occlusive episodes. At these times, rest and immobilization are encouraged, and analgesic treatments range from aspirin or acetaminophen for less severe episodes to parenterally administered (intramuscular or intravenous) narcotics given during hospitalizations (Cole, Sprinkle, Smith, & Buchanon, 1986; Scott, 1982). In the latter situation, a fixed dosing schedule adjusting for dosage of analgesic is much preferred to either p.r.n. or variable-schedule dosing. Fixed dosing facilitates the maintenance of therapeutic levels of the analgesic, thereby reducing the severe peaks and valleys experienced as the drug is metabolized. This facet, in tandem with the fact that the patient receives the analgesic without having to ask for it, reduces the tendency of constantly attending to one's level of discomfort. In addition, recent data indicate that in adolescents with sickle cell disease, patient-controlled analgesia is an efficient means of delivering therapeutic doses of narcotic analgesics (Schechter, Berrien, & Katz, 1988).

Self-regulatory techniques have been shown to be of benefit to adolescent and young adult patients experiencing painful episodes. Zeltzer, Dash, and Holland (1979) described two cases in which a combination of hypnosis and thermal biofeedback was used to reduce the frequency and intensity of pain crises, the need for heavy analgesia, the frequency of emergency room visits, and the frequency and length of hospitalizations. Similar techniques and results were obtained in a larger within-subjects design study conducted with 15 adults between 22 and 35 years of age (Thomas, Koshy, Patterson, Dorn, & Thomas, 1984). Finally, in a study with eight patients between the ages of 10 and 20 years, Cozzi, Tryon, and Sedlacek (1987) demonstrated the immediate short-term effectiveness of biofeedback training (e.g., frontalis muscle tension, digital temperature, frequency of headache as a crisis symptom, analgesic use, perceived pain intensity), but no significant effect on emergency room or inpatient utilization. Clearly much more systematic research is needed on the efficacy of both pharmacologic and nonpharmacologic interventions for pain in sickle cell disease.

Sickle Cell Disease and Chronic Pain

The key assumption underlying an acute pain model of intervention is that the pain is principally peripheral in its origin (Crue, 1985). That is, vaso-occlusion, a pathophysiological condition, leads to nociception. Implicit here is the notion that once the condition resolves, the pain will dissipate, and the patient will return to a normal routine. Also implicit is that psychological factors play a relatively small part in the patient's pain experience and thus these issues are often ignored. For most pediatric and adolescent sickle cell disease patients, the acute pain model is valid (Dampier et al., in review). There is a minority, however, for whom psychological and social issues play a major role in affecting their pain experience, and thus these issues should not be ignored. As discussed by Walco and Dampier (1987), these patients are typically adolescents whose life-styles are marked by maladaptive coping patterns, poor psychological adjustment, inadequate family and social support, and school absenteeism and failure. Clearly to ignore these factors and continue hospitalizing such patients for pain only contributes to the cycle of dependency on the medical system and withdrawal from prosocial activities.

Although it seems that these psychological factors parallel those found in adults with chronic pain syndromes, devising appropriate assessment and treatment strategies is difficult. For example, when such a patient presents in the emergency room complaining of severe pain, medical professionals are faced with the truly impossible task of determining the extent to which that pain is due to vaso-occlusion or to psychosocial factors. For many professionals, this distinction carries the incorrect implication that the former is "real" pain, whereas the latter is "all in the patient's head." As a result, antagonistic relationships develop between patients and caregivers that often lead to manipulation and malingering. Furthermore, because treatment of pain follows from assessment, medical professionals are faced with another conflict. As mentioned above, if pathophysiologic factors are emphasized and psychological and social issues are ignored, the maladaptive pattern is reinforced. On the other hand, if one assumes that the pain is purely psychological, there is a strong chance of undertreating a severe vaso-occlusive episode.

As described by Walco and his colleagues (Varni et al., 1990; Walco & Dampier, 1987), in order to treat such patients adequately, biomedical, psychological, and social factors must be addressed. Behaviorally based interventions have been used, including protocols specifying the frequency and duration of hospitalizations (for uncomplicated painful episodes), inpatient analgesic dosing schedules, frequency of emergency room visits, and availability of narcotics for outpatient use. Each of these variables are modified over time to successively approximate norms for matched peers, and all medical personnel are provided with these protocols so that responses are standardized and few relevant decisions are made on a subjective basis.

This strategy has been successful in curbing inappropriate health care utilization and the frequency and intensity of manipulative or malingering behavior has decreased. Quality of life outside of the hospital, however, does not improve dramatically until psychological interventions are introduced to specifically address psychological maladjustment. This may include facilitating reentry to school, building social skills, working to improve the family system, and in some cases psychopharmacologic interventions.

Summary

In contrast to acute pain, the assessment and management of pain associated with chronic illness in children requires increased attention to factors such as psychological adjustment and family environment in addition to disease-related parameters. Because the pain experience is not finite, coping strategies must be mobilized by children and their families. Thus, a high degree of flexibility is required in the comprehensive assessment and treatment of chronic and recurrent pain. As a result, an interdisciplinary, multidimensional approach is essential to address these patients' needs adequately.

References

Achenbach, T. M., & Edelbrock, L. S. (1983). *Manual for the Child Behavior Checklist and Revised Child Behavior Profile*. Burlington, VT: University of Vermont.

Aradine, C. R., Beyer, J. E., & Tompkins, J. M. (1988). Children's pain perception before and after analgesia: A study of instrument construct validity and related issues. *Journal of Pediatric Nursing, 3*, 11–23.

Beales, J. G., Keen, J. H., & Lennox Holt, P. J. (1983). The child's perception of the disease and experience of pain in juvenile chronic arthritis. *Journal of Rheumatology, 10*, 61–65.

Beyer, J. E., & Knapp, T. R. (1986). Methodologic issues in the measurement of children's pain. *Children's Health Care, 14*, 233–241.

Bibace, R., & Walsh, M. (1980). Development of children's concepts of illness. *Pediatrics, 66*, 912–917.

Bonica, J. J. (1977). Neurophysiologic and pathologic aspects of acute and chronic pain. *Archives of Surgery, 112*, 750–761.

Cole, T. B., Sprinkle, R. H., Smith, S. J., & Buchanon, G. R. (1986). Intravenous narcotic therapy for children with severe sickle cell pain crisis. *American Journal of Diseases of Children, 140*, 1255–1259.

Cozzi, L., Tryon, W. W., & Sedlacek, K. (1987). The effectiveness of biofeedback-assisted relaxation in modifying sickle cell crisis. *Biofeedback and Self-Regulation, 12*, 51–61.

Crue, B. L. (1985). Multidisciplinary pain treatment programs: Current status. *Clinical Journal of Pain, 1*, 31–38.

Dampier, C. D., Walco, G. A., & Zimo, D. A. (in review). Therapy of pain syndromes in children and adolescents with sickle cell disease. Submitted for publication.

Fordyce, W. E. (1976). *Behavioral concepts in chronic pain and illness*. St. Louis: C. V. Mosby.

Huskisson, E. C. (1983). Visual analogue scales. In R. Melzack (Ed.), *Pain measurement and assessment* (pp. 33–37). New York: Raven Press.

Karayalcin, G., Lanzkowsky, P., & Kazi, A. B. (1981). Serum alpha-hydroxybutyrate dehydrogenase levels in children with sickle cell disease. *American Journal of Pediatric Hematology/Oncology, 3*, 169–171.

Laaksonen, A. L., & Laine, V. (1961). A comparative study of joint pain in adult and juvenile rheumatoid arthritis. *Annals of the Rheumatic Diseases, 20*, 386–387.

Lawrence, C., & Fabry, M. E. (1986). Erythrocyte sedimentation rate during steady state and painful crisis in sickle cell anemia. *American Journal of Medicine, 81*, 801–809.

Levine, J. D., Gordon, N. C., Smith, R., & Fields, H. L. (1981). Analgesic responses to morphine and placebo in individuals with post-operative pain. *Pain, 10*, 379–389.

Lovell, D. J., & Walco, G. A. (1989). Pain associated with juvenile rheumatoid arthritis. *Pediatric Clinics of North America, 36*, 1015–1027.

McGrath, P. A. (1986). The measurement of human pain. *Endodontics and Dental Traumatology, 2*, 124–129.

McGrath, P. A. (1987a). The management of chronic pain in children. In G. D. Burrows, D. Elton, & G. V. Stanley (Eds.), *The handbook of chronic pain management* (pp. 205–216). Amsterdam: Elsevier Press.

McGrath, P. A. (1987b). The multidimensional assessment and management of recurrent pain syndromes in children. *Behaviour Research and Therapy, 25*, 251–262.

McGrath, P. A., & deVeber, L. L. (1986). The management of acute pain evoked by medical procedures in children with cancer. *Journal of Pain and Symptom Management, 1*, 145-150.

McGrath, P. A., deVeber, L. L., & Hearn, M. T. (1985). Multidimensional pain assessment in children. In H. L. Fields, R. Dubner, & F. Cervero (Eds.), *Advances in pain research and therapy, Vol. 9* (pp. 387-393). New York: Raven Press.

McGrath, P. J. (1986). The clinical measurement of pain in children: A review. *Clinical Journal of Pain, 1*, 221-227.

McGrath, P. J., Johnson, G., Goodman, J. T., Schillinger, J., Dunn, J., & Chapman, J. (1985). The Children's Hospital of Eastern Ontario Pain Scale (CHEOPS): A behavioral scale for rating post-operative pain in children. In H. L. Fields, R. Dubner, & F. Cervero (Eds.), *Advances in pain research and therapy, Vol. 9* (pp. 395-402). New York: Raven Press.

Melzack, R. (1975). The McGill Pain Questionnaire: Major properties and scoring methods. *Pain, 1*, 277-299.

Merskey, H. (1973). The perception and measurement of pain. *Journal of Psychosomatic Research, 17*, 251-255.

Moos, R. H., & Moos, B. S. (1981). *Family Environment Scale.* Palo Alto, CA: Consulting Psychologists Press.

O'Hara, M., McGrath, P. J., D'Astous, J. D., & Vair, C. A. (1987). Oral morphine versus injected meperidine (Demerol) for pain relief in children after orthopedic surgery. *Journal of Pediatric Orthopedics, 7*, 78-82.

Price, D. D., McGrath, P. A., Rafii, A., & Buckingham, B. (1983). The validation of visual analogue scales as ratio measures of experimental and chronic pain. *Pain, 17*, 45-56.

Reading, A. E. (1983). The McGill Pain Questionnaire: An appraisal. In R. Melzack (Ed.), *Pain measurement and assessment* (pp. 55-61). New York: Raven Press.

Schechter, N. L., Berrien, F. B., & Katz, S. M. (1988). The use of patient controlled analgesia in adolescents with sickle cell pain crisis. *Journal of Pain and Symptom Management, 3*, 1-5.

Scott, P. J., & Huskisson, E. L. (1979). Vertical and horizontal visual analogue scales. *Annals of the Rheumatic Diseases, 38*, 560.

Scott, P. J., Ansell, B. M., & Huskisson, E. C. (1977). Measurement of pain in juvenile chronic polyarthritis. *Annals of the Rheumatic Diseases, 36*, 186-187.

Scott, R. B. (1982). The management of pain in children with sickle cell disease. In R. B. Scott (Ed.), *Advances in the pathophysiology, diagnosis, and treatment of sickle cell disease* (pp. 47-58). New York: Alan R. Liss.

Seymour, R. A., Simpson, J. M., Charlton, J. E., & Phillips, M. E. (1985). An evaluation of length and end-phrase of visual analogue scales in dental pain. *Pain, 21*, 177-185.

Shapiro, B. S. (1989). The management of pain in sickle cell disease. *Pediatric Clinics of North America, 36*, 1029-1045.

Sternbach, R. A. (1975). Psychophysiology of pain. *International Journal of Psychiatry in Medicine, 6*, 63-73.

Taenzer, P. (1983). Post-operative pain: Relationships among measures of pain, mood, and narcotic requirements. In R. Melzack (Ed.), *Pain measurement and assessment* (pp. 111-118). New York: Raven Press.

Teske, K., Dart, R. L., & Cleeland, L. S. (1983). Relationships between nurses' observations and patients' self-reports of pain. *Pain, 16*, 289-296.

Thomas, J. E., Koshy, M., Patterson, L., Dorn, L., & Thomas, K. (1984). Management of pain in sickle cell disease using biofeedback therapy: A preliminary study. *Biofeedback and Self-Regulation, 9*, 413–420.

Thompson, K. L., & Varni, J. W. (1986). A developmental cognitive-biobehavioral approach to pediatric pain assessment. *Pain, 25*, 282–296.

Thompson, K. L., Varni, J. W., & Hanson, V. (1987). Comprehensive assessment of pain in juvenile rheumatoid arthritis: An empirical model. *Journal of Pediatric Psychology, 12*, 241–255.

Varni, J. W. (1981a). Behavioral medicine in hemophilia arthritic pain management. *Archives of Physical Medicine and Rehabilitation, 62*, 183–187.

Varni, J. W. (1981b). Self-regulation techniques in the management of chronic arthritic pain in hemophilia. *Behavior Therapy, 12*, 185–194.

Varni, J. W. (1983). *Clinical behavioral pediatrics: An interdisciplinary biobehavioral approach.* New York: Pergamon Press.

Varni, J. W., Bessman, C. A., Russo, D. C., & Cataldo, M. F. (1980). Behavioral management of chronic pain in children. *Archives of Physical Medicine and Rehabilitation, 61*, 375–379.

Varni, J. W., & Gilbert, A. (1982). Self-regulation of chronic arthritic pain and long-term analgesic dependence in a hemophiliac. *Rheumatology and Rehabilitation, 22*, 171–174.

Varni, J. W., Gilbert, A., & Dietrich, S. L. (1981). Behavioral medicine in pain and analgesia management for the hemophilic child with factor VIII inhibitor. *Pain, 11*, 121–126.

Varni, J., & Jay, S. M. (1984). Biobehavioral factors in juvenile rheumatoid arthritis: Implications for research and practice. *Clinical Psychology Review, 4*, 543–560.

Varni, J. W., Jay, S. M., Masek, B. J., & Thompson, K. L. (1986). Cognitive-behavioral assessment and management of pediatric pain. In A. D. Holzman & D. C. Turk (Eds.), *Pain management: A handbook of psychological treatment approaches* (pp. 168–192). New York: Pergamon.

Varni, J. W., Katz, E. R., & Dash, J. (1982). Behavioral and neurochemical aspects of pediatric pain. In D. C. Russo & J. W. Varni (Eds.), *Behavioral pediatrics: Research and practice* (pp. 177–224). New York: Plenum Press.

Varni, J. W., Thompson, K. L., & Hanson, V. (1987). The Varni/Thompson Pediatric Pain Questionnaire: I. Chronic musculoskeletal pain in juvenile rheumatoid arthritis. *Pain, 28*, 27–38.

Varni, J. W., Walco, G. A., & Wilcox, K. T. (1990). Cognitive-biobehavioral assessment and treatment of pediatric pain. In A. M. Gross & R. S. Drabman (Eds.), *Handbook of clinical behavioral pediatrics* (pp. 83–109). New York: Plenum Press.

Varni, J. W., Wilcox, K. T., Hanson, V., & Brik, R. (1988). Chronic musculoskeletal pain and functional status in juvenile rheumatoid arthritis: An empirical model. *Pain, 32*, 1–7.

Walco, G. A., & Dampier, C. D. (1987). Chronic pain in adolescent patients. *Journal of Pediatric Psychology, 12*, 215–225.

Walco, G. A., & Dampier, C. D. (1990). Pain in children and adolescents with sickle cell disease: A descriptive study. *Journal of Pediatric Psychology, 15*, 643–658.

Walco, G. A., Dampier, C. D., & Djordjevic, D. (1987, September). *Pain assessment in children and adolescents with sickle cell disease.* Presented at "Sickle Cell Disease in the Next Decade: Innovative Therapeutic Approaches," Washington, D. C.

Walco, G. A., Dampier, C. D., Hartstein, G., Djordjevic, D., & Miller, L. (1990).

The relationship between recurrent clinical pain and pain threshold in children. In D. C. Tyler & E. J. Krane (Eds.), *Advances in pain research and therapy: Volume 15. Pediatric pain* (pp. 333–340). New York: Raven Press.

Walco, G. A., Varni, J. W., Hartstein, G., & Ilowite, N. T. (1988, November). *Cognitive-behavioral interventions for pain in children with juvenile rheumatoid arthritis: A preliminary report.* Paper presented at the Canadian and American Pain Societies Joint Meeting, Toronto.

Warth, J. A., & Rucknagel, D. L. (1984). Density ultra centrifugation of sickle cells during and after pain crisis: Increased dense erythrocytes in crisis. *Blood, 64,* 507–515.

Wolff, B. B. (1983). Laboratory methods of pain assessment. In R. Melzack (Ed.), *Pain measurement and assessment* (pp. 7–13). New York: Raven Press.

Zeltzer, L. K., Dash, J., & Holland, J. P. (1979). Hypnotically induced pain control in sickle cell anemia. *Pediatrics, 64,* 533–536.

Appendix.   The Varni/Thompson Pediatric Pain Questionnaire: Forms C, A, and P

Form C (Child)

Name: _____

Age: _____

Date: _____

What words would you use to describe pain or hurt?

_____

_____

_____

From the words listed below, circle the ones that best describe the way it feels when you hurt or are in pain.

cutting	pounding	tingling	tiring	deep
beating	squeezing	throbbing	horrible	stabbing
burning	pulling	sickening	biting	screaming
scraping	aching	uncomfortable	cold	tugging
pricking	cruel	warm	miserable	stretching
pinching	unbearable	sad	itching	terrible
stinging	cool	sore	flashing	pressing
fearful	pins & needles	sharp	jumping	tight
hot	spreading	punishing	scared	lonely
				bad

From the words you circled, which three words best described the pain you are feeling right now?

_____

_____

Put a mark on the line that best shows *how you feel now*. If you have no pain or hurt, you would put a mark at the end of the line by the happy face. If you have some pain or hurt, you would put a mark near the middle of the line. If you have a whole lot of pain or hurt, you would put a mark by the sad face.

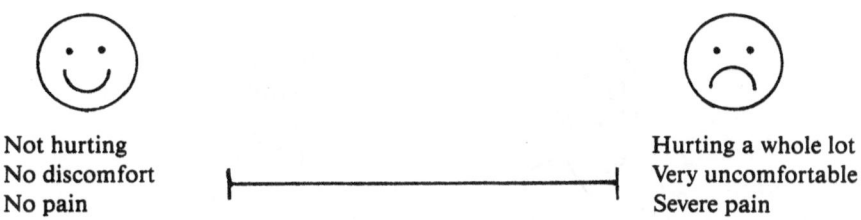

Not hurting   Hurting a whole lot
No discomfort   Very uncomfortable
No pain   Severe pain

Put a mark on the line that best shows what was the *worst pain you had this week*. If you had no pain or hurt this week, you would put a mark at the end of the line by the happy face. If the pain or hurt you had was some hurting, you would put a mark by the middle of the line. If the worse pain you had was a whole lot of pain or hurt, you would put a mark by the sad face.

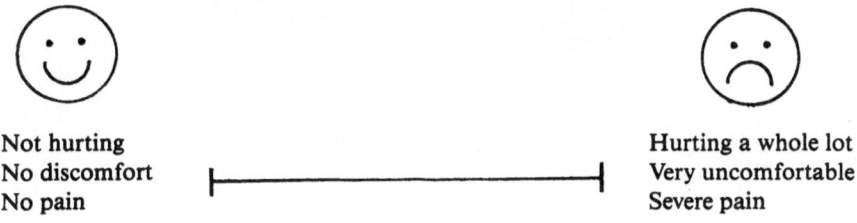

Not hurting   Hurting a whole lot
No discomfort   Very uncomfortable
No pain   Severe pain

No pain	Mild pain	Moderate pain	Severe pain
No hurt	A little hurt	More hurt	A lot of hurt

Pick the colors that mean *No hurt*, *A little hurt*, *More hurt*, and *A lot of hurt* to you and color in the boxes. Now, using those colors, color in the body to show how you feel. Where you have no hurt, use the *No hurt* color to color in your body. If you have hurt or pain, use the color that tells how much hurt you have.

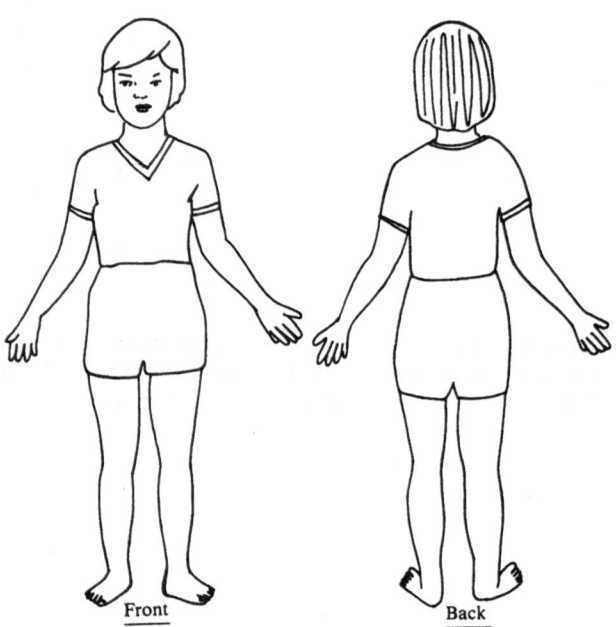

Front   Back

Form A (Adolescent)

The purpose of this questionnaire is to help us to obtain a comprehensive history of your pain problems. All information obtained from this questionnaire and in interviews will remain strictly confidential. If you do not wish to answer a particular question, for any reason, please write "Do not wish to answer" in the space provided. Please print or write clearly.

Today's date: _____

Your name: _____

Age: _____   Date of birth: _____

Grade in school: _____   Place of work: _____

Address: _____

_____

Phone number: _____

When did your present pain problem begin? Please also explain the symptoms, exact locations of pain and whether the pain has been on or off over the months and years?

_____

_____

_____

_____

_____

What was your reaction to the pain at that time? Please explain.

_____

_____

Were any major changes in your life occurring then? Please explain.

_____

_____

Is your current pain constant or does it appear to come and go?

_____

_____

Is your pain accompanied by nausea, vomiting, dizziness, feeling faint, anxiety, rapid breathing or other symptoms? If so, please list the symptoms.

_____

_____

If your pain were suddenly to disappear, how would it change your life?

_____

_____

_____

How would it change your family relationships? _____

_____

_____

_____

Assuming that the pain continues, what kinds of things do you think you should do *now*, which will help you later on?

_____

_____

_____

Is there anything else you would like to tell us about your pain and the effect it has on yourself or your family?

_____

_____

_____

What words would you use to describe your pain?

_____

_____

_____

From the words listed below, circle the ones that best describe the way it feels when you hurt or are in pain.

cutting	pounding	tingling	tiring	deep
beating	squeezing	throbbing	horrible	stabbing
burning	pulling	sickening	biting	screaming
scraping	aching	uncomfortable	cold	tugging
pricking	cruel	warm	miserable	stretching
pinching	unbearable	sad	itching	terrible
stinging	cool	sore	flashing	pressing
fearful	pins & needles	sharp	jumping	tight
hot	spreading	punishing	scared	lonely
				bad

From the words you circled, which three words best describe the pain you are feeling right now?

_____

_____

What day of the week do you have the most pain? _____

What week of the month do you have the most pain? _____

What season or month do you have the worst pain? _____

Have you ever noticed something that tells you that you are about to experience a pain episode (e.g., stiffness, particular thoughts or statements, physical sensations or irritability)?

_____

_____

_____

How many hours a day do you have pain now? _____

How long does a single pain episode last (minutes, hours)? _____

What do you call your pains? (For example, "headache," "joint pain," "stomach-ache," "backache," etc.) Please list them in order of severity, #1 being the most severe pain.

Pain problem #1: _____

Pain problem #2: _____

Pain problem #3: _____

On a scale of 0–10	6 a.m. _____	6 p.m. _____
(0 = no pain, 10 = severe pain),	9 a.m. _____	9 p.m. _____
how severe is your pain	12 noon _____	12 midnight _____
at the following times	3 p.m. _____	3 a.m. _____
of the day?		

What is the worst time of the day? _____

What is the best time of the day? _____

Are you currently taking medication for pain?
        Yes_____ No_____
If yes, please complete the following information.

Medication	Dose	#Times/day	When	How effective (0 = not effective, 10 = very effective)
_____				
_____				
_____				
_____				
_____				

What medications or other treatments have you tried in the past? On a scale of 0–10 (0 = not effective, 10 = very effective), how effective has each one been?

_____

_____

_____

_____

_____

What do you currently do, besides taking medication, to relieve your pain?

_____

_____

_____

Does your pain seem worse when your are?

	Yes	No		Yes	No
tired			angry		
anxious			busy		
bored			lonely		
happy			arguing		
unhappy			upset		

Are there any other situations in which your pain is worse?
If yes, what are they?

_____

_____

_____

Does your pain interfere with any of the following? Please circle the most correct number.

	Never	Rarely	Sometimes	Often	Always
Enjoying the family	1	2	3	4	5
Eating/appetite	1	2	3	4	5
Seeing friends	1	2	3	4	5
Sports	1	2	3	4	5
Sleeping	1	2	3	4	5
Watching T.V.	1	2	3	4	5
Reading	1	2	3	4	5
Schoolwork	1	2	3	4	5
Attending school	1	2	3	4	5
Going to the movies	1	2	3	4	5
Favorite activities	1	2	3	4	5
Unliked activities	1	2	3	4	5

Comments?_____

_____

_____

_____

During the past 3 months, did your pain limit you from doing things which you wanted to do?
1. _____ Yes
2. _____ No

If yes, please explain _____

_____

_____

_____

During the past 3 months of the school year, how often did your pain keep you from going to school?

0. _____ Not at all
1. _____ 1 day only
2. _____ 2–3 days
3. _____ 4–7 days
4. _____ more than 1 week
5. _____ more than 2 weeks
6. _____ more than 3 weeks
7. _____ more than 1 month

During the past 3 months, how often did your pain limit you from *vigorous* activities such as running, bicycling, lifting heavy objects, or participating in strenuous sports?

0. _____ Not at all
1. _____ 1 day only
2. _____ 2–3 days
3. _____ 4–7 days
4. _____ more than 1 week
5. _____ more than 2 weeks
6. _____ more than 3 weeks
7. _____ more than 1 month

During the past 3 months, how often did your pain limit you from *moderate* activities such as climbing several flight of stairs, bending, walking several blocks, lifting or stooping?

0. _____ Not at all
1. _____ 1 day only
2. _____ 2–3 days
3. _____ 4–7 days
4. _____ more than 1 week
5. _____ more than 2 weeks
6. _____ more than 3 weeks
7. _____ more than 1 month

During the past 3 months, how often did your pain limit you from *mild* activities such as walking one block, climbing one flight of stairs, sitting, or standing?

0. _____ Not at all
1. _____ 1 day only
2. _____ 2–3 days
3. _____ 4–7 days
4. _____ more than 1 week
5. _____ more than 2 weeks
6. _____ more than 3 weeks
7. _____ more than 1 month

Please rate how much pain you are *having at the present time* by placing a mark somewhere on the line.

Not Hurting   Hurting a whole lot
No discomfort   _____   Very uncomfortable
No pain   Severe pain

Please rate how much pain you have *on an average* each day by placing a mark somewhere on the line.

Not hurting		Hurting a whole lot
No discomfort	_____	Very uncomfortable
No pain		Severe pain

Please rate how severe the *worst pain* you had *in the past week* (7 days) by placing a mark somewhere on the line.

Not hurting		Hurting a whole lot
No discomfort	_____	Very uncomfortable
No pain		Severe pain

Please mark an "X" on the *exact* place where you are having pain now. If there is more than one painful place, mark them "1," "2," "3," etc., starting with the most painful place as "1."

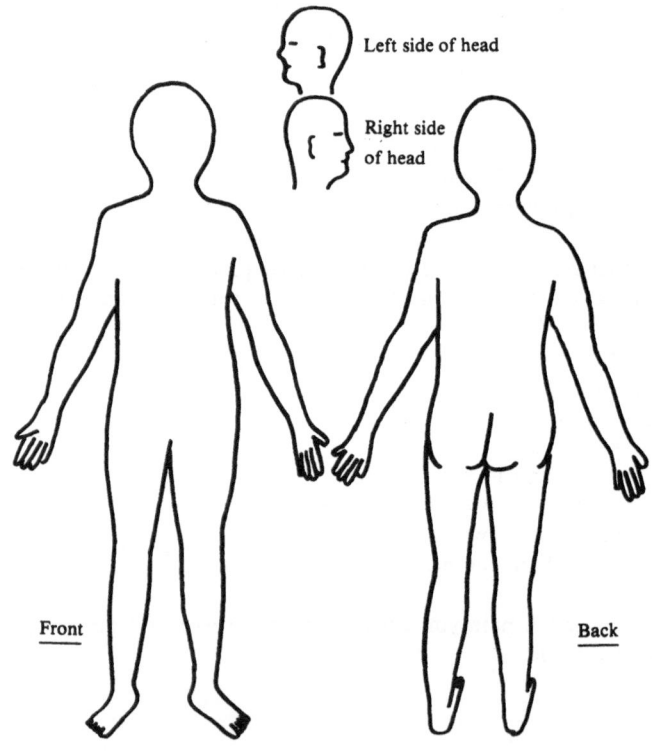

Form P (Parent)

The purpose of this questionnaire is to help us to obtain a comprehensive history of your child's pain problems. All information obtained from this questionnaire and in interviews will remain strictly confidential. If you do not wish to answer a particular question, for any reason, please write "Do not wish to answer" in the space provided. Please print or write clearly.

Today's Date: _____

Your name: _____

Address: _____

_____

Phone number: _____

Relationship to child of person completing this form: _____

Child Information

Name:_____

Age:_____   Date of birth:_____

Sex:_____

Grade in school:_____

Home Information

Please list the name, age and sex of all individuals living in the home.

Name	Age	Sex

Please list any health problems that your child has.

_____

_____

_____

If anyone else in the family has health problems please list the person and the health problem. Example: son with asthma, husband with arthritis.

_____

_____

_____

Please list all severe or chronic family illnesses that your child has been aware of.

Family member	Dates	Type of illness	Outcome

Please list all severe and/or chronic pain problems experienced by other family members that your child has observed.

Family member	Dates	Type of pain	Outcome

Are there currently any major life stresses in the family situation (e.g. divorce, separation, difficult financial burden, illness)? If yes, please list.

_____

_____

_____

_____

When did your child's present pain problem begin? Please also explain the symptoms, exact locations of pain and whether the pain has been on or off over the months and years?

_____

_____

_____

_____

_____

What was your reaction to the pain at that time? Please explain.

_____

_____

Were any major changes in yours or your child's life occurring then? Please explain.

_____

_____

Is your child's current pain constant or does it appear to come and go?

_____

_____

Is your child's pain accompanied by nausea, vomiting, dizziness, feeling faint, anxiety, rapid breathing or other symptoms? If so, please list the symptoms.

_____

_____

When your child has pain how do you react? Please explain.

_____

_____

_____

If your child's pain were to suddenly disappear, how would it change his/her life?

_____

_____

_____

How would it change your life?_____

_____

_____

How would it change family relationships?_____

_____

_____

_____

Assuming that the pain continues, what kinds of things do you think your child should do *now*, which will help him/her later on?

_____

_____

_____

Is there anything else you would like to tell us about your child's pain and the effect it has on your child, yourself or the family?

_____

_____

_____

_____

What words would you use to describe your child's pain?

_____

_____

_____

Please circle any of the words listed below that you feel describe your child's pain.

cutting	pounding	tingling	tiring	deep
beating	squeezing	throbbing	horrible	stabbing
burning	pulling	sickening	biting	screaming
scraping	aching	uncomfortable	cold	tugging
pricking	cruel	warm	miserable	stretching
pinching	unbearable	sad	itching	terrible
stinging	cool	sore	flashing	pressing
fearful	pins & needles	sharp	jumping	tight
hot	spreading	punishing	scared	lonely
				bad

What day of the week does your child have the most pain? _____

What week of the month does your child have the most pain? _____

What season or month does your child have the worst pain? _____

Have you ever noticed something that tells you that your child is about to exerience a pain episode (e.g., stiffness, particular thoughts or statements, physical sensations or irritability)?

_____

_____

_____

How many hours a day does your child have pain now? _____

How long does a single pain episode last (minutes, hours)? _____

What do you label your child's pains as (e.g., "headache," "joint pain," "stomach-ache," "backache," etc.)? Please list them in order of severity, #1 being the most severe pain.

Pain problem #1: _____

Pain problem #2: _____

Pain problem #3: _____

On a scale of 0–10	6 a.m. _____	6 p.m. _____
(0 = no pain, 10 = severe pain),	9 a.m. _____	9 p.m. _____
how severe is your child's	12 noon _____	12 midnight _____
pain at the following	3 p.m. _____	3 a.m. _____
times of the day?		

What is the worst time of the day? _____

What is the best time of the day? _____

Is your child currently taking medication for pain?
        Yes _____   No _____
If yes, please complete the following information.

Medication	Dose	#Times/day	When	How effective (0 = not effective, 10 = very effective)
_____	_____	_____	_____	_____
_____	_____	_____	_____	_____
_____	_____	_____	_____	_____
_____	_____	_____	_____	_____
_____	_____	_____	_____	_____

What medications or other treatments have been tried in the past? On a scale of 0–10 (0 = not effective, 10 = very effective), how effective has each one been?

_____

_____

_____

_____

_____

What do you currently do, besides giving medication, to relieve your child's pain?

_____

_____

_____

Does your child's pain seem worse when he/she is?

	Yes	No		Yes	No
tired			angry		
anxious			busy		
bored			lonely		
happy			arguing		
unhappy			upset		

Other situations in which your child's pain is worse? Please describe.

_____

_____

_____

Does your child's pain interfere with any of the following? Please circle the most correct number.

	Never	Rarely	Sometimes	Often	Always
Enjoying the family	1	2	3	4	5
Eating/appetite	1	2	3	4	5
Seeing friends	1	2	3	4	5
Sports	1	2	3	4	5
Sleeping	1	2	3	4	5
Watching T.V.	1	2	3	4	5
Reading	1	2	3	4	5
Schoolwork	1	2	3	4	5
Attending school	1	2	3	4	5
Going to the movies	1	2	3	4	5
Favorite activities	1	2	3	4	5
Unliked activities	1	2	3	4	5

Comments?_____

_____

_____

_____

During the past 3 months, did your child's pain limit him/her from doing things which he/she wanted to do?

1. _____ Yes
2. _____ No

If yes, please explain _____

_____

_____

_____

During the past 3 months of the school year, how often did your child's pain keep him/her from going to school?

0. _____ Not at all
1. _____ 1 day only
2. _____ 2–3 days
3. _____ 4–7 days
4. _____ more than 1 week
5. _____ more than 2 weeks
6. _____ more than 3 weeks
7. _____ more than 1 month

During the past 3 months, how often did your child's pain limit him/her from *vigorous* activities such as running, bicycling, lifting heavy objects, or participating in strenuous sports?

0. _____ Not at all
1. _____ 1 day only
2. _____ 2–3 days
3. _____ 4–7 days
4. _____ more than 1 week
5. _____ more than 2 weeks
6. _____ more than 3 weeks
7. _____ more than 1 month

During the past 3 months, how often did your child's pain limit him/her from *moderate* activities such as climbing several flights of stairs, bending, walking several blocks, lifting or stooping?

0. _____ Not at all
1. _____ 1 day only
2. _____ 2–3 days
3. _____ 4–7 days
4. _____ more than 1 week
5. _____ more than 2 weeks
6. _____ more than 3 weeks
7. _____ more than 1 month

During the past 3 months, how often did your child's pain limit him/her from *mild* activities such as walking one block, climbing one flight of stairs, sitting, or standing?

0. _____ Not at all
1. _____ 1 day only
2. _____ 2–3 days
3. _____ 4–7 days
4. _____ more than 1 week
5. _____ more than 2 weeks
6. _____ more than 3 weeks
7. _____ more than 1 month

Please rate how much pain you think your child is *having at the present time* by placing a mark somewhere on the line.

Not Hurting   Hurting a whole lot
No discomfort   _____   Very uncomfortable
No pain   Severe pain

Please rate how much pain you think your child has *on an average* each day by placing a mark somewhere on the line.

Not hurting   Hurting a whole lot
No discomfort   _____   Very uncomfortable
No pain   Severe pain

Please rate how severe was the *worst pain* your child had *in the past week* (7 days) by placing a mark somewhere on the line.

Not hurting   Hurting a whole lot
No discomfort   _____   Very uncomfortable
No pain   Severe pain

Please mark an "X" on the *exact* place where you think your child is having pain now. If there is more than one painful place, mark them "1," "2," "3," etc., starting with the most painful place as "1."

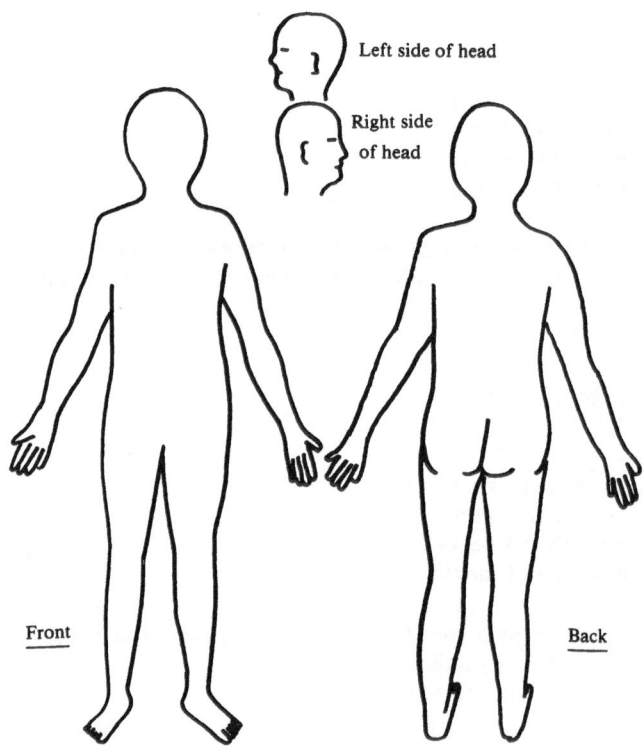

Physician's Report

Patients's name _____   Date _____
                                          Time _____

Directions

Please rate your perception of the patient's pain at the present time by placing a mark at a point along the line.

No pain   _____   Severe pain

13
Pain and Pain-Related Distress in Children With Cancer

Sharon L. Manne and Barbara L. Andersen

Cancer in children is relatively rare, accounting for slightly less than 1% of the 1 million cases of cancer diagnosed annually in the United States (Silverberg, Boring, & Squires, 1990). When it occurs, however, it can be fatal. Cancer is the second leading cause of death among individuals 14 years of age or less, and accounts for 10 to 12% of the annual childhood deaths (Silverberg et al., 1990). Although there are cardinal signs and symptoms of cancer in children (Fernbach, 1984), including fever, a tumor mass, pallor, changes in balance, gait, or personality, or changes in the eye, pain is perhaps the most classic sign or symptom. For example, bone pain has been found in 15 to 52% of children presenting with leukemia (Fernbach, 1984; Miser, McCalla, Dothage, Wesley, & Miser, 1987), the most common form of childhood cancer. Pain often accompanies the remaining prevalent sites of disease, including brain tumors (headache), kidney tumors (abdominal pain), and soft tissue disease (a painful mass with rhabdomyosarcoma) (Miser et al., 1987). Thus, it is often the child's complaint of pain or their parents' suspicion that the child is in pain, from seeing changes in his/her behavior or affect, that prompts a visit to a physician.

Our focus is on the psychological and behavioral aspects of pediatric oncological pain. To facilitate understanding, we first provide a brief overview of the common pediatric cancers and their treatments and highlight their painful aspects. This section is intended for behavioral scientists naive to the nature of pediatric disease; those familiar with these issues may prefer to note the epidemiologic summaries in Tables 13.1, 13.2, and 13.3 and move to the following section. Cancer for a child or adolescent may include a variety of other disease characteristics (e.g., seizures or personality changes with brain tumors) or treatment toxicities (e.g., nausea/vomiting with chemotherapy or neuropsychological sequelae with cranial irradiation) that are as difficult or more difficult for the child as the experience of pain. Thus, although we necessarily focus on pain, this presentation is to be viewed within the context of this potentially debilitating disease and the difficult treatment and recovery experiences.

The second section discusses children's understanding of disease and

TABLE 13.1. Frequency of major cancers in children less than 15 years of age by race.

	Percentage of total	
Site	White	Black
Leukemia	31	24
Central nervous system	18	22
Lymphoma	14	11
Sympathetic nervous system	8	7
Soft tissue	6	9
Kidney	6	9
Bone	5	4
Retinoblastoma	3	4
Gonadal and germ cell	2	4
Miscellaneous	8	7

Note. From "Incidence of malignant tumors in U.S. children" by J. L. Young and R. W. Miller, 1975, *Journal of Pediatrics, 86*, pp. 254–258. Copyright by the American Academy of Pediatrics. Adapted by permission.

TABLE 13.2. Trends in survival by type of cancer for children less than 15 years at diagnosis.

	Relative 5-year survival rate (%)		
Type	1967–73	1974–76	1977–83
Leukemia	15	45	61
Acute lymphocytic	18	53	68
Acute granulocytic	0	16	26
Acute, unspecified	14	43[a]	42[a]
Brain and central nervous system	45	56	54
Hodgkin's disease	78	80	88
Non-Hodgkin's lymphomas	24	43	54
Sympathetic nervous system	42	[b]	[b]
Soft tissue sarcomas	44	57	67
Rhabdomyosarcoma	34	53[a]	64
Kidney — Wilms' tumor	65	74	82
Bone	28	52[a]	45
Osterosarcoma	26	55[a]	38
Ewing's sarcoma	23	38[a]	46[a]
Retinoblastoma	82	89[a]	92

Note. From "Cancer statistics, 1990" by B. S. Silverberg, C. C. Boring, and B. A. Squires, 1990, *Ca—A Cancer Journal for Clinicians, 40*, pp. 9–26. Copyright by American Cancer Society. Reprinted by permission.
[a]Standard error of 5 to 10%.
[b]No longer calculated separately.

TABLE 13.3. Long-term survival rates for the five most frequent childhood cancers by age group.

| Age | Site | Relative survival rates (%) | |
		5 year	10 year
<5	Acute lymph. leukemia	65	57
	Brain	44	39
	Kidney	77	75
	Soft tissue	64	59
	Eye	90	88
5–9	Acute lymph. leukemia	62	52
	Brain	51	44
	Non-Hodgkin's lymphomas	50	46[a]
	Kidney	81	81
	Hodgkin's disease	89	82[a]
10–14	Brain	58	50
	Hodgkin's disease	76	76
	Acute lymph. leukemia	46	33
	Bone	48	45
	Non-Hodgkin's lymphoma	52	49
15–19	Hodgkin's disease	89	79
	Brain	59	53
	Bone	47	42
	Thyroid	99	99
	Testis	71	72

Note. From "Cancer statistics, 1990" by B. S. Silverberg, C. C. Boring, and B. A. Squires, 1990, *Ca—A Cancer Journal for Clinicians, 40*, pp. 9–26. Copyright by the American Cancer Society. Reprinted by permission.
[a]Standard error of 5 to 10%.

pain-related phenomena from a cognitive-developmental perspective. Although much of this literature is centered around Piagetian notions of cognitive development applied to children's understanding of the causes of illness and pain, there are some data that focus on children's perceptions of cancer, per se.

The majority of the assessment strategies developed thus far quantify a child's distress and/or pain prior to, during, and following painful diagnostic or treatment monitoring procedures (e.g., bone marrow aspirations). Assessments have sampled three domains: cognition/emotion, behavior, and physiological correlates. As many children with cancer may be too young to provide reliable evaluations of their emotions or their pain, behavioral observations (e.g., frequency measures of crying, clinging, etc., during painful procedures) have been important. Evaluations of the child's affect and/or behavior by significant others (e.g., parent, nurse, physician) have provided a supplementary perspective. Finally, some investigators have also gathered physiological data, such as heart rate, and examined their relationship with other self-report and observational ratings. Other than the narrow context of procedural pain, fewer methods are available for the assessment of a child's pain from the disease itself, its treatment, treatment side effects, or the combination of these factors. We will conclude this section by discussing assessment strategies within a developmental perspective.

The remainder of the chapter reviews the literature on psychological interventions for acute pain with diagnostic or treatment monitoring procedures, including venipuncture and lumbar puncture or bone marrow aspiration. Interventions usually include multiple components, such as using relaxation or relaxation-like procedures (e.g., hypnosis), providing sensory and procedural information to the child, and teaching the child coping strategies. As these interventions have not been developed as substitutes for appropriate medical management of pain by oncologists, anesthesiologists, or other medical personnel, this section begins with a brief overview of current medical "standard" care practices.

Common Cancers of Childhood and Adolescence

Childhood cancers usually involve the hematologic system, the central nervous system (CNS), or connective tissue. Table 13.1 provides a frequency distribution of the major cancers in children less than 15 years of age by race. We will provide a site-by-site description of the common diseases, including information on incidence, presentation, common diagnostic and treatment regimens, and prognoses.

Leukemias

These diseases are the most common childhood cancers. Acute lymphocytic leukemia (ALL) is the most common subtype, with six new cases per 100,000 individuals annually (Pui & Rivera, 1990). The modal age of incidence is 4 years, followed by a rapid decline, with only infrequent incidence after 15 years. The disease is slightly more prevalent among males. Symptoms are rarely present more than 6 weeks prior to diagnosis and include lethargy, fatigue, anorexia, abdominal discomfort, hemorrhagic signs (e.g., easy bruising), and headache. Bone and joint pain are more frequent in ALL than in the other leukemias and are often the chief complaint (Silverstein & Kelly, 1963; Simmons, Harle, & Singleton, 1968). In addition to painful symptoms, the diagnostic procedures including blood draws and bone marrow aspirations (BMA) are often difficult for children. The latter is performed to detect leukemic cells in blood, marrow, and spinal fluid.

Treatment of ALL for the majority of children consists of multiagent chemotherapy to induce remission, followed by cranial irradiation combined with intrathecal administration of chemotherapy (e.g., methotrexate) to prevent recurrence in the central nervous system. Maintenance chemotherapy may also be offered to prevent relapse. This maintenance therapy is typically discontinued after 2 to 3 years if the child remains free of disease. During the entire treatment period, blood draws and BMAs are performed on a regular basis to monitor the course or remission of the disease. A common pain scenario for a 4-year-old child following chemotherapy might be the following: severe mouth pain related to mucositis from the chemotherapy; mild bone pain related to invasion of the bone marrow; anxiety related to the pain; reduced eating secondary to mouth pain; bone pain related to chemotherapy toxicity (Schechter, 1988).

ALL was once a fatal disease. Table 13.2 provides the data on the dramatic turnaround that has occurred within the last 25 years, with 5-year survival rates improving from 18 to 61%. The primary reason for this change has been the inclusion of the CNS treatment component to prevent relapse in the brain (which was previously the most frequent site for disease relapse). When maintenance chemotherapy ends in the 3rd year, approximately 75% of the children will remain in remission and are considered "cured" (Baum, Suther, & Nachman, 1979). Of the 25% who relapse, approximately 80% can be treated successfully with combination chemotherapy (e.g. vincristine, prednisone, and L-asparaginase). If a second remission occurs, the subsequent disease-free interval is shorter than the first, and long-term survival with successive remissions is rare. For recurrent ALL patients who have a histocompatible sibling, allogeneic bone marrow transplantation is considered.

Although ALL is the most common leukemia found in the pediatric population, there are others. These diseases are collectively referred to as acute nonlymphoblastic leukemia (ANLL) and include acute undifferentiated leukemia, myeloblastic leukemia, promyelocytic leukemia, acute monocytic leukemia, acute myelomonocytic leukemia, and several other rare forms of the disease.

Central Nervous System Tumors

The annual incidence of brain tumors in children younger than 15 years in the United States is 2.4 per 100,000, or 1,200 to 1,500 new diagnoses per year (Young & Miller, 1975). The most common tumor is astrocytoma, accounting for 40 to 50% of all diagnoses (Duffner, Cohen, & Freeman, 1985). With this disease, specific problems can be caused by direct invasion or irritation of regions of the brain, which produces symptoms/signs characteristic of that region (e.g., occipital lobe tumors can produce loss of vision). More often, tumors produce increased intracranial pressure from their growth, swelling of the surrounding tissue, or obstruction of cerebrospinal fluid pathways. The symptoms/signs of increased intracranial pressure include irritability, lethargy, headache, vomiting, decreased appetite, and withdrawn behavior. A classic scenario for a child may be that he or she wakes up several mornings with headache and vomiting. The symptoms usually resolve within a week or so and parents may attribute the episode to the flu (this temporary cessation of symptoms may be attributable to move-ment in the sutures of the child's skull) (Duffner et al., 1985). Several weeks later, the symptoms recur and progress. Computed tomography (CT) of the brain is the most common procedure used for diagnosing and localizing tumors.

Although brain tumors are the second most common cancer in children, advances in treatment have lagged behind those for other forms of child-hood cancer. Survival has remained in the 50% range for the last 25 years (see Table 13.2) due to factors unique to brain tumors. First, the inability to safely debulk (surgically remove the tumor with disease-free margins) limits the possibility of cure. Second, the toxicity of high dose cranial radiation therapy can produce secondary tumors. Third, factors unique to pediatric brain tumors (e.g., small numbers of patients seen annually at a single cancer center) make it difficult to conduct clinical trials.

Surgery is the primary modality of treatment. However, complete resec-tion is often not possible because of damage to normal tissue and proximity to vital structures. Radiation therapy to the local area, the whole brain, or the entire CNS, may follow. Large dosages are normally required to destroy brain tumors, and the treatment is complicated further by the potential of the tumor to seed surrounding tissues. The long-term effects of radiation therapy (combined with surgery) are considerable. Difficulties include grad-ual intellectual deterioration (often resulting in functioning in the retarded range), endocrine disturbances (growth hormone deficiency is most com-mon), and development of secondary cancers (other CNS tumors or non-CNS tumors, such as thyroid carcinomas). Chemotherapy is receiving in-creased use because its long-term effects may be less severe; however, its short-term effects may be comparable (or somewhat greater) than those of radiation therapy. The location of the tumor, its growth rate, mitotic activi-ty, and the ability of the drug to enter the CNS influence the choice of agents and the route of administration (e.g., drug administration directly into the tumor cavity or intra-arterial infusion).

Survival rates for children with brain tumors vary with the tumor's loca-tion and histology. In view of the possibility of secondary disease, longer term estimates, such as 10-year rates, may be more appropriate survival end points.

Lymphomas

Approximately 40% of lymphomas are Hodgkin's disease and the remaining 60% are non-Hodgkin's lymphoma (NHL). The latter is rare among children under 5 years, with the majority appearing between 5 and 15 years (median age of diagnosis is 9 years) (see Table 13.3). Two thirds of these children are male. NHL encompasses a heterogeneous group of malignancies, and the presenting symptoms are varied. Children with supradiaphragmatic involve-ment typically have malaise, cough, and dyspnea. Disease of this sort has also often metastasized to the bone marrow (80 to 90% of the cases), the CNS, or the gonads (30%). Children may also present with an abdominal mass or a malnutrition syndrome with colitis-like symptoms; abdominal disease of this sort frequently metastasizes to the CNS (Ziegler, Bluming, Morrow, Fass, & Carbone, 1970). As with other types of pediatric cancers, diagnostic procedures include surgical (lymph node) biopsy, laboratory studies, BMA, lumbar puncture (LP), and/or radiographic studies.

Treatment plans are individualized but are influenced by the patient's age and general condition as well as the sites of involvement, stage, and histologic subtype. Treatment may include all three major modalities. In the past, local surgery and radiation treatment resulted in only 25% survival rates for children (Glatstein et al., 1974). Current multimodal treatment regimens achieve remission in 80 to 90% of patients (Carabell, Cassady, Weinstein, & Jaffe, 1978). Most recurrences occur within the first 12 months posttreatment and only rarely after 24 months (Carabell et al., 1978; Wollner et al., 1976).

Less than 10% of all Hodgkin's disease (HD) cases occur before the age of 10 years (see Table 13.3). The typical presentation includes painless lymph node enlargement with or without fever, sweating, itching, weight loss, and/ or malaise. Diagnostic procedures of lymph node biopsy and blood findings and chemistries are used. Radiation therapy is the treatment of choice for localized HD, and chemotherapy is used for generalized forms. The initial staging of the disease and decision regarding treatment are particularly important, as radiation therapy can potentially be curative if the treatment fields encompass all disease. As Table 13.2 notes, survival rates for HD are significantly more favorable that those for NHL.

Neuroblastoma

These virulent tumors can arise anywhere along the sympathetic nervous system, but the most common sites are the adrenal gland (40%) and the paraspinal ganglion (25%). They account for only 7% of all the cases of childhood cancer but 15% of the deaths. The incidence of these tumors is estimated to be 1 in 10,000 to 40,000 live births. The peak age of diagnosis is 2 years, and incidence declines dramatically after the age of 6 (Swank, Fetterman, Sieber, & Kiesewetter, 1971). The disease accounts for 50% of all neonatal malignancies and 30% of all infant cancers. For the family with a child diagnosed with this disease there is the potential of added burden — there is a tendency for this disease to occur in more than one sibling and it is associated with other hereditary disorders (e.g., von Recklinghausen's disease). The disease commonly presents with a fixed mass in the chest, abdomen, or neck. Though uncommon, the mass may be painful, or pain may occur with bony metastases. A less common presenting syndrome includes fever, weakness, pallor, weight loss, shortness of breath, and cough. A range of diagnostic procedures can be used including lab studies, radiographic exams, CT scans, ultrasound, surgical biopsy, chest x-rays, bone scans, and BMA to detect metastatic spread.

The first step in treatment is total excision (or as much as possible) of the primary tumor. This strategy is sufficient for localized disease. For those with metastatic disease, chemotherapy (e.g., cyclophosphamide, cisplatin, doxorubicin) is often given. Unfortunately, cure is rarely achieved and chemotherapy appears only to lengthen the disease-free interval. Spontaneous regression has been documented more frequently in this disease than in any other malignancy (Everson & Cole, 1966). When it occurs, the child is usually under 2 years of age. The processes that underlie regression are unknown, but may involve the interaction of spontaneous maturation and the immunologic destruction of malignant cells. The prognosis largely depends on the age at diagnosis and the stage of disease. Infants younger than 1 year have a better prognosis than older infants and children, and 80% of patients with disseminated disease will die despite aggressive therapy.

Rhabdomyosarcoma

This disease is the most common pediatric soft tissue sarcoma (Young & Miller, 1975). The incidence in the United States is 4.5 per million/year in whites and 1.3 per million/year in blacks, a 3 : 1 ratio. The disease is most often diagnosed in early childhood or late adolescence (Miller & Dalager, 1974). Rhabdomyosarcoma arises in the embryonic mesenchyme, and commonly presents as an asymptomatic mass with poorly defined margins. Specific presentations relate to the disease site. In early childhood, the primary sites are the head and neck and the genitourinary tract, with symptoms/signs that may include, respectively, polyps, decreased hearing, and cranial nerve abnormalities, or urethral, vaginal, or other perineal masses, blood in the urine, or other urinary problems. In adolescence, primary sites are often the extremities or the testes, both of which may present with painful or asymptomatic masses. Distant disease is present in 20% of the cases (Okamura, Sutow, & Moon, 1977). Specific diagnostic procedures are dependent upon the site of the disease.

Most subtypes of rhabdomyosarcoma are soft, fleshy tumors that vary in the depth and volume of invasion into the surrounding tissue, and spread to adjacent structures, such as the regional nodes. Wide excision of the primary tumor and the surrounding normal tissue, if possible, has offered good local control of the disease. However, because of the sites of the disease and extent of surgery that may be required, surgical excision is often tailored and coupled with radiation and chemotherapy to reduce morbidity and cosmetic deformity. Survival, obviously, is dependent upon the extent of disease at diagnosis. In general, patients with the most favorable stage at diagnosis have survival rates in the range of 83%, whereas estimates are 20% (with a median survival time of 12 months) for children with the least favorable stage at diagnosis (Maurer et al., 1981).

Wilms' Tumor (Nephroblastoma)

This tumor is the most common renal malignancy found in children (Pui & Crist, 1990). The incidence in children under 15 years of age is 7.55 per million per year in Caucasians, with a slightly higher incidence (7.80 per million per year) in blacks. The peak ages at diagnosis are 1 to 3 years, with 90% under 7 years at diagnosis (Knudson & Strong, 1973) (see Table 13.3). In 83% of the cases the presenting sign is an abdominal mass, with about a third of the children complaining of abdominal pain from distention of the kidney. Diagnostic and disease staging procedures include blood counts, liver and kidney function tests, chest x-rays and CT scans of the chest and abdomen. If metastases are found, BMA and bone scans are performed. Surgery may also be performed for diagnosis and staging.

Within oncology, the concept of multimodal therapy began with the successful treatment of Wilms' tumor. In this context, treatment incorporates all primary modalities. Surgery typically includes removal of the ipsilateral kidney and tumor, with the surrounding structures biopsied or taken, depending on the spread. Radiation therapy is tailored to the extent of the disease, but may be given to the tumor bed or whole abdomen, for example, to prevent local regional recurrences. Combination chemotherapy (e.g., vincristine, actinomycin D, and doxorubicin) is more effective than single agents. The increase in survival rate with multimodal therapy has been dramatic, with a shift during the 20th century from 8% following surgery alone to 92% with multimodal therapy (D'Angio et al., 1984).

Bone Tumors

These tumors account for only 3 to 4% of all malignancies in childhood, but are second only to brain tumors in children over the age of 10 (Pui & Crist, 1990). Osteogenic sarcoma is the most common and appears to arise from the bone-forming mesenchyme. Most tumors occur in children ranging in age from 10 to 15 (see Table 13.3). A relationship between the adolescent growth spurt and the tumor development suggests that rapid growth increases the risk of somatic mutation, leading to neoplasm formation. The disease usually presents as a bone pain, with or without a palpable overlying mass. Other signs may include pain with increased activity, a limited range of motion, swelling, or (rarely) a pathological fracture. Approximately 70% of the tumors occur around the knee. Diagnostic procedures include x-rays, CT scan, bone scans, and tumor biopsy.

Osteogenic sarcoma is relatively radioresistant. Treatment consists of complete surgical removal of the tumor, with the possibility of adjuvant chemotherapy to prevent recurrence in the stump left by amputation and/or metastatic disease (particularly to the lungs). To reduce the psychological and functional morbidity of amputation (Marcove & Rosen, 1980), limb salvage procedures have been used and appear to offer the same disease-free survival rate (Henderson & Dahlin, 1963). In this case, the tumor-bearing bone is removed and replaced with a cadaver allograft or a custom-made prosthesis. Many patients undergoing this procedure require amputation at a later date because of frequent complications (e.g., infection, local tumor recurrence, breaking of the inserted rod from metal fatigue). Historically only 10 to 20% of children survived. There has been some improvement with the addition of adjuvant therapy and the aggressive treatment of pulmonary metastases.

Ewing's sarcoma is the most common bone tumor in children under the age of 10 years and the second most common (following osteogenic sarcoma) in 11- to 20-year-olds (Pui & Crist, 1990). The median age at diagnosis is 13 years. Ewing's sarcoma is a highly malignant, nonosseous tumor thought to originate from immature reticulum cells in the bone marrow cavity. In 40% of the cases the disease arises in the flat bones, such as the pelvis, ribs, or hands. The disease presents much like osteogenic sarcoma, with localized pain and swelling, and symptoms are frequently present for several months before diagnosis. As many as one third of the children may have metastatic disease in the lungs or other bones at diagnosis. Systemic symptoms such as weight loss, fatigue, and fever, are common. Primary tumors of the rib can be massive and result in breathing difficulties for the adolescent.

Fortunately, amputation is not necessary for Ewing's tumors as the disease is sensitive to both radiation and chemotherapy. Treatment may begin with multiagent therapy (e.g., cyclophosphamide, doxorubicin, vincristine, and actinomycin-D) to reduce tumor bulk, and then radiation can follow to a smaller area, sparing normal tissue, and, if possible, employing a lower dosage. For expendable bones (e.g., a rib) complete surgical resection may be preferred. Current survival estimates are 70% for localized disease and 40% with metastatic disease. Unfortunately, late relapses (e.g., after 10 years) can occur.

Retinoblastoma

This is a relatively rare tumor that arises from neuroectodermal tissue within the nuclear layer of the retina in the eye (Pui & Crist, 1990). Approximately 200 children per year are diagnosed in the United States, usually prior to the age of 2 years. The mean age at diagnosis is 8 months for bilateral cases and 26 months for unilateral cases. There are two forms of the disease, one sporadic (60%) and the other inherited. When it is detected, parents typically first notice an eye abnormality, such as cat's eye reflex (a whitish appearance of the pupil) or strabismus. Ophthalmoscopic examinations under anesthesia are used for diagnosis.

Regarding treatment, efforts are made to preserve sight by irradiation or cryotherapy. When the tumor is advanced or extended, chemotherapy (e.g., cyclophosphamide, doxorubicin, vincristine) may be given with radiotherapy. Prognosis depends on size and location of the tumor(s) and presence and degree of ocular and extraocular involvement. Survival rates can be quite favorable (see Table 13.2), but once the tumor has extended to the optic nerve, for example, cure rates decrease to about 50%.

Summary

For the behavioral scientist interested in the pain problems of children with cancer, one may be initially impressed with the diversity of pediatric diseases. However, there are epidemiologic aspects of the disease, such as the differing prevalence rates within age groups, that simplify the picture. Of all children, those with hematologic malignancies have received the most attention in the psychological study of pain. Few data are available on the pain problems of children with soft tissue or solid tumors. This situation has occurred primarily because the painful procedures studied (e.g., BMAs and lumbar punctures) are more commonly used to monitor hematologic malignancies.

Children's Understanding of Pain, Cancer, and Cancer-Related Pains

Pain is subjective. As such, it falls within the domain of psychology. Efforts to understand the cognitive, affective, behavioral, and psychophysiological aspects of pain are recent. This volume notwithstanding, even fewer efforts have been made to understand pain phenomena in infants, children, and adolescents. We will attempt to organize the available data within age groupings. Although imperfect, this categorization may lend greater specificity to children's initial interpretations and understanding of cancer and cancer-related pain. Children's understanding may become more accurate and elaborate as they learn about their disease and its treatment from their parents, other patients, physicians, and nurses. There are few studies investigating how children with cancer explain how they got the disease. Thus, the discussion regarding cancer explanations that follows is based mostly upon generalizations from the literature on healthy children's understanding of illness.

Infancy to Five years

For decades, researchers and clinicians have believed, and behaved as if, pain was not a sensory experience of infants. Owens (1984) notes that some (e.g., Merskey, 1970) assert that circumcision would produce little or no reaction in the newborn. When physicians prescribed postoperative analgesics for children, the dosages would frequently be insufficient (Schechter, Allen, & Hanson, 1986). To make the situation worse, the nursing staff would often administer less medication than was prescribed. Research on emotions supports the inference of subjective distress in nonverbal infants (Izard & Buechler, 1979) and other data indicate behavioral and physiological signs of distress (e.g., Poznanski, 1976). It is now accepted that pain is a real phenomenon in infants that can be accompanied by a variety of responses, including facial expression (Eckman & Oster, 1979), motor responses (Craig, McMahon, Morison, & Zaskow, 1984), crying (Johnston & Strada, 1986), cardiac activity (Wolff, 1969), and endocrine activity (Talbert, Kraybill, & Potter, 1975), among other responses.

On the basis of these data, we could infer that if a growing tumor or disease process (e.g., leukemia, eye tumor) produced pain in the infant, the infant would express these sensations to the caretaker with some overt action, such as constant crying (as with head pain from a brain tumor) or acute episodes of crying with specific episodes of pain. We may also conclude that pain-producing diagnostic procedures such as BMA would produce significant distress for the unanesthetized infant. Thus, pediatric oncologists need to provide local anesthesia as well as general anesthesia to infants during such procedures (Schechter, 1988).

It has been suggested that children's understandings of illness etiology and cure parallel Piaget's stages of cognitive development (Bibace & Walsh, 1980). If so, the approximate period of 2 to 6 years would be characterized by preoperational explanations of illness and/or pain. During this period, the child gives explanations for events (e.g., a cold, the measles) that are currently dominating his/her experience, spatially or temporally. The earliest of explanations may be in the form of phenomenism, i.e., the cause of illness is something that co-occurs with the illness but is spatially and/or temporally remote. A child in this stage would not understand the causal link between the source of the illness and the illness itself. For example, a child may give an answer, "from the bees," to the query, "How did you get a cold this summer?" A slightly more mature response would be a contagion explanation, when the cause of an illness is located in objects or people that are in the vicinity of the child. A child offering this type of preoperational explanation might say, "I got my cold from the outside."

For children diagnosed with cancer during this age range, the most frequent types/sites would be leukemia, or tumors of the brain, kidney, soft tissue, or eye. These sites are potentially characterized by diffuse symptoms, some of which are pain related. A child's initial hypotheses about the reasons for his/her cancer or the pain accompanying it would likely be of the same type as those for illness or sickness in general. For example, a child might say, "Cancer comes from other kids."

To assess pain in infants, toddlers, and preschoolers, behavioral data have been the mainstay. An important investigation describing the developmental aspects of behavioral distress in children undergoing bone marrow aspirations was conducted by Katz, Kellerman, and Siegel (1980). Observational data were reported for 115 children undergoing BMA, ranging in age from 8 months to 17 years, 9 months. Data were obtained prior to (waiting room and entry into the treatment room), during the BMA, and following (the immediate rest period in treatment room). Thirty-eight children were in the youngest sample and included children from 8 months to 6 years, 4 months (M = 3 years, 10 months). Data indicated that these young children evidenced a wider range of behavioral distress. They were most likely to express their fear and pain by crying, screaming, needing to be physically restrained, and verbalizing their pain (e.g., "ouch," "it hurts," "you are hurting me"). These children also exhibited their distress over the longest period of time. For example, while in the waiting room some children began to cry, request emotional support, and cling. During the procedure, their behavior was more disruptive and their distress continued longer during the postprocedure rest period.

Five to Nine Years

Continuing with the Piagetian conceptualization, concrete-operational reasoning characterizes this period. Illness hypotheses of contamination and internalization predominate. In the former, illness is believed to be caused by external events (e.g., person, object, or action) that have attributes that are "bad" or harmful to the body. The child understands him/herself to be "contaminated" either through physical contact (e.g., touching a person) or by engaging in a harmful action. For example, to the query, "Christina, how did you get your earache?" she replies, "from Jason." And to the question, "How did Jason give it to you?" she adds, "He shooted me with his gun."

A child who provides an internalization explanation still believes that illness is located in the body, although the cause, as before, is outside. However, now illness is seen as occurring through a process of internalizing the causative agent (e.g., swallowing, breathing). Although illness resides within the body, it remains confusing and vague and not linked to specific organs or functions. Bibace and Walsh (1980) provide an example of a child's internalized understanding of how she got her cold. She states that colds come from breathing too much air in the wintertime, and she adds that "bacteria get in by breathing and then the nose is blocked up."

For children in this age range, the most common types/sites for cancer are leukemia, lymphoma, and brain and kidney tumors. A child's contamination explanation for cancer or the pain from a tumor when it is diagnosed might be, for example, that it was due to eating something she or he didn't like or from smoking without a parent's permission (Bibace & Walsh, 1979). One aspect of this type of understanding for the child is that although the caregiver can provide disconfirming information about causal hypotheses, providing accurate, understandable explanations for the child with cancer may be difficult. Research suggests that children with cancer in this or prior developmental stages may perceive their illness or painful medical procedures as punishment for misdeeds (Perrin & Gerrity, 1981). Other researchers (Ross & Ross, 1984) examining children's causal hypotheses for pain have reported that common responses include accidents (36% of the explanations), environmental and nonsocial factors (e.g., heat and noise) (11%), illness (8%), surgery (7%), and aggressive acts of others (6%).

Returning to the Katz et al. (1980) behavioral observation investigation noted earlier, data from 38 children ranging in age from 6 years, 6 months to 9 years, 11 months (M = 7 years, 5 months) were also reported. This group resembled the youngest children in their fear and pain responses during the aspiration period. However, prior to and following BMA, they exhibited only as much distress as the oldest group of children (see discussion below). Thus, these children began to exercise some verbal and body control over their anticipatory fears, and they regained control more quickly.

Ten to Nineteen Years

At this stage (formal operations), the child has presumably become able to understand that illness is located within the body, and that external and internal forces may be causative. At this point explanations may be physiologic (e.g., germ theory) or psychophysiologic (e.g., psychosomatic hypotheses).

For the younger children in this group (e.g., 10 to 14 years), physiologic explanations may predominate. Prevalent sites for these children, in descending order, include the brain, lymphomas, leukemia, and bone tumors. As cancer is one of the less understood diseases, this may cause additional distress for the child. Survey data indicate that children of this age range view cancer as a more severe illness that is more difficult to recover from than comparisons such as heart disease, diabetes, or mental illness (Michielutte & Diseker, 1982).

Psychophysiologic explanations would suggest that the teenager might have some understanding that emotions, behavior, or social factors may play a role in illness. If such hypotheses were raised by the teenager with cancer, it would be important to provide disconfirming information as there are no data linking such factors to the incidence or etiology of pediatric cancers. It should also be noted that even older children may regress to an earlier level of reasoning when they feel frightened by their disease.

The oldest group of children participating in the Katz et al. (1980) BMA investigation ranged in age from 10 years to 17 years, 9 months (M = 12 years, 7 months). In comparison to the younger groups, these teens evidenced the least behavioral distress. When it occurred, however, it was primarily confined to the BMA period and consisted of verbalizations of pain and muscular rigidity. Crying and requests for emotional support also occurred.

Summary

Piagetian frameworks have been applied to children's understandings of illness and pain. This view suggests that children increasingly differentiate internal from external causative agents as the source of their illness and/or pains. Behavioral observation data have provided a vivid picture of children with cancer as they anticipate, undergo, and recover from painful BMA procedures. These studies show how children evidence fewer signs of behavioral distress as they age. Behavioral data provide an alternative for children too young to introspect and provide self-report data. Another finding from this investigation was that female children, in general, evidenced greater behavioral distress, particularly during the postprocedural period, when they were more likely to continue crying, requesting support, and clinging. Boys, on the other hand, were more likely to "stall" during the anticipatory periods. These data are consistent with a variety of other data on sex differences in reports of distress and pain (e.g., Bush & Holmbeck, 1987; Lollar, Smits, & Patterson, 1982).

Assessment Strategies

Self-report measures, including the McGill Pain Questionnaire (Melzack, 1975) or simple visual analogue scales (VAS), are often used with adults. The latter have demonstrated their utility and validity with adults (Scott & Huskisson, 1976) and they have occupied a central place in the assessment of pain in children as well (e.g., Sanders et al., 1989; Scott, Ansell, & Huskisson, 1977). In some cases, however, assessment of child pain is hindered by the child's cognitive or developmental level, verbal or spatial ability, or his/her ability to monitor physical symptoms. In such contexts, behavioral observations of the child and/or observer ratings of the child's pain and/or distress have been useful. Some researchers have also used psychophysiologic measures and inferred greater distress (or heightened arousal) from these data. (See chapter 3 for general descriptions of these three assessment methods.) We will limit this discussion to their utility thus far for pediatric cancer.

Self-Report Methods

The aspect of pain most commonly assessed via self-report is intensity. Visual analogue scales, usually presented in the form of a 100-mm line (often portrayed as a "pain thermometer") with the anchors of "no hurt at all" and "the most hurt possible," are used (see Jay, Elliott, Katz, & Siegel, 1987; Katz, Kellerman, & Ellenberg, 1987). To use such a scale, children must have the ability to conceptualize their pain experience along a continuum and translate that understanding to the visual representation of the line and anchors.

Similar strategies, such as Likert scales with anchor points of 1 ("no pain") and 5 ("extreme pain"), have also been used (LeBaron & Zeltzer, 1984). Again, children would need to interpret their pain using the descriptors and numerals. Rather than numbers paired with the descriptors, other investigators have used visual cues, such as different pictures of a child's face which are graded from happy or neutral expressions (no pain) to sad/distressed expressions (extreme pain). Some investigators (Kuttner, Bowman, & Teasdale, 1988; LeBaron & Zeltzer, 1984) also use number cues under each face, whereas others do not (Manne et al., 1990). As there are data indicating the universality of facial expressions (e.g., Eckman, 1984), this strategy has "face" validity, and face scales have been successfully used in several studies (Kuttner et al., 1988; Manne et al., 1990).

Other self-report strategies (e.g., self-monitoring using pain diaries, projective measures) that have been used with pediatric pain to assess the localization and frequency of pain episodes as well as affective components of the child's pain (see chapter 3) have not yet been used to assess pediatric cancer pain.

Behavioral Observation

Researchers studying procedural pain in children with cancer have been at the forefront in the development of observational methods to assess pain in children. Two observational schemes have emerged from two research programs (Jay & Elliott, 1984; Katz et al., 1980; LeBaron & Zeltzer, 1984) that have studied children's distress during BMA or LPs. The first scale developed was the Procedure Behavior Rating Scale (PBRS: Katz et al., 1980) to assess pain associated with LP and BMAs in children ranging in age from 8 months to 18 years. Observers noted the occurrence of 13 behaviors prior to, during, and following the procedure. The behaviors monitor anticipatory fears and behaviors (e.g., flail, clinging, refuse position, stalling, verbal fear) as well as pain behaviors (e.g., cry, muscular rigidity, request termination, verbal pain). As noted above, this scale has been sensitive to important developmental trends in pain expression and the scores correlate significantly with nurse ratings of child anxiety.

This scale was revised by Jay and her colleagues (Jay & Elliott, 1984) and renamed the Observational Scale of Behavioral Distress (OSBD). Three changes were made: categories were rated continuously rather than for presence/absence, intensity ratings of each category were also used, and some items were added and others revised or deleted. Validity data indicated that OSBD total scores were significantly correlated with trait anxiety, pain thermometer ratings of anticipated or experienced pain, and parent ratings of child anxiety. Subsequent study (Jay & Elliott, 1984) noted significant correlations of the OSBD with children's self-rated pain, nurse evaluations, and pulse rates. Further analyses of the scale indicated that no additional sensitivity was achieved by using continuous scales or the intensity ratings, suggesting that the less cumbersome presence/absence scheme of the PBRS is sufficient to detect important differences in pain and distress among children. Additional psychometric study has replicated the correlation of the OSBD with the measures of pain and distress; however, correlations with psychophysiologic measures (heart rate and blood pressure) may be unstable and in the low range (.30 to .40 range) (Elliott, Jay, & Woody, 1987).

LeBaron and Zeltzer (1984) have developed a simple and short rating system, the Procedure Behavior Checklist (PBCL). Eight behaviors (muscle tension, screaming, crying, restraint used, pain verbalized, anxiety verbalized, verbal stalling, physical resistance) are rated on 5-point scales. Validity data indicate that the scores are significantly correlated with children's self-rated pain and with observer ratings of pain and anxiety. Other data suggest that the PBCL may more accurately reflect child anxiety rather than pain. Similar methodologies have been applied to coding children's distress during venipuncture. Dahlquist, Gil, Armstrong, Ginsberg, and Jones (1985) have used the OSBD, whereas we (Manne et al., 1990) have used a revision of the PBRS. In both studies, satisfactory reliability was demonstrated.

The purpose of the above measures has been to quantify the occurrence, intensity, and range of child pain and distress during traumatic procedures. A new direction for behavioral observation researchers is to examine the child's interactions with others during these procedures. This strategy is common to other research areas (e.g., marital interactions and their relationship to marital distress and relationship change; mother-infant interactions and their relationship to the attachment process), but it is novel for pain research. This newer strategy utilizes continuous coding of child and adult interactions during painful procedures, with sequential data analysis to examine the relationship among behaviors rather than their absolute levels. Blount and his colleagues (Blount et al., 1989) code children's pain and distress behaviors as well as coping efforts during BMAs. This system, the Child-Adult Medical Procedure Interaction Scale (CAMPIS), includes aspects common to both marital interaction (Hops, Wills, Patterson, & Weiss, 1972) and child distress (Jay, Ozolins, Elliott, & Caldwell, 1983) coding schemes. For example, child content codes contain 16 categories, including child distress behaviors, nondistress verbalizations (e.g., normal talk occurring during the procedure such as the child informing others about his/her status), and child coping behaviors (e.g., humor). Despite the complexity of the system, initial reliability estimates appear good (e.g., inter-rater reliability for the child and adult codes is .80 to .90).

We have developed a similar coding system for use during venipuncture (Manne, Bakeman, Jacobsen, Gorfinkle, Bernstein, & Redd, in review) that focuses on child and adult distress and coping behaviors. Our system includes the same dimensions as Blount's coding scheme but also adds categories to assess child compliance and noncompliance to adult commands. In this manner, we can examine the relationship between child distress and specific adult behaviors such as providing explanations, coping suggestions (e.g., distraction), or commands necessary for the procedure (e.g., sitting still) and discover the processes by which child distress may be moderated by adult interactions.

Gauvain-Piquard, Rodary, Rezvani, and Lemerle (1987) have designed the only behavioral observation scale that can be employed to evaluate pain that lasts several days (in this case, tumor-related pain), with children 2 to 6 years of age. The scale consists of 17 items. Seven items concern pain (e.g., spontaneous protection of painful areas, child points out painful areas), six items concern depression (e.g., child retires into his shell, lack of expressiveness), and four items assess anxiety (e.g., nervousness, moodiness/irritability). Each child was scored at the same time by four independent observers (two nurses and two aides). The observational period was 4 hours. Weighted kappa coefficients analyzed for pairs of observers (pairs of nurses and pairs of aides) were quite low, ranging from .24 to .60. Factorial correspondence analyses indicated that pain and depression items both contributed to the first factor, accounting for 51% of the variance, whereas anxiety items contributed to a second factor, accounting for 13% of the variance. Although this study is important because assessment of disease-related pain is the focus, the low kappa coefficients and the lack of operationalization of scale items (e.g., what behaviors constitute "retiring in his shell" or "social withdrawal") suggests that the scale's reliabililty is questionable.

Global Adjustment Ratings

Observer ratings of child pain in pediatric oncology studies have included three categories of raters: a parent who might accompany their child during the procedure, the nurse or physician conducting the invasive procedure or providing the child's care, and independent observers such as research assistants (e.g., Kuttner et al., 1988; LeBaron & Zeltzer, 1984), although ratings made by the parent are less frequently used (Kuttner et al., 1988; Manne, Jacobsen, & Redd, in press). Likert scales are the most frequently employed response formats in these studies.

It has appeared that these ratings have had lower reliability and validity than other strategies. However, this circumstance may be due to the lack of quality control in implementation rather than by design. For example, training raters prior to data collection is a routine and necessary aspect of behavioral observation data collection, yet investigators seldom note that such training has been conducted prior to use of rating schedules. Similarly, operationalization of the rating categories is necessary to keep inference to a minimum. Even if accomplished, rater objectivity is difficult because of the emotional distress that the rating environment engenders for all: viewing children in pain and/or emotional distress is upsetting to most people. Parent ratings may be most vulnerable to bias as parents have the greatest concern for the child's welfare. Validity of global ratings is usually assessed by examining correlations with behavioral observation or the child's self-report data. Studies have found significant correlations between either parent or nurse ratings and behavior-coded child distress and the child's self-reported pain, although the nurse correlations tend to be higher than the parent ones (Katz et al., 1980; LeBaron & Zeltzer, 1984; Manne, Jacobsen, & Redd, in press). Not surprisingly, parent and nurse ratings are correlated (Manne et al., in press).

Observer ratings have not been used in studies examining chronic pain in children with cancer (disease and treatment-related pain). The lack of studies using observer ratings is probably because there are few controlled studies intervening with these types of pain.

Psychophysiological Measures

Although considered an important component in comprehensive pain assessment, psychophysiological measures have not been used to measure pediatric oncology pain. Two studies have used psychophysiological methods to assess anxiety or global arousal immediately prior to invasive medical procedures. Jay et al. (1987) measured heart rate and blood pressure prior to BMA, and Smith, Ackerman, and Blotcky (1989) measured heart rate prior to BMA. In both studies, these measures were significantly correlated with other methods of assessing pain, although the lack of synchrony between different domains is not uncommon (e.g., Abu-Saad, 1984). Investigators have not gathered parallel data during and after procedures to study the psychophysiological correlates of pain or painful stimuli.

Summary

Important advances have been made in the last 10 years in the assessment of pain in children with cancer. This research suggests several issues to be addressed in the future. First, it is unclear what exactly is being assessed by these instruments, pain or anxiety. Although some investigators have attempted to have observers and the child him/herself rate pain and anxiety separately, it is not clear that the child (particularly the very young child) is able to discriminate between the two feelings.

Second, what factors influence differences between the various methods of pain assessment is an issue that is not frequently addressed. Most researchers examine correlations between different measures as a validation strategy. However, this does not help to explain why the observers' perspectives may differ. We (Manne, Jacobsen, & Redd, in press) examined this issue by employing a set of demographic, medical, and psychological variables to predict behavior code distress (coded by trained raters), self-reported pain, parent and nurse-rated child pain. We found that the factors associated with behavior-coded distress and nurse ratings were similar. In addition, nurse ratings were predicted to a great degree by behavior-coded distress, suggesting that the nurse was basing her ratings on how much overt distress the child was exhibiting. Parents appeared to make their ratings based less on how much overt distress the child was exhibiting and more on their own judgment of the child's pain and their own expectations about the child's experience. The child's self-report was the most difficult to predict; it was affected by how much distress the child exhibited and the child's age. This study helps to elucidate the basis for different sources of pain ratings, and these data suggest that the variability between different pain ratings may provide an opportunity to understand different perspectives on the child's pain experience.

A third issue is the relative lack of assessment devices for disease and treatment-related pain. Other than the Gauvain-Piquard et al. (1987) observation system, there have been no scales developed for this population. Recent evidence has suggested that this type of pain may be underdiagnosed and labeled as a psychiatric disturbance rather than viewed as pain related. For example, Steif and Heiligenstein (1989) found that pain problems in children were frequently misdiagnosed as psychiatric problems such as depression, anxiety, behavioral problems, or cognitive/perceptual disturbances. In this study, approximately 20% of the referrals to consultation/liaison psychiatry resulted in the consultant assessing pain as the major problem. These results suggest that the assessment of cancer and/or treatment-related pain is complex. Medical staff overlook pain problems and attribute symptoms to psychological problems. Pain may also present as psychological symptoms such as depression or anxiety.

Differentiating the presenting problem may be particularly difficult in children, who may not be as able to describe their symptoms. The adaptation of multidimensional pain assessment instruments used in other pediatric populations such as the Pediatric Pain Questionnaire (Varni, Thompson, & Hanson, 1987) would provide a more comprehensive method for assessing pain and also address the affective component of the cancer pain. Cognitive factors such as the child's verbal ability and developmental level, as well as the child's understanding of pain and disease are all important to take into account when assessing the child's pain experience. McGrath and his colleagues have described a taxonomy that takes into account developmental factors in the selection of pain measures (McGrath, Beyer, Cleeland, Eland, McGrath, & Portenoy, 1990). This taxonomy is shown in Table 13.4. According to McGrath and colleagues, self-report is not usually appropriate in children under 30 months, and pain should be inferred from physiological and behavioral measures (the PBCL and a new scale developed by Mills, 1989, have been used with children younger than 3 years of age). By age 3, the child is able to provide ratings of "greater" and "lesser" pain intensity, so self-report measures are an important source of information. However, behavioral and physiological measures are important additional sources of information for children in this age range. For children over 6 years of age, Schechter recommends self-report measures as the primary source of pain assessment. In particular, self-report should be the primary means of assessing pain when a noxious stimulus is present (according to McGrath, behav-

TABLE 13.4. Age and most appropriate measures of pain intensity.

Age	Behavioral measures	Physiological measures	Self-report
Birth to 3 years	Few specialized scales available	Of primary importance	Not appropriate
3 to 6 years	Of primary importance; specialized scales available	Primary if behavioral scales not available	Important source
Over 6 years	Important source	Important source	Primary source

Note. From "Report of the Subcommittee on Assessment and Methodologic Issues in the Management of Cancer" by P. J. McGrath, J. Beyer, C. Cleeland, J. Eland, P. A. McGrath, and R. Portenoy, 1990, *Pediatrics, 86*, supplement. Copyright by American Academy of Pediatrics. Reprinted by permission.

ioral indicators are less valid indicators of pain in this situation). However, behavioral indicators should be employed as a primary source of information when self-report is not available due to disability or disease.

Efforts to Reduce Pain and Distress

The clinical management of pain in children with cancer is a significant problem. As noted in the introduction, there are data indicating that it is often not recognized, and, even if noticed, its severity may be underestimated (and therefore undertreated) or interpreted as due to psychologic factors (Steif & Heiligenstein, 1989). For the purposes of clarity, we will discuss two contexts for intervention, one of acute pain caused by distressing medical procedures or brief treatments (e.g., venipuncture) and the other for pain of longer duration from disease or treatment. Within each section, we will summarize pharmacologic and psychologic strategies, in keeping with the view that comprehensive cancer care incorporates both medical and psychological/behavioral management. We begin each section with a brief view of medical management strategies as these efforts may be the first and only efforts needed for some children and contexts.

Acute Pains and Distress

The majority of these pains are caused by the frequently performed procedures: venipuncture, bone marrow aspirations, and lumbar punctures. For venipuncture, pharmacological studies to investigate the efficacy of a topical lignocaine mixture (EMLA) have been carried out. Clarke and Radford (1986) investigated the efficacy of EMLA with 15 children, ages 1 to 14 years. Children received either lignocaine or a placebo cream and were assessed over the course of four venipunctures. Each child was given four tubes (two lignocaine, two placebo) administered in an alternating crossover design (i.e., drug/placebo/drug/placebo and the reverse). Cream was applied at home 1 hour before venipuncture. Pain was assessed using a 100-mm VAS and a four-category verbal scale. In addition, a nurse blind to the drug condition rated the ease of performing venipuncture on a 3-point scale. Results indicated a significant difference between EMLA and placebo cream on VAS and verbal response scale ratings. There was no difference with respect to the nurse's rating of the ease of venipuncture. Clinical efficacy was also demonstrated (11 of the 15 children wanted to continue using the cream). Similar efficacy of EMLA has been demonstrated earlier by Wahlstedt, Kollberg, Moller, and Uppfeldt (1984). They conducted a double blind placebo controlled study of 60 children, ages 5 to 15 years (it was not reported whether the children had cancer or not). Child pain ratings ("none," "slight," or "severe") were significantly lower for the EMLA group and the staff rated the procedure as easier to perform. In sum, these data indicate that the pain from venipuncture may be reduced with a mild and easy-to-use treatment such as topical cream.

There are fewer pharmacologic studies for the more severe pain of BMA or LP procedures. The most common method of treatment is an injection of lidocaine to anesthetize the skin surface and the bone, but, unfortunately, this does not lessen the pain from marrow suctioning. General anesthesia is employed less frequently because of the possible short- and long-term effects of repeated anesthesia inductions. Heavy sedation with injections of Demerol, Phenergan, and/or Thorazine have also been used, although the necessity of an intramuscular injection to administer the medication makes it less desirable for children. Orally administered sedative agents are less invasive and have fewer side effects, though they require forethought and medical support to be optimally effective and safe.

The earliest investigations employing psychological efforts for children's acute pains used hypnosis during BMA or LP. Hilgard and LeBaron (1982) were the first to report reductions in pain and anxiety with hypnosis for 24 children undergoing BMAs. The hypnotic induction was individualized but included induction, imagery, and rehearsal components. Dependent measures included judges' ratings based on observer notes of child behavior during the procedure and child self-reported pain immediately after the procedure. The design included a baseline assessment and two intervention treatments. Results indicated that hypnosis was effective in reducing self-reported and observer-rated pain during the first BMA, as compared with baseline ratings. This study provided an important first demonstration of the potential efficacy of hypnosis; however, the lack of a control group allows for the possibility of alternative interpretations for the effects (e.g., nonspecific or placebo effects).

Kellerman, Zeltzer, Ellenberg, and Dash (1983) used a multiple baseline design to investigate the efficacy of hypnosis with adolescents undergoing BMA, LP, or injection. Hypnosis was again individualized, but generally included induction, progressive relaxation, visualization, and additional hypnotic suggestions during the procedure. Self-reports of discomfort and anxiety before, during, and after the procedure were obtained. Analysis of multiple baseline data in the absence of treatment indicated no significant reductions in discomfort or anxiety across time (i.e., children evidenced no habituation to the painful procedures), however, with hypnosis, 89% of the children showed a significant reduction in both anxiety and discomfort during all assessment periods.

Two controlled investigations of hypnosis have been conducted. In the first, Zeltzer and LeBaron (1982) compared hypnosis administered during the procedure with a "supportive" intervention that included a combination of deep breathing, distraction, and rehearsal. Patients and independent observers provided pain and anxiety ratings before, during, and after the procedure. Although both interventions resulted in lowered pain and anxiety when compared with preintervention ratings, the reductions for the hypnosis group were significantly greater. No significant age differences in patient response to the intervention were found.

The second controlled study of hypnosis examined the generalization of therapeutic effect across repeated BMAs. Katz et al. (1987) compared hypnosis during BMA with a "nondirective session" control condition. The hypnosis condition included hypnotic inductions and training in self-hypnosis and the nondirective intervention included nondirective play sessions in which rapport and nonmedical play were initiated. Measures were obtained at baseline and three subsequent BMAs. Dependent measures included observed behavior (BPRS-R), nurse ratings of anxiety, child self-reports of fear and pain, and therapist ratings of rapport with the child and response to hypnosis. Both nurses and behavioral observers were blind to experimental condition. Results indicated generalization of treatment effects across time, with self-reported pain and fear decreasing from baseline to subsequent BMAs in both groups. However, no significant decreases were found on the observational measures, with the BPRS-R actually increasing over the course of the postintervention procedures. Analyses of individual differences revealed a gender by treatment interaction, with females evidencing greater reductions in distress with hypnosis than males.

In contrast to the hypnosis literature, the efficacy of cognitive-behavioral interventions has received more investigative attention. Multicomponent "packages," which may include preparatory information, relaxation, pleasant imagery, positive coping statements, modeling, and/or behavioral rehearsal are used. Such clinical investigations are patterned, for example, on the work of Melamed (Melamed & Siegel, 1975) on preparation of children for surgery and the stress inoculation model described by Turk (1978).

Dahlquist et al. (1985) conducted an early study with pediatric cancer patients. A single subject, multiple baseline design was used with three adolescents (ages 11, 12, and 13 years) receiving venipuncture for chemotherapy. Dependent measures included observational measures, patient self-reports, and parent and medical personnel adjustment ratings. Four intervention sessions were conducted and incorporated cue-controlled relaxation, imagery, positive coping statements, and rewards for practicing relaxation between chemotherapy procedures and for using coping statements during the procedure. Observed and self-reported distress decreased for all three subjects. However, parent ratings were not reduced, and medical personnel ratings declined only slightly. Although many variables remained uncontrolled, this report provided an early demonstration of the potential clinical efficacy of these techniques.

Another multicomponent clinical study was conducted by McGrath and DeVeber (1986). Fourteen children were provided intervention consisting of four 45-minute sessions scheduled 6 weeks prior to their next LP. Intervention included procedural information, desensitization (role playing LPs with a stuffed animal), training in distraction (e.g., squeezing the parent's hand), imagery techniques, and cognitive restructuring for pain sensations. Baseline measures were devised by "averaging" parent and nurse ratings of child pain and anxiety obtained after each procedure the child underwent for 24 months prior to the first intervention. These ratings included separate VAS pain and anxiety ratings and a behavior checklist (the contents of this scale were not described in the report). Children's pain and anxiety decreased significantly when the average preintervention rating was compared with ratings taken after the procedure when intervention was employed. These reductions remained at 3- and 6-month follow-ups. Although the authors report significant reductions, the measures and methods are not described in sufficient detail to permit conclusions with regard to the efficacy of the intervention.

As noted above, Jay and her colleagues (Jay et al., 1987; Jay, Elliott, Ozolins, Olson, & Pruitt, 1985) have contributed to the development of observational techniques for the assessment of pain-related behaviors. In addition, they have developed a multicomponent "package" to reduce children's distress during BMAs and LPs. Their Cognitive Behavioral Therapy Package includes five components: filmed modeling (watching a child use the techniques during a BMA), breathing exercises, positive reinforcement (receiving a trophy for lying still and doing breathing exercises), imagery (the child pretends that he or she is a "Superhero"), and behavioral rehearsal (the child role-plays a BMA). The intervention is provided in the hour preceding the BMA. An initial clinical report with five patients (ages 3.5 to 7 years) reported significant reductions in observed distress (Jay et al., 1985). The second study by Jay and colleagues is significant in that it compared the efficacy of the multicomponent package with both pharmacologic therapy (Valium) and an attention control (Jay et al., 1987). A counterbalanced crossover design was used in assigning 56 children to one of three experimental conditions. Results indicated that the cognitive-behavioral intervention was significantly more effective than attention-control in reducing behavioral distress, self-reported pain, and physiological arousal in the anticipatory period (i.e., prior to cleansing the BMA site). In the group administered Valium, these signs of distress were not significantly different from the attention-control condition, although Valium did reduce diastolic blood pressure and observed distress during the anticipatory phase. These results suggest that the drug effects may be specific to physiological arousal. Unfortunately, physiologic data were gathered only during the anticipatory period; physiological indices may have been lower during the procedure as well. Follow-up analyses of individual differences in age, gender, ethnicity, and prior experience with BMA revealed no interactions with outcome. This study is important because it is unique in comparing pharmacological with psychological intervention.

Several investigators have examined the role of distraction in reducing children's distress. Kuttner and colleagues (Kuttner et al., 1988) compared distraction to "imaginative involvement" (a procedure presumably similar to hypnosis). Distraction procedures were behavioral ones, including activities (e.g., blowing bubbles or playing with objects) and discussion of nonprocedural topics. Imaginative involvement by the therapist incorporated hypnotic-like suggestions and storytelling. Results indicated that the effectiveness of the interventions varied with the children's age. In the first treatment session, imaginative involvement was more effective in reducing observed distress in younger children (3 to 6 years), and it was equally effective as distraction for the older group (7 to 10 years). However, by the second session, these differences disappeared. Pain self-reports and observer measures of anxiety and distress decreased in all groups, including the control group. In commenting on their effects, the authors suggest that the distraction task required the child to take on an active role in managing his/her distress, such as initiating breathing when anxious. This active role may be more difficult for a younger child, which explains why distraction was less effective with the younger child.

In studying children undergoing venipuncture, we use a simple distraction technique (Manne et al., 1990). A child blows into a party blower while the parent actively coaches the child to blow by counting out loud to pace the child's blowing. Reward stickers are given to the child contingent upon the child's paced blowing and for holding his/her arm still during needle insertion. In an initial study, data were collected on 23 children during venipuncture. After baseline assessment, children and their parents were randomly assigned to an intervention or an attention-control group. The intervention was provided during the next three venipunctures. Before the first intervention trial, a psychologist taught the parent and child the intervention techniques. During the procedure, the psychologist aided the parent in coaching the child. The amount of active encouragement provided to the parent by the psychologist decreased over the course of the next two intervention trials. By the third session, he or she was present only as an observer while the parent conducted the intervention. Dependent measures included child self-reported pain (using the Faces Scale), parent and nurse ratings, observational measures including whether or not restraint was employed and the PBRS-R and parent and nurse self-reports of anxiety and distress. Results indicated significantly lowered levels of distress on the behavioral measures and parent ratings of child pain, and reductions in parents' anxiety reports across the three sessions. The remaining measures did not indicate significant reductions. These findings suggest that parents can be taught simple, effective strategies to help their children through venipuncture. These procedures are effective in reducing the children's behavioral distress and lowering the parent's anxiety.

Smith et al. (1989) investigated the interaction of two behavioral interventions, distraction and procedural information, with coping style (repression versus sensitization). The distraction intervention included discussing favorite topics with the child; the procedural information intervention included providing information about the bone marrow aspiration or lumbar puncture. Children were categorized as either "sensitizers" or "repressors" based upon their responses to an interview. Dependent measures included observational measures, self-reports of pain, and heart rate prior to the procedure. Results indicated that there were no differences in treatment outcome between the two intervention groups on any of the measures. Unfortunately, the sensitizer and repressor groups differed on important disease and treatment variables (i.e., repressors had been diagnosed for a shorter period of time and had fewer BMAs), which complicates interpretation of the coping style differences. In fact, findings contrary to prediction were revealed: repressors taught distraction had the highest experienced pain ratings, and sensitizers given information had the second highest pain ratings. Other details of the analyses (e.g., the efficacy of the interventions compared with a control group) are not provided.

Factors Influencing Treatment Efficacy

Given the important role that developmental, psychological, medical and sociodemographic variables play in the child's pain experience and the expression of pain, it is important to examine the effect of these factors in intervention outcome. Jay et al. (1987) examined the influence of age, gender, ethnicity, and prior experience with the medical procedure upon the efficacy of their cognitive-behavioral and pharmacologic interventions. No effects of any of these variables were found. However, Kuttner et al. (1988) found that age was related to the most effective type of treatment. Coping style (sensitizer or repressor) has also been found to relate to the effectiveness of interventions (Smith et al., 1989). These studies suggest that the child's age along with other variables such as coping style may influence the outcome of psychological interventions. However, the exact role of these factors cannot be clarified until they are included in the analyses of a greater number of intervention studies.

Summary

Several clinically useful techniques have been studied to help children with cancer undergoing repeated painful procedures. Hypnosis appears to be successful in reducing the immediate pain and distress during a single procedure, and the therapeutic effects appear to persist across multiple procedures. However, these promising results may not be due to any active ingredient of hypnosis per se, since the same positive effects (though possibly less robust ones) are found with nonspecific and supportive interventions.

The multicomponent interventions appear as clinically useful as the hypnotic techniques. In addition, the controlled comparison with Valium and the attention control in the Jay et al. (1987) investigation suggests that there may be some specificity for the effects from multicomponent efforts. However, it is unknown which component or combination of components is responsible for these effects. Distraction, including both behavioral and cognitive engagement of the child during the painful procedures, has been suggested as the treatment component fundamental to the efficacy of multicomponent interventions.

The notion of attentional distraction is complex and raises many interesting research questions. One could hypothesize that the extent to which the child is active (or passive) in the distraction efforts might be one variable that could co-vary with outcome. The child's amount of responsibility has ranged across investigations, from total responsibility (Kuttner et al., 1988), wherein the child was left to his/her own devices to generate distracting cognitions, to a more passive role (Manne et al., 1990), in which the parent was responsible for engaging the child in a behavioral task. The child's degree of involvement in the distraction task may also exert an effect on its effectiveness. Similarly, the use of cognitive versus behavioral distraction may be an important variable. The effectiveness of the intervention may be moderated by the ability of the child to perform the task. That is, it may be easier for young children to perform behavioral distraction tasks, whereas older children may find some cognitive tasks more engaging. The effectiveness of the interventions may also vary with aspects of the medical stressor. For example, it may be more difficult to maintain distraction during long procedures or when the child cannot see the procedure progress from step to step (e.g., venipunctures are in view whereas BMAs are not).

Another important issue is the effectiveness of interventions in reducing the signs and symptoms of pain and distress. All of the interventions reviewed appear to be effective in reducing behavioral distress. However, changes in the children's self-reports of pain are less common. Some attribute the lack of pain reduction to the method of measurement. Frequently, 5-point scales are used, and declines in pain are not found (Manne et al., 1990; Siegel & Peterson, 1981). Investigators using 100-mm pain thermometer scales have reported decreases in pain (Dahlquist et al., 1985; Jay et al., 1987; Katz et al., 1987). Whether or not measurement issues are contributory requires further study. This review suggests that more consistent reductions in self-reported pain result from interventions incorporating hypnosis or multicomponent packages. In addition, the Kuttner study (Kuttner et al., 1988), comparing a hypnotic-like intervention with distraction, indicated that hypnosis may be more effective than distraction with younger children.

Several other therapeutic components that may contribute to treatment effectiveness are preparation for the procedure (e.g., watching a film about the procedure), learning self-management skills, increasing the child's sense of mastery and control over an aversive experience, and parent involvement in the intervention (a reduction of parent anxiety may lead to reductions in child distress). No studies have analyzed the contribution of these components, so conclusions regarding their roles are not possible at this time.

Finally, there has been only preliminary study of individual differences that may moderate intervention effectiveness. Such variables include age and developmental level as well as psychological variables such as coping style.

Disease and Treatment Side Effect Pains

Appropriate medical management of disease and treatment-related pains is essential. A primary method for treating disease-related pain is the cancer treatment itself, particularly chemotherapy and radiation. For example, a child whose disease is disseminated may not be a candidate for maximal chemotherapy or radiation therapy. Palliative radiotherapy to painful sites may provide pain relief even when it does not provide cure. As described previously, the etiology of cancer and cancer treatment pains can be heterogeneous. Examples include pain caused by infection (e.g., aching pain from septicemia) or mucositis, pain from peripheral neuropathy from chemotherapy such as vincristine, phantom limb pain, prolonged postlumbar puncture pain, headache, abdominal pain from chemotherapy-induced vomiting, radiation dermatitis, and radiation-induced nerve damage. Indeed, it would be difficult to conduct controlled studies with such a heterogeneous group of pain etiologies.

The main approach used in the treatment of pain due to cancer has been analgesic medication tailored to the child's condition. One current organizing principle for such management is the analgesic "ladder" (see Berde, Albin, Glazer, Miser, Shapiro, Weisman, & Zeltzer, 1990 for a description). Three general categories are specified. For "mild" pain, initial management usually uses nonopiates, such as acetaminophen. For "moderate" pain, children often continue to receive acetaminophen with the addition of a weak opiate agonist such as codeine. For severe pain, patients often continue with the "moderate" regimen with the addition of an opiate, often morphine or methadone may be selected. Dilaudid is a more potent choice, particularly for children with disseminated disease or in the terminal stages.

Miser and her colleagues have published a series of studies investigating the use of opioid analgesics with pediatric cancer patients. One study (Miser, Miser, & Clark, 1980) reported on the use of morphine sulfate given via continuous intravenous infusion ranging from 1 to 16 days for eight children with terminal stage metastatic disease. Pain was assessed by children's self-reports and pain ratings from the physician, nurse, and parent (it is unclear if numeric scales were given). Pain relief was defined as "freedom from pain" and the absence of pain complaints more than 95% of the time. As with adults, morphine infusion provided adequate and consistent pain relief (i.e., fewer periods of uncontrolled pain). In a related report, Miser, Davis, Hughes, Mulne, and Miser (1983) treated 17 children with malignant cancer pain using continuous subcutaneous infusion of morphine. Pain relief was assessed in the same fashion. All patients achieved satisfactory pain control with drowsiness as the major side effect. In 5 out of 15 patients, respiratory depression, a (possibly lethal) side effect of morphine, did occur.

The efficacy of oral methadone has also been studied by Miser and Miser (1986). Methadone was administered in a fixed 4- or 6-hour schedule to 22 patients with tumor or treatment-related pain. Therapy duration varied from 5 to 267 days. A single VAS pain rating for each patient was made by a physician (Miser) on the basis of observation, physical examination, and questioning of the patient. For children 8 years of age or older, the child also completed a VAS rating. Physician-rated pain levels of less than 20 mm on the VAS were achieved in 12 patients and from 20 mm to 50 mm in 9 patients. Only one patient did not achieve satisfactory pain control. Results regarding the child's self-report ratings were not presented.

Despite the uncontrolled nature of these reports (e.g., varying dosages and duration of treatment, inadequate pain assessment, no comparison groups, absence of pretreatment ratings), Miser's clinical reports illustrate the effectiveness and importance of drugs, particularly opiates, for cancer-related pain. However, there are many misconceptions regarding these drugs and their use with children that impede many physicians from effectively incorporating them into their treatment regimens (see Berde et al., 1990; Schechter, 1985; or Yaster & Deshpande, 1988 for discussions). One misconception regards the development of drug tolerance. Many physicians assume they must continuously escalate dosages to obtain effective pain management. Data suggest that this is not the case; the development of tolerance, a diminished drug effect in the context of continuous administration, is variable. For many patients, once an adequate analgesic dose is achieved, it may remain stable for extended period of time. Physical dependence, the need to continue drug administration in order to avoid the occurrence of symptoms associated with withdrawal, is common among patients receiving opiates for pain. However, when pain medication is no longer necessary, withdrawal symptoms are usually avoided by tapering opiate administration over 5 to 10 days (Schechter, 1985). The behavioral syndrome of addiction is rare (Berde et al., 1990). Finally, a side effect of opiate administration, respiratory depression, is often cause for much concern. The fears may be worsened by the "air hunger" associated with terminal disease. However, many feel that patients have a right to receive adequate analgesia and sedation for the pain and distress of terminal disease (Berde et al., 1990).

Other methods of controlling pain, such as neurosurgery, nerve blocks and transcutaneous electrical nerve stimulation (TENS) units have not been investigated in this population.

There are only two reports of psychological analgesic interventions for chronic pain associated with cancer or its treatment. The available studies are clinical descriptions of intervention programs. LaBaw, Holton, Tewell, and Eccles (1975) used a broad-band hypnosis intervention with 27 children. Suggestions were given in twice-a-month group sessions for improving sleep, increasing food and fluid intake, and increasing tolerance for diagnostic procedures. Of the 12 cases described, pain control was a presenting problem among 5 children. The authors described a decrease in pain in 3 children. However, the only objective data presented was a reported decrease in the number of analgesics taken by one of the children, and one child going through a BMA using only hypnosis rather than anesthesia. Olness (1981) reported on the use of self-hypnosis with 25 pediatric cancer patients. Intervention included individual training in imagery, four practice sessions and an optional twice monthly group session. Each patient was also offered a cassette tape of individual exercises to use at home. Children participating in the study were referred for reasons other than pain associated with the disease process (e.g., children with anticipatory nausea and vomiting and procedural pain were also included). The authors observed that several children in relapse who were no longer receiving chemotherapy tolerated pain without the need for pharmacological pain medication. These children also reported "feeling better" as a result of the imagery intervention.

Summary and Future Directions

Assessment and treatment of pain in children with cancer has focused mostly upon pain associated with invasive medical procedures. Results of these studies suggest that pain and distress can be reliably assessed and effectively reduced during these procedures. Although there is evidence to suggest that pain related to the disease and its treatment are prevalent, there are few controlled studies investigating pharmacological and psychological interventions for these types of pain. Future studies need to focus on developing assessment methods and interventions for these chronic pains. The influence of developmental factors and individual differences upon the selection of appropriate assessment instruments and upon treatment outcome are also important; these factors should be taken into account in a greater number of studies.

Cancer pain is a complex phenomenon with cognitive, evaluative, and affective components, creating a challenging research area. It is hoped researchers and clinicians alike will recognize the need for better management of pediatric cancer pain and address this important issue.

Acknowledgments. Barbara L. Andersen's work was supported by Grant PBR #27 from the American Cancer Society to Barbara L. Andersen. Sharon Manne's work was supported by Grant PBR #17 from the American Cancer Society. The authors would like to thank Mary Walling for early assistance and Sharon Melnick for her editorial comments.

References

Abu-Saad, H. (1984). Assessing children's responses to pain. *Pain, 19,* 163–171.

Baum, E., Suther, H., & Nachman, J. (1979). Relapse rates following cessation of chemotherapy during complete remission of ALL. *Medical Pediatric Oncology, 1,* 25–34.

Berde, C., Albin, A., Glazer, J., Miser, A., Shapiro, B., Weisman, S., & Zeltzer, P. (1990). Report of the Subcommittee on Disease-Related Pain in Childhood Cancer. In N. Schechter, A. Altman, & S. Weisman (Eds.), *Report of the Consensus Conference on the Management of Pain in Childhood Cancer. Pediatrics, 86(5),* supplement.

Bibace, R., & Walsh, M. (1979). Developmental stages in children's conceptions of illness. In G. Stone, F. Cohen, & N. Adler (Eds.), *Health psychology.* Washington: Jossey-Bass.

Bibace, R., & Walsh, M. (1980). Development of children's concepts of illness. *Pediatrics, 66,* 912–917.

Blount, R., Corbin, S., Sturges, J., Wolfe, V., Prater, J., & James, L. (1989). The relationship between adults' behavior and child coping and distress during BMA/ LP procedures: A sequential analysis. *Behavior Therapy, 20,* 585–601.

Bush, J., & Holmbeck, G. (1987). Children's attitudes about health care: Initial development of a questionnaire. *Journal of Pediatric Psychology, 12,* 429–443.

Carabell, S. C., Cassady, J. R., Weinstein, H. J., & Jaffe, N. (1978). The role of radiation therapy in the treatment of pediatric non-Hodgkin's lymphomas. *Cancer, 42,* 2193–2205.

Clarke, S., & Radford, M. (1986). Topical anesthesia for venipuncture. *Archives of Disease in Childhood, 61,* 1132–1134.

Craig, K., McMahon, R., Morison, J., & Zaskow, C. (1984). Developmental changes in infant pain expression during immunization injections. *Social Science and Medicine, 19,* 1331–1337.

Dahlquist, L., Gil, K., Armstrong, F., Ginsberg, A., & Jones, B. (1985). Behavioral management of children's distress during chemotherapy. *Journal of Behavior Therapy and Experimental Psychiatry, 16,* 325–329.

D'Angio, G. J., Evans, A. E., Breslow, N., Beckwith, B., Baum, E., DeLorimier, A., Farewell, V., Fernbach, D., Hrabovsky, E., & Jones, B. (1984). Results of the Third National Wilms' Tumor Study: A preliminary report. *Proceedings of the Annual Meeting of the American Association of Cancer Research, 25,* 183–185.

Duffner, P., Cohen, M., & Freeman, A. (1985). Pediatric brain tumors: An overview. *Ca — A Cancer Journal for Clinicians*, *35*, 287-301.

Eckman, P. (1984). Expression and the nature of emotion. In K. Scherer & P. Eckman (Eds.), *Approaches to emotion* (pp. 319-343). Hillsdale, NJ: Erlbaum.

Eckman, P., & Oster, H. (1979). Facial expression of emotion. *Annual Review of Psychology*, *30*, 527-554.

Elliott, C., Jay, S., & Woody, P. (1987). An observational scale for measuring children's distress during medical procedures. *Journal of Pediatric Psychology*, *12*, 543-551.

Everson, T. C., & Cole, W. H. (1966). *Spontaneous regression of cancer*. Philadelphia: W. B. Saunders.

Fernbach, D. J. (1984). Natural history of acute leukemia. In W. W. Sutrow, D. J. Fernbach, & T. J. Vietti (Eds.), *Clinical pediatric oncology* (pp. 332-377). St. Louis: C. V. Mosby.

Gauvain-Piquard, A., Rodary, C., Rezvani, A., & Lemerle, J. (1987). Pain in children aged 2-6 years: A new observational rating scale elaborated in a pediatric oncology unit-preliminary report. *Pain*, *31*, 177-188.

Glatstein, E., Kim, H., Donaldson, S. S., Dorfman, R. F., Gribble, T. J., Wilbur, J. R., Rosenberg, S., & Kaplan, H. S. (1974). Non-Hodgkin's lymphomas. VI. Results of treatment in childhood. *Cancer*, *34*, 204-211.

Henderson, E. D., & Dahlin, D. C. (1963). Chondrosarcoma of bone — A study of 288 cases. *Journal of Bone and Joint Surgery*, *45A*, 1450-1458.

Hilgard, J., & LeBaron, S. (1982). Relief of anxiety and pain in children and adolescents with cancer: Quantitative measures and clinical observations. *International Journal of Clinical and Experimental Hypnosis*, *30*, 417-442.

Hops, H., Wills, T., Patterson, G., & Weiss, R. (1972). *Marital interaction coding system*. Unpublished manuscript, University of Oregon and Oregon Research Institute, Eugene, Oregon.

Izard, C. E., & Buechler, S. (1979). Emotion expressions and personality integration in infancy. In C. E. Izard (Ed.), *Emotions in personality and psychopathology* (pp. 445-472). New York: Plenum.

Jay, S., & Elliott, C. (1984). Behavioral observation scales for measuring children's distress: The effects of increased methodological rigor. *Journal of Consulting and Clinical Psychology*, *52*, 1106-1107.

Jay, S., Elliott, C., Katz, E., & Siegel, S. (1987). Cognitive-behavioral and pharmacologic interventions for childrens' distress during painful medical procedures. *Journal of Consulting and Clinical Psychology*, *55*, 860-865.

Jay, S., Elliott, C., Ozolins, M., Olson, R., & Pruitt, S. (1985). Behavioral management of children's distress during painful medical procedures. *Behaviour Research and Therapy*, *5*, 513-520.

Jay, S., Ozolins, M., Elliott, C., & Caldwell, S. (1983). Assessment of children's distress during painful medical procedures. *Health Psychology*, *2*, 133-147.

Johnston, C., & Strada, M. (1986). Acute pain response in infants: A multidimensional description. *Pain*, *24*, 373-382.

Katz, E., Kellerman, J., & Ellenberg, L. (1987). Hypnosis in the reduction of acute pain and distress in children with cancer. *Journal of Pediatric Psychology*, *12*, 379-394.

Katz, E., Kellerman, J., & Siegel, S. (1980). Behavioral distress in children with cancer undergoing medical procedures: Developmental considerations. *Journal of Consulting and Clinical Psychology, 48*, 356-365.

Kellerman, J., Zeltzer, L., Ellenberg, L., & Dash, J. (1983). Adolescents with cancer: Hypnosis for the reduction of the acute pain and anxiety associated with medical procedures. *Journal of Adolescent Health Care, 4*, 85-90.

Knudson, A. G., & Strong, L. C. (1973). Mutation and cancer: A model for Wilms' tumor of the kidney. *Journal of the National Cancer Institute, 48*, 313-324.

Kuttner, L., Bowman, M., & Teasdale, M. (1988). Psychological treatment of distress, pain and anxiety for young children with cancer. *Developmental and Behavioral Pediatrics, 9*, 374-381.

LaBaw, W., Holton, C., Tewell, K., & Eccles, D. (1975). The use of self-hypnosis by children with cancer. *American Journal of Clinical Hypnosis, 17*, 233-238.

LeBaron, S., & Zeltzer, L. (1984). Assessment of acute pain and anxiety in children and adolescents by self-reports, observer reports, and a behavior checklist. *Journal of Consulting and Clinical Psychology, 52*, 729-738.

Lollar, D., Smits, S., & Patterson, D. (1982). Assessment of pediatric pain: An empirical perspective. *Journal of Pediatric Psychology, 7*, 267-277.

Manne, S., Bakeman, R., Jacobsen, P., Gorfinkle, K., Bernstein, D., & Redd, W. H. (in press). Adult and child interaction during invasive medical procedures: A sequential analysis.

Manne, S., Jacobsen, P., & Redd, W. H. (in press). Assessment of acute pediatric pain: Do child self-report, parent ratings, and nurse ratings measure the same phenomenon? *Pain*.

Manne, S., Redd, W. H., Jacobsen, P., Gorfinkle, K., Schorr, O., & Rapkin, B. (1990). Behavioral intervention to reduce child and parent distress during venipuncture. *Journal of Consulting and Clinical Psychology, 58*, 565-572.

Marcove, R. C., & Rosen, G. (1980). En bloc resections for osteogenic sarcoma. *Cancer, 45*, 3040-3044.

Maurer, H. M., Donaldson, M., Gehan, E. A., Hammond, D., Hays, D. M., Lawrence, W., Lindberg, R., Newton, W., Ragab, A., Raney, B., Ruymann, F., Soule, E., Sutow, W., & Tefft, M. (1981). The intergroup rhabdomyosarcoma study. Update, November, 1978. Journal of the National Cancer Institute Monograph, *56*, 61-68.

McGrath, P. J., Beyer, J., Cleeland, C., Eland, J., McGrath, P. A., & Portenoy, R. (1990). Report of the Subcommittee on Assessment and Methodologic Issues in the Management of Pain in Childhood Cancer. In N. Schechter, A. Altman, & S. Weisman (Eds.), *Report of the Consensus Conference on the Management of Pain in Childhood Cancer. Pediatrics, 86(5)* suppl.

McGrath, P. A., & deVeber, L. (1986). The management of acute pain evoked by medical procedures in children with cancer. *Journal of Pain and Symptom Management, 1*, 145-150.

Melamed, B., & Siegel, L. (1975). Reduction in anxiety in children facing hospitalization and surgery by use of filmed modeling. *Journal of Consulting and Clinical Psychology, 43*, 511-521.

Melzack, R. (1975). The McGill Pain Questionnaire: Major properties and scoring methods. *Pain, 1*, 277-299.

Merskey, H. (1970). On the development of pain. *Headache, 10*, 116-123.

Michielutte, R., & Diseker, R. A. (1982). Children's perceptions of cancer in comparison to other chronic illnesses. *Journal of Chronic Diseases, 35*, 843-852.

Miller, R. W., & Dalager, N. A. (1974). Fatal rhabdomyosarcoma among children in the United States 1960–69. *Cancer, 34,* 1897–1900.

Mills, N. (1989). Pain behaviors in infants and toddlers. *Journal of Pain and Symptom Management, 4,* 184–190.

Miser, A., Davis, D., Hughes, C., Mulne, A., & Miser, J. (1983). Continuous infusion of morphine in children with cancer. *American Journal of Diseases in Children, 137,* 383–385.

Miser, A., McCalla, J., Dothage, J., Wesley, M., & Miser, J. (1987). Pain as a presenting symptom in children and young adults with newly diagnosed malignancy. *Pain, 29,* 85–90.

Miser, A., & Miser, J. (1986). The use of oral methadone to control moderate and severe pain in children and young adults with malignancy. *Clinical Journal of Pain, 1,* 243–248.

Miser, A., Miser, J., & Clark, B. (1980). Continuous intravenous infusion of morphine sulphate for control of severe pain in children with terminal malignancy. *Journal of Pediatrics, 96,* 930–932.

Okamura, J., Sutow, W. W., & Moon, T. E. (1977). Prognosis in children with metastatic rhabdomyosarcoma. *Medical Pediatric Oncology, 3,* 243–251.

Olness, K. (1981). Imagery (self-hypnosis) as adjunct therapy in childhood cancer. *American Journal of Pediatric Hematology/ Oncology, 1,* 313–321.

Owens, M. E. (1984). Pain in infancy: Conceptual and methodological issues. *Pain, 20,* 213–230.

Perrin, E., & Gerrity, P. (1981). There's a demon in your belly: Children's understanding of illness. *Pediatrics, 67,* 841–849.

Poznanski, F. O. (1976). Children's reactions to pain: A psychiatrist's perspective. *Clinical Pediatrics, 15,* 1114–1119.

Pui, C., & Crist, W. M. (1990). Pediatric solid tumors. In A. Holleb & D. Fink (Eds.), *Clinical oncology.* Atlanta, GA: American Cancer Society.

Pui, C., & Rivera, G. K. (1990). Childhood leukemia. In A. Holleb & D. Fink (Eds.), *Clinical oncology.* Atlanta, GA: American Cancer Society.

Ross, D. M., & Ross, S. A. (1984). Childhood pain: The school-aged child's viewpoint. *Pain, 20,* 179–191.

Sanders, M., Rebgetz, M., Morrison, M., Bor, W., Gordon, A., Dadds, M., & Shepherd, R. (1989). Cognitive-behavioral treatment of recurrent nonspecific abdominal pain in children: An analysis of generalization, maintenance, and side effects. *Journal of Consulting and Clinical Psychology, 57,* 294–300.

Schechter, N. L. (1985). Pain and pain control in children. *Current Problems in Pediatrics, 15,* 1–67.

Schechter, N., Allen, D. A., & Hanson, K. (1986). Status of pediatric pain control: A comparison of analgesic usage in children and adults. *Pediatrics, 77,* 11–15.

Scott, P., Ansell, B., & Huskisson, E. (1977). Measurement of pain in juvenile chronic polyarthritis. *Annals of Rheumatic Diseases, 36,* 186–187.

Scott, P., & Huskisson, E. (1976). Graphic representation of pain. *Pain, 2,* 175–184.

Siegel, L., & Peterson, L. (1981). Maintenance effects of coping skills and sensory information on young children's response to repeated dental procedures. *Behavior Therapy, 12,* 530–535.

Silverberg, B. S., Boring, C. C., & Squires, B. A. (1990). Cancer statistics, 1990. *Ca–A Cancer Journal for Clinicians, 40,* 9–26.

Silverstein, M. N., & Kelly, P. J. (1963). Leukemia with osteoarticular symptoms and signs. *Annals of Internal Medicine, 59*, 637-645.

Simmons, C. R., Harle, T. S., & Singleton, E. B. (1968). The osseous manifestations of leukemia in children. *Radiologic Clinics of North America, 6*, 115-130.

Smith, K., Ackerman, J., & Blotcky, A. (1989). Reducing distress during invasive medical procedures: Relating behavioral interventions to preferred coping style in pediatric cancer patients. *Journal of Pediatric Psychology, 14*, 405-419.

Steif, B., & Heiligenstein, E. (1989). Psychiatric symptoms of pediatric cancer pain. *Journal of Pain and Symptom Management, 4*, 191-196.

Swank, R. L., Fetterman, G. H., Sieber, W. K., & Kiesewetter, W. B. (1971). Prognostic factors in neuroblastoma. *Annals of Surgery, 174*, 428-435.

Talbert, L. M., Kraybill, E. N., & Potter, H. D. (1975). Adrenal cortical response to circumcision in the neonate. *Obstetrics and Gynecology, 48*, 208-210.

Turk, D. (1978). Cognitive behavioral techniques in the management of pain. In J. P. Foreyt & D. P. Rathjen (Eds.), *Cognitive behavior therapy* (pp. 199-227). New York: Plenum.

Varni, J., Thompson, K., & Hanson, V. (1987). The Varni/Thompson Pediatric Pain Questionnaire. I. Chronic musculoskeletal pain in juvenile rheumatoid arthritis. *Pain, 28*, 27-38.

Wahlstedt, C., Kollberg, H., Moller, C., & Uppfeldt, A. (1984). Lignocaine-Prilocaine cream reduces venipuncture pain. *Lancet,*

Wolff, P. H. (1969). The natural history of crying and other vocalizations in early infancy. In B. Foss (Ed.), *Determinants of infant behavior* (Vol. 4, pp. 81-115). London: Methuen.

Wollner, N., Burchenal, J. H., Lieberman, P. H., Exelby, P., D'Angio, G., & Murphy, M. L. (1976). A comparative study of 2 modalities of therapy. *Cancer, 37*, 123-134.

Yaster, M., & Deshpande, J. (1988). Management of pediatric pain with opioid analgesics. *Journal of Pediatrics, 113*, 421-429.

Young, J. L., & Miller, R. W. (1975). Incidence of malignant tumors in U.S. children. *Journal of Pediatrics, 86*, 254-258.

Zeltzer, L., & LeBaron, S. (1982). Hypnosis and nonhypnotic techniques for reduction of pain and anxiety during painful procedures in children and adolescents with cancer. *Journal of Pediatrics, 101*, 1032-1035.

Ziegler, J. L., Bluming, A. Z., Morrow, R. H., Fass, L., & Carbone, P. (1970). Central nervous system involvement in Burkitt's lymphoma. *Blood, 36*, 718-728.

14
Migraine in Childhood: Developmental Aspects of Biobehavioral Treatment

MARIE ANNE B. VIEYRA, NANCY L. HOAG, AND BRUCE J. MASEK

Description of Pediatric Migraine Syndromes

Pediatric psychologists are treating increasing numbers of children and adolescents with headache disorders. In recent years, biobehavioral approaches to the treatment of headache in children have proliferated. Research has shown that these approaches are highly effective in managing headache as well as other pain disorders. Currently, a growing number of neurologists are viewing them as treatment of choice (Rapoff, Walsh, & Engel, 1988).

Biobehavioral approaches to pediatric migraine, including self-regulation training, contingency management of pain behavior, and cognitive behavior therapy strategies, have received a great deal of attention since 1980 (Varni, Jay, Masek, & Thompson, 1986). Despite the emphasis on children as patients, the literature has not addressed developmental concerns in the biobehavioral treatment of migraine. The focus of this chapter is on the developmental issues relevant to clinical treatment and research in pediatric migraine. A review of pertinent medical information is provided as background. Developmental considerations are discussed, and various biobehavioral treatment procedures are reviewed as they apply to children and adolescents. Future research directions from a developmental perspective are proposed. Finally, clinical considerations relevant to different age groups are illustrated in case examples.

Epidemiology

It is estimated that 5% of children between the ages of 7 and 15 suffer from some sort of migraine disorder (Bille, 1962; Sillanpaa, 1976). The incidence of migraine is slightly higher in boys before age 10, but by adolescence, girls outnumber boys three to two (Bille, 1962). This shift is alternately understood either as a decrease in migraine in males with the onset of adolescence or as an increase in female migraine in the same developmental period (E. Oppenheimer, personal communication, January 1989). Although the average onset of childhood migraine is reported to be 7 years (Guidetti, Ottaviano, Pagliarini, Paolella, & Seri, 1983), others have reported onset as early as ages 1 to 4 years (Vahlquist & Hackzell, 1949). Vahlquist and Hackzell described 31 cases in which migraine first appeared at this young age and noted that the symptom picture is similar to that of older children. They also noted that the diagnosis of migraine is more difficult to make in this age group because of the difficulty young children have in clearly communicating symptomatology.

The short-term prognosis for childhood migraine is excellent. Prensky and Sommer (1979), Forsythe, Gillies, and Sills (1984), and Noronha (1985) all reported that approximately half the children they studied improved significantly within 6 months of a visit to a neurologist, independent of type of treatment. Long-term prognosis for the children whose headaches do not resolve quickly has been examined through longitudinal investigation and is not as optimistic. Bille (1981) conducted a 23-year follow-up of 73 children who were subjects in his original work. He reported that 60% of the more severe headache sufferers were still reporting migraines as adults, although they reported the attacks to be less severe and less frequent. Sillanpaa (1983) reported that 78% of his school-age sample were still experiencing migraine at 7-year follow-up. Hockaday (1978) found that 73% of her original sample of 102 children and adolescents reported continued migraines in adulthood.

Morbidity has been little studied in relation to childhood migraine. Infrequent mild migraines may not produce adverse consequences, and can usually be managed with rest and nonprescription analgesics. Chronic severe migraine in children, however, has been associated with a greater number of somatic complaints, depression, behavior problems, high rates of school absenteeism, and increased family conflict (Masek & Hoag, 1990). These personality and behavioral characteristics have also been noted in children with recurrent abdominal pain, chronic musculoskeletal pain, and other pain conditions. It has yet to be understood which children are vulnerable to such negative outcomes and if more adaptive functioning can be achieved with these children (Andrasik, Blake, & McCarran, 1986; Masek & Hoag, 1990).

Clinical Characteristics

Migraine headaches are recurrent paroxysmal attacks of throbbing head pain. Classic migraines are preceded by an aura that is usually visual, but may also involve other senses, in the form of paresthesia or an olfactory aura (Barlow, 1984). The pain is unilateral and pounding in a sharply defined location. Common migraine, the most frequent type of migraine suffered by children, is typically frontal and bilateral, with no prodromal aura. Complicated migraine, including basilar artery, confusional, "Alice in Wonderland" syndrome, and hemiplegic migraine are more rare in childhood. Family history of migraine is a factor in approximately 90% of pediatric cases (Barlow, 1984). Compared with adult migraines, which may last up to several days, the duration of migraine pain in children is typically shorter (Barlow, 1984), usually lasting several hours.

Pathophysiology of Migraine

The pathogenesis of migraine is not well understood and has been the subject of a variety of unconfirmed explanations. In fact, there is disagreement as to whether migraine is a unitary disorder or a set of related disorders. Migraine is considered by some to be an inherited disorder characterized by vasomotor instability of cranial arteries leading to excessive vasoreactivity (Barlow, 1984). McGrath and Unruh (1987) point out, however, that virtually no research on the pathogenesis of migraine has used pediatric subjects, and thus speculations are based on research with adults. Adult migraine patients have usually been subject to years of taking powerful medications and years of repeated migraine, potentially causing changes in vascular immunology and biochemical reactivity.

Both extracranial and intracranial arteries are involved in a process of dilation and pulsation in migraine, but vasoconstriction and vasodilation alone do not fully explain the throbbing quality of the pain (Edmeads, 1979). More current theories posit the release of a vasoactive neurohumoral substance that triggers the painful vascular phenomenon; recently substance P has been implicated in this process (Moskowitz, 1984). Other theories have suggested immunological mechanisms (Lord, Duckworth, & Charlesworth, 1972) and platelet dysfunction (Hannington, 1986), but have received little confirmatory evidence. Psychological factors have also been cited in the etiology of migraine. These factors include operant conditioning (McGrath & Unruh, 1987), stress, depression, personality variables, and family factors (Masek & Hoag, 1990). Although the role that these factors play in aggravating the severity, duration, or frequency of migraine in children is unquestioned, there is little evidence to support the etiological role of these factors in the development of migraine disorders.

Medical Therapies

Pharmacological treatments for migraine in children are most frequently palliative or prophylactic. Occasionally, abortive therapy in the form of ergotamine preparations is indicated. Nonprescription analgesics, such as acetaminophen or ibuprofen, are used with children, since they can be taken safely. In less severe forms of migraine, these medications combined with rest can usually provide adequate symptom relief.

Prophylactic medications, taken to prevent the occurrence of migraine, are considered for children who have not responded to palliative treatment and whose headaches are debilitating. The cardiovascular drug, propranolol, and the tricyclic antidepressant, amitriptyline, are the two most widely prescribed prophylactic medications for pediatric migraine. Antiepileptics, such as Dilantin, have gradually fallen into disfavor. Calcium channel blockers are being investigated as an alternative to propranolol (Spierings, 1988). There have been notably few well-controlled clinical trials of these medications with children. The most widely cited is that of Ludvigsson (1974), who studied the effectiveness of propranolol, using a double blind crossover design with 28 children, 7 to 16 years of age. He found that the medication resulted in a substantial reduction in headache (20 children with excellent improvement) compared to responses to a placebo (3 children with complete remission). However, Forsythe et al. (1984) conducted a similarly designed study with children from 9 to 15 years of age and reported no difference in headache improvement between propranolol and placebo groups.

Biobehavioral Treatment of Pediatric Migraine

In view of the scant supportive evidence for pharmacological treatment, side effects of medication, parental concerns about long-term drug treatment, and the growing acceptance of migraine as a stress-induced and physically triggered phenomenon, great interest has been stimulated in biobehavioral treatment for pediatric migraine. It is now routinely recommended by many pediatric neurologists. There is a substantial literature on this approach and its efficacy (e.g., Fentress, Masek, Mehegan, & Benson, 1986; Hoag & Masek, in review; Labbe & Williamson, 1984; Larsson & Melin, 1986). These writings have for the most part, however, grouped together children of widely divergent ages and have neglected to examine how developmental issues impact upon and influence treatment strategies. We will (a) outline some important developmental considerations, (b) review biobehavioral treatment modalities, (c) discuss clinical considerations for different age groups with case examples, and (d) discuss future areas of research from a developmental perspective.

Developmental Considerations

For the most part, behavioral treatment of headache in children has borrowed from the methods of adult treatment (Andrasik et al., 1986) and adapted them to the emotional, cognitive, and environmental considerations of childhood. The nature of these adaptations and the theoretical framework guiding treatment decisions with pediatric populations are quite general and lack a developmental focus. The following are developmental factors we consider salient to treatment.

Age of Child

Clinical evaluation and treatment of approximately 1,000 children in the Behavioral Medicine Programs of The Children's Hospital in Boston and North Shore Children's Hospital in Salem, Massachusetts, has led us to conclude that the minimum age for effective biobehavioral treatment of migraine is around 7 years. Below age 7, children do not appear to have the cognitive and emotional maturity to appreciate the subtleties of treatment and therefore rarely become motivated to participate actively in the treatment plan. For children under 7, parents are the primary participants in treatment, which focuses on operant pain behavior management (see chapters 4 and 8).

Cognitive Development

The age of 7 years as minimally desirable for effective biobehavioral migraine treatment was primarily determined through clinical trial. The literature on cognitive development in childhood supports this age as also theoretically logical (see chapter 8). According to Piagetian theory (Ginsberg & Opper, 1969), 7 years is around the end of the preoperational stage and the beginning of concrete operations. Piagetian stage theory of intellectual development has been used in conceptualizing children's understanding of illness phenomena (Bibace & Walsh, 1980; Perrin & Gerrity, 1981). A few studies have expanded this work into the study of pediatric pain by demonstrating that children's perceptions of pain are consistent with these developmental stages (Gaffney & Dunne, 1986, 1987).

Accurate assessment of pain, an essential first step in behavioral treatment, is difficult with young children. In preoperational reasoning (ages 2 to 7), children perceive the world in terms of what they are able to see, touch, or manipulate. In terms of pain, they attend to the perceptually dominant features of a painful experience. They tend to define pain as something in the tummy or the head or as something that hurts. Preoperational thought is characterized by egocentrism; the child views the world entirely from his or her own perspective. Time is present centered, "consisting of a series of succeeding 'nows'" (Whitt, 1982). Verbal skills are not yet fully developed. The combination of limited verbal capacity and the above-mentioned cognitive limitations result in great difficulty for these young children in giving an accurate verbal report of pain occurrence, quality, intensity, or duration.

The quality of reasoning in the preoperational stage makes it difficult for children to understand the rationale for behavioral treatment of migraine. Reasoning at this level is transductive; children put two events together without defining their causal relationship so that cause and effect may be interchangeable. Syncretistic thinking refers to the tendency of children at this stage to group events together into one schema without considering how they are related to each other. Finally, they tend to view the state of reality as static, and are not sensitive to concepts of fluency, process, and change. It is logical therefore that children in this stage of cognitive development do not perceive the relationship between pain and illness or think of pain as a symptom of more serious pathophysiology (Gaffney & Dunne, 1987). It follows, too, that complex causation of migraine pain and the relationship between the mind and the body would be beyond the grasp of children at this age:

Concrete operational (approximately 7 to 11) and formal operational (approximately 12 and older) modes of thinking are much more conducive to effective cognitive intervention. Children in concrete operations are able to focus on several aspects of a situation simultaneously, recognize sequences of events that result in perceptual changes, and verify their logical judgment. Gaffney and Dunne (1986) found that at the level of concrete operations, children were able to use more generalized and abstract conceptualizations of pain and were thus capable of forming analogies or mentioning psychological effects of pain ("pain makes me feel unhappy or like crying"). By the onset of formal operations, the ability for introspection with more abstract thinking enabled children to define pain in physical, psychological, and psychosocial terms. It is possible at this level to form multiple hypotheses about events and to develop tests of their validity. It therefore follows that children in concrete and formal operations are more developmentally ready to understand the rationale of stress-triggered physiological reactivity and to incorporate behavioral strategies for pain control.

While keeping these stages and the chronological age of the child in mind during assessment, the approximate intelligence level of the child should be noted as well as other individual differences in cognitive development. Assessment of individual differences in intelligence, causal reasoning, and cognitive ability should guide the clinician in choosing appropriate language and treatment modalities.

Perceptions of Causality of Pain

In the pediatric literature there have been frequent observations, mostly through individual case histories and clinical impressions, that children tend to interpret pain as punishment for past misdeeds (Langford, 1948; Varni, Katz, & Dash, 1982). There has been some research indicating that children tend to view the development of illness as a result of the violation of rules or regulations. In a carefully designed study, Gaffney and Dunne (1987) found that, in response to a sentence completion item, "A person gets pain because . . . ," transgression of many kinds was a very common response in all age groups studied (5 to 14 years). Forty-four percent of their sample responded to the inquiry with transgressions involving eating too much, other activities (e.g., running too much, watching too much television), general transgressions (e.g., is careless, doesn't look after himself), or transgressions involving punishment (e.g., they are bold, they disobeyed the doctor). It was noted that objective, physical explanations for pain increased with age, as did abstract psychological explanations. However, transgression explanations continued to occur even at later developmental stages. These authors refer to the heteronomous, rule-and-punishment oriented nature of children's reasoning about moral issues described by Kohlberg (1969) and

Piaget (1977), as theoretical explanation for these findings. As discussed by these theoreticians, children tend to have an absolute belief in the externally imposed rules of adults. If something is punished it is therefore wrong. Since cause and effect are often confused by children, the occurrence of a "bad thing" (pain) presupposes the existence of a prior misbehavior. Therefore, "I got a headache because I was bad" or "I hit my brother so I got a headache" are, for a child, plausible arguments. Young children have complete belief in their own perception of events and do not check for errors in their logic. It is therefore very important to elicit beliefs about the causation of pain from all children and particularly younger ones, because these beliefs may be quite different from an adult view, and may impede treatment. The adult literature supports the view that attributions and cognitive factors affect behavioral treatment outcomes (Holzman, Turk, & Kerns, 1986).

According to Whitt (1982), a child's understanding of illness may also vary according to the perceptual cues provided by the affected organ system. For example, it would be easier for a young child to understand adequately a broken arm than an internal organ disease such as a dysfunctional pancreas in diabetes or abnormal electroencephalogram (EEG) activity in seizure disorder. Migraine, being a complex interaction of neurohumoral, skeletal muscular, and cerebral vascular reactivity would therefore, from this perspective, be quite difficult for a child to understand. In addition, the routine tests ordered by pediatric neurologists, such as an EEG, magnetic resonance imaging (MRI), or computerized tomography (CT) scan, to make a definitive diagnosis of migraine and to rule out other disorders, frequently confuse and can frighten children, leaving them with the impression that there is something awful going on in their brains.

The only known study examining children's beliefs about headaches was conducted by Ross and Ross (1984), who investigated pain beliefs among a large sample of healthy and ill children. One group of subjects were 44 children suffering from chronic headache requiring medical attention. The mean age of this group of 21 boys and 23 girls was 9.5 with a standard deviation of 1.4 years. Of these 44 children, 41 attributed their headaches to tension and reported that their pediatricians had recommended a more relaxed daily routine. Although this study appears to indicate rather realistic views of pain causality, only three of these children were diagnosed as having migraine, and six others had migraine-like symptomatology; the rest of the sample had tension headaches. With so little relevant data and much theoretical work explaining the prevalence of erroneous causal beliefs, it appears important to explore fully children's beliefs about their pain, in order to detect the existence of such faulty assumptions.

Experience of Pain

Another factor that must be assessed in the behavioral treatment of pediatric migraine is the amount of experience and contact these children have had with pain and pain models. These contacts may develop over time with increased exposure to older relatives and to a widening circle of friends and acquaintances. Some work has been done on the family's role in teaching children to respond to painful experiences; however, most discussions of these influences are anecdotal and retrospective (McGrath & Unruh, 1987). Craig (1983) discussed the requisite developmental skills for pain modeling to occur. These include the ability to attend to the observation of painful events and to remember what has been observed and what the child has him or herself experienced in similar painful situations. Sufficient motor skills to repeat the behavior observed in family members with pain is also required. It was noted that experiences of pain are often salient, easily drawing attention and thus facilitating learning by a child about what causes pain, how others react, and the consequences of those reactions. It is hypothesized, based upon social learning theory concepts of imitation and rehearsal (Bandura, 1977), that if a child observes important people such as parents showing frequent verbal or behavioral expressions of pain, reacting strongly to low levels of painful stimuli, or restricting activities due to pain, the child will be more likely to react with poor coping skills to pain and to exhibit exaggerated pain responses. This is increasingly likely if the child observes positive consequences for pain behaviors in adults, such as increased spouse support and closeness, special privileges, or escape from undesirable activities or responsibilities.

Few studies have examined this issue in a thorough or prospective manner with children. Apley (1975) noted that abdominal pain was six times more likely to occur in siblings and parents of abdominal pain patients than in controls. Edwards, Zeichner, Kuczmierczyk, and Boczkowski (1985) reported that college students who disclosed that they had a number of relatives with chronic pain were more likely to report pain complaints. Christensen and Mortensen (1975) provided support for the vicarious learning hypothesis in their observation that children were very likely to have the same pain symptoms as their parents at the present time but less likely to have the same symptoms as their parents had when they were children. The strong contribution of a genetic component to migraine confounds these observations in the study of headache modeling. However, given that many young patients have a parent with migraine, it is clinically useful to understand how the parent copes with his or her own pain, and what the child has observed of these coping efforts.

Coping Strategies

Because a significant portion of behavioral treatment of migraine involves the teaching of coping strategies for pain control, it is important to consider the nature and development of spontaneous coping strategies used by children when they are confronted with stressful or painful situations. Spontaneous coping strategies used by 487 children in stressful and painful situations were studied by Brown, O'Keeffe, Sanders, and Baker (1986). Children in this sample ranged in age from 8 to 18 years and were 52% female and 43% male, with 5% not reporting gender. Dependent measures included the State-Trait Anxiety Inventory (Spielberger, 1970) and a questionnaire about stressful situations, including getting an injection at the dentist. The coping strategies reported by children in this hypothetical situation were (a) positive self-talk (e.g., I can take this), (b) attention/diversion by thinking of something else or listening to music, (c) relaxation, and (d) thought stopping. Self-talk was used at all ages, but its frequency increased with age, whereas thought stopping was rarely used at any age. It was found that the number of strategies used by children to cope with dental pain and the number of children who were considered "copers" (used coping strategies in two out of three situations) increased with age. Catastrophizing strategies included: (a) dwelling on the negative aspects of the dental situation, (b) thoughts of escape or avoidance, (c) concerns about an unlikely consequence (e.g., excessive bleeding), and (d) concerns about the dentist or negative feelings about the dentist. None of the four types of catastrophizing strategies increased or decreased with age; however, the number of children who were considered "catastrophizers" decreased with age. Despite this decrease in catastrophizing and increase in coping, 79% of children aged 8 to 9 years and 54% of children aged 16 to 18 years were judged to be catastrophizers. Less anxiety was reported by copers of all ages compared to the catastrophizers.

Similarly, Ross and Ross (1984) found that only 213 of the 994 children in their study of children's perception of pain (ages 5 to 12 years) used self-initiated coping strategies. The most commonly used strategies were distraction (93 children) and physical activity such as clenching fists (91 children). The remaining 29 children used strategies such as thought stopping, relaxation/imagery, and fantasy. The ages of these children, and the types of pain they had experienced were not reported, thus it cannot be determined from this investigation if spontaneous coping followed a developmental progression or if coping strategies are specific to certain types of pain.

Spirito, Stark, and Williams (1988) have developed a 10-item checklist (Kidcope) designed to assess common cognitive and behavioral coping strategies used by children and adolescents: distraction, social isolation, cognitive restructuring, self-blame, blaming others, problem solving, emotional regulation, wishful thinking, social support, and resignation. The Kidcope has been administered to healthy children (Stark, Spirito, Williams, & Guevremont, 1989), and to pediatric patients with a variety of diagnoses, such as abdominal pain, headaches, cancer, hemophilia, encopresis, sleep disorders, and seizures (Spirito et al., 1988). Nevertheless, the authors have not yet reported developmentally relevant results from a large sample of pediatric pain patients.

Environmental Changes

Several developmentally related environmental changes occur in the lives of young migraine patients that must be assessed. For example, it is important to keep track of major shifts in schedules or in time with important caretakers, which may correspond to the onset of pain complaints. These might include a shift from a half-day kindergarten schedule to full-day first grade, a previously full-time caretaker returning to work and thus spending less time with the child, or a change in schools because of promotion or relocation. It is not uncommon to discover the onset of migraine pain to be related to the discovery of a previously undiagnosed learning disability (Bille, 1962), since such learning problems frequently only manifest themselves when the task demands at school become more complex and taxing. Therefore, it is important to determine if the child has had increased difficulty at school around the time of pain onset. In addition, the complexity and pressure of social interactions with peers increase with age. Children who may have gotten along with other children relatively well when social rules were simpler and more time was spent at home, may have increasing trouble when peer acceptance becomes more central and self-esteem is more linked to social success. Peer difficulty may contribute to migraine pain as a stressor, or by maintaining pain behaviors through the reinforcement provided by escape from uncomfortable social situations.

Biobehavioral Treatment Modalities

Biobehavioral treatment strategies for pediatric migraine and other chronic pain disorders in children fall into three general categories: self-regulation training such as relaxation with or without biofeedback, contingency management of pain behavior, and cognitive behavior therapy. A review of 18 efficacy studies of behavioral approaches to the treatment of pediatric migraine revealed reductions in headache activity following treatment ranging from 60 to 100% (Masek & Hoag, 1990). For a comprehensive review and critique of the literature prior to 1984, the reader is referred to Hoelscher and Lichstein (1984).

Self-Regulation

Self-regulation training is the most widely employed intervention for both adult and pediatric headache disorders. Typically, the treatment combines some form of biofeedback training with relaxation instructions. The goal of this intervention is to teach children to monitor their physiological state and to produce a relaxation response when overly aroused. It is hypothesized that the mechanism by which this reduces headache pain is through attenuating sympathetic outflow and "short circuiting" cerebral vasomotor hyperactivity that is capable of triggering migraine activity.

Relaxation techniques include meditative breathing (Benson, 1975), progressive muscle relaxation (Jacobson, 1938), and autogenic training (Schultz & Luthe, 1969). All of these techniques have four basic elements in common: (a) a mental device similar to a mantra to aid concentration; (b) a passive attitude; (c) decreased muscle tonus and awareness of other sensations (e.g., numbness, heaviness, or warmth); and (d) a comfortable resting position in a quiet environment. Often, visual imagery is used in association with these relaxation instructions. As the patient practices relaxation and the use of imagery together, the physiological relaxation response becomes classically conditioned to soothing images. Eventually, conjuring up these images alone produces relaxation, without a long relaxation procedure.

Biofeedback training involves the presentation of information in the form of an analogue signal about a physiological function such as heart rate, skin temperature, or muscle tension (surface electromyogram, EMG). The analogue signal is usually a line graph output on a television screen or a variably pitched tone. The feedback is paired with instructions to increase or decrease physiological reactivity through mental activity. Change in the desired direction is presumed to be reinforcing and is the basis for establishing control of the physiological function.

Thermal biofeedback with autogenic phrases has been employed in the treatment of pediatric migraine. Autogenic training teaches the patient to concentrate on repeated phrases that describe a heaviness in the limbs, a sense of warmth, or of cooling and lightness. Simultaneously, the patient is provided with analogue feedback of finger temperature and is instructed to gradually increase it. EMG biofeedback combined with progressive muscle relaxation has also been used with children. This approach combines instructions to systematically reduce muscle tension in various muscle groups while being provided with analogue feedback of EMG activity, usually recorded from the forehead area. Although originally thought to be useful only for muscle contraction headaches, recent studies have indicated its utility in the treatment of migraine (Mehegan, Masek, Harrison, Russo, & Leviton, 1987). It has been argued that facial muscle hyperactivity is a prominent symptom before and during a migraine episode (Pickoff, 1984).

With children, these self-regulation techniques appear to be effective after the age of 7 years, for a variety of cognitive developmental reasons described in the preceding section. With children in the lower end of this range, we have found it important to make both the relaxation instruction and the feedback as concrete, dynamic, and accessible as possible. Thus, relaxation procedures (and the tapes that children bring home to practice after the first treatment session) are shorter than those used by adults, and more use is made of vivid, concrete imagery. For example, warming of hands is produced through the image of warming hands before a fire, or putting hands in warm water or around a cup of hot cocoa. Good results have been obtained using imagery instructions for progressive muscle relaxation. Images such as "squeezing lemons" to tighten hand and arm muscles, a fly landing on the child's nose or forehead that must be gotten off without touching, to tighten muscles in the face, and pretending to be a turtle with his head in his shell, to tighten shoulder and neck muscles, are useful for this purpose. Imagery of restful beach scenes is often used, but frequently children become bored with these images more quickly than would their adult counterparts. Therefore, more imaginative and fluid images are preferred, such as climbing on a magic cloud or floating down a gentle, magic stream that travels to far away and mystical lands. The child's active assistance in providing new images and scenes provides continued interest and motivation. With younger children, it is sometimes beneficial to provide other external incentives for practicing these skills. This can be in the form of either a sticker chart or some token system at home, or short periods of video game play with the therapist at the end of each biofeedback session.

Similarly, it is helpful for the analogue feedback to be as captivating and concrete as possible. There are a variety of software packages that provide children with the opportunity to select their own colors for feedback channels, where auditory and visual feedback is simultaneous and where different games are provided to create a more interesting process for children. An example of this is a software program (J & J Instruments, Poulsbo, WA) that has a brightly colored graphics display of a black box on a table and a bat, flying around the room, representing the analogue feedback. The goal is for the child, by controlling arousal, to place and keep the bat in the box. This is achieved at a certain threshold, set by the clinician.

Pain Behavior Management

Contingency management of pain behavior is based on Fordyce's (1976) theory that pain behaviors such as grimacing, verbal complaints, gestures, and retreat from activity are learned responses that are maintained by parental and social attention and/or by the avoidance of unpleasant situations or responsibilities. Pain behavior management treatment involves instructions to parents and other caregiving figures (a) to minimize attention to pain behaviors such as excessive complaining, pain gestures, and requests for special treatment; (b) to avoid questioning about the presence or status of a headache; and (c) if they ascertain that the child is avoiding something, to minimize this occurrence or provide an unappealing alternative (e.g., bed rest). Parents are directed to provide positive reinforcement for healthy behaviors and for the child's attempts to engage in normal activities and other coping behaviors. Parents are assisted in encouraging daily school attendance and staying in school despite the occurrence of a migraine (Masek, Russo, & Varni, 1984).

Parents are often unaware that their behavior is reinforcing pain behaviors in their children. Even when they are aware of providing attention to pain behaviors, it is often difficult for parents to change their existing behavior patterns, since they often associate these behaviors with nurturance, caring, and love for their child. It is essential, therefore, that parents be provided with a persuasive rationale for making the indicated changes based on "teaching your child to cope with pain" and with alternative suggestions and opportunities to provide their children with understanding and nurturance.

Pain behavior management is important for patients of all ages. However, the relative importance of this treatment modality decreases as the child increases in age. For children under seven who present with migraine symptoms, this parental work is usually used exclusively. It remains primary, along with other modalities, in the treatment of school-aged children. In adolescence, the role of reinforcement of pain behaviors must be assessed; care must also be given, however, to maintaining the relationship between the adolescent and therapist, in order to maximize motivation and compliance. Permission is generally elicited from the adolescent to speak with his or her parents, and often these directions are provided in the presence of the adolescent. If these issues can be addressed as a conversation among family members with mutually agreed-upon changes, the chances for follow-through on recommendations and treatment success are heightened.

Research in support of this approach is provided by Ramsden, Friedman, and Williamson (1983) and Lake (1981) who reported single case studies on using contingency management procedures successfully to reduce pain reports in a 6-year-old girl and school absenteeism in an 11-year-old boy, respectively. Yen and McIntire (1971) successfully reduced headache reports in a 14-year-old girl by applying a response cost contingency. In these studies, the researchers were not concerned with the actual reduction in headache activity, but were exclusively interested in altering the child's level of dysfunction. Other studies have used contingency management in conjunction with other treatments, but have not isolated this modality's effectiveness.

Cognitive Behavioral Treatment

Cognitive behavior therapy focuses on the modification of negative, arousal-inducing cognitions associated with headache activity that can trigger or exacerbate headache symptoms. Patients are helped by the therapist to identify these negative cognitions and to substitute problem solving and reassuring self-statements. For example, on first noting the prodrome of a headache, a child may experience anticipatory anxiety and think "Oh, I can tell a headache is coming on; it's going to be terrible; I'll probably throw up and have to lie in my room all day." This statement can be replaced with a more positive statement such as, "I can do my relaxation and sleep some and this headache will be over soon." Attitudes and beliefs about pain and the control that the child has over his or her pain are explored and modified. With the help of self-monitored headache diaries, children are also taught to identify stressful situations that often trigger headaches, such as exams or difficult social situations, and to use imagery, problem solving, and other stress-reducing techniques to abort a headache episode. Such techniques may involve assertiveness training, social skills training, or time management as appropriate, based on the discovered environmental triggers.

In the treatment of children, language for these types of cognitive interventions must be kept simple and direct. For younger children, verbal strategies may be less useful, and drawings or the use of pictorial analogies (What color/animal is your headache?) are useful in order to communicate about pain cognitions in a more compelling manner. For both children and adolescents, it may be helpful to frame negative self-statements as an "audiotape that automatically goes on in your head at certain stressful times." The therapeutic task then becomes to rerecord the message or to change the cassette. Because of the nature of children's reasoning discussed above, it is particularly important to elicit younger children's beliefs about the causes of their headaches and about their understanding of the neurologist's tests and diagnosis. For adolescents with more advanced reasoning skills, this information is also important since they are more likely to have gotten the same inadvertent and inaccurate message that is frequently seen in adult populations: "The doctor thinks that I'm making it up and it's all in my head." For adolescents in particular, cognitive-behavioral interventions may appeal to the newly developing sense of independence and mastery typical of this developmental period.

Research

A number of recent controlled investigations provide data on the efficacy of biofeedback and relaxation training, and other treatment modalities for the treatment of pediatric migraine (Fentress et al., 1986; Hoag & Masek, in review; Labbe & Williamson, 1984; Larsson & Melin, 1986; McGrath et al., 1988; Mehegan et al., 1987; Richter et al., 1986). None of these investigations reported the effects of age on outcome, so that no conclusions about developmental appropriateness of treatment can be made on the basis of these data. Labbe and Williamson (1984) used a waiting list control group design to study the effect of autogenic training with thermal feedback on 28 children ranging in age from 7 to 16 years. Using a criterion of 50% headache reduction as clinical improvement, they found that 93% of the treatment group had improved at the end of treatment and at 1 month follow-up, compared with only 7% of the control group at the end of treatment and 14% at follow-up. Similarly, Fentress et al. (1986) reported that, in 18 children with migraine between the ages of 8 and 12 years, those provided with relaxation training alone or in combination with EMG biofeedback were significantly improved at the end of treatment, whereas the waiting list control subjects were unchanged. Treatment effectiveness was maintained at 1 year follow-up. Mehegan et al. (1987) employed a multiple baseline across subjects design to evaluate the effectiveness of a treatment package consisting of EMG biofeedback, relaxation training, and operant pain behavior management. Subjects were 18 children between the ages of 7 and 12 years, who were diagnosed with migraine. At the conclusion of treatment, 14 of 18 patients experienced a greater than 90% reduction in headache activity; two other subjects reduced their headaches by more than 50%. Headache improvement was maintained at 6- and 12-month follow-up.

Studies that have employed placebo control groups have yielded contradictory findings. Larsson and Melin (1986) and Richter et al. (1986) employed attention placebo control groups and found that nonspecific or placebo factors did not result in significant headache improvement, whereas the active treatments of cognitive restructuring and progressive muscle relaxation resulted in significant improvement in children aged 9 to 18 years. In contrast, Hoag and Masek (in review) found that a credible placebo control treatment was nearly as effective as relaxation training alone or in combination with EMG biofeedback in a group of 24 children aged 6 to 12 years with migraine. By the end of treatment, 71% of the placebo group had clinically improved compared to 85% of the relaxation group and 88% of the relaxation plus EMG biofeedback group. However, the placebo group had not maintained treatment gains at 12-month follow-up whereas the other two groups did. Finally, McGrath et al. (1988) reported similar findings in their study of 62 children aged 9 to 17 years with migraine. They were treated with either relaxation training, psychological placebo (individual therapy sessions in which children were taught to recognize and label their emotions, to relate them to their life situation, and to discuss their feelings daily with a friend or parent), or "own best efforts" treatment, consisting of a single session to discuss triggers for headache attacks and suggestions for strategies to reduce the impact of these possible triggers. Results indicated that all three treatment groups showed significant reductions in headaches following treatment. Furthermore, all three groups maintained this reduction at 3- and 12-month follow-up. Relaxation was not found to be superior to the two other groups. The authors suggest that a "credible treatment method which includes suggestions of techniques for self-control of headaches" (p. 629) may be the salient factor in effective psychological treatment of pediatric migraine.

Research Issues

Given the number of studies and overall favorable results for "package" biobehavioral treatments for pediatric migraine, it appears to be of limited utility to continue to test for the global effectiveness of this treatment modality for a wide range of age groups. However, the recent findings implicating nonspecific variables in treatment efficacy point to the need for carefully designed component analyses of biobehavioral treatment. Although it is widely accepted that behavioral treatment approaches are effective in reducing and controlling migraine episodes in children, future research should address the issue of isolating the various components of treatment to determine the relative contribution or combined contributions of self-regulation, pain behavior management, cognitive behavioral treatment, and nonspecific variables. Also, the issue of developmental level has not yet been addressed in relation to these treatment variables. As the above review suggests, clinical observations based on developmental theory lead clinicians to emphasize different treatment components depending upon age. However, there is a need for empirical support for these treatment choices. Do children of certain ages or cognitive developmental levels respond differentially to treatment, or to different components of treatment? Work in this area would allow clinicians to make more informed treatment choices, maximizing treatment efficacy.

Another area of research involves the question of whether biobehavioral treatment is effective with severe forms of migraine in children. Most efficacy studies have not controlled for severity of migraine as defined by intensity and duration of head pain and number and type of associated symptoms. It may be the case that behavioral treatment is more effective with certain subtypes of migraine and is indicated in combination with medication for other subtypes. With this information the pediatric neurologist could more effectively triage and sequence the treatment effort.

Finally, there is need for continued research into the psychosocial impact of chronic headache in childhood. There are no epidemiological or prospective studies of this population, and therefore it remains unclear if children with migraine are at increased risk for developmental delays or long-term psychosocial consequences. Although most research uses a criterion such as pain report or missed school days as an indicator of present psychosocial disruption, there are many children who miss much school but whose grades do not suffer, and other children go to school but are not able to concentrate and therefore do not achieve as well as prior to headache onset. Similarly, some children report much pain but remain active, whereas others withdraw from social activities at the onset of mild pain. Therefore more sophisticated measures of pain impact are needed. For example, one might measure disruption of a variety of activities, school absences, and achievement test scores rather than relying on a single criterion measure.

Case Illustrations

Case Study 1: Younger Child

J., a 5-year, 8-month-old female, was referred by her pediatric neurologist for behavioral treatment of migraine headache. J.'s medical record revealed that she was also diagnosed with Dandy-Walker syndrome, a hydrocephalus of infancy, and was being treated with a well-functioning shunt. According to her mother, J.'s headaches became more frequent and more severe when the shunt was replaced 2 years ago. Other pertinent historical information includes the fact that J.'s parents separated when she was an infant and she had had no contact with her father since that time. J.'s mother was not employed and spent little time outside of the home. Her stated reason was that J.'s recurrent headaches required her attention and care.

At the time of the referral, J. was reporting an average of two headaches per day. Her mother estimated the typical duration to be 3 hours. The headaches were described as episodes of severe, throbbing pain. Accompanying nausea was also reported. Information obtained from a headache diary revealed that J.'s headaches tended to coincide with meals, chores, and her mother's social activities. J.'s mother generally managed her daughter's headaches by giving her analgesic medication, decreasing demands placed on J., and encouraging J. to rest.

The obtained baseline headache data suggested that J.'s headache activity was functionally reinforced by increased attention from her mother and avoidance of undesirable activities. This finding, combined with an assessment that J. was not developmentally ready for relaxation and biofeedback instruction (she did not respond to relaxation imagery and did not comprehend the association between relaxation and pain control), indicated that a behavioral treatment focusing on the use of operant strategies would be most beneficial. Accordingly, J.'s mother was instructed to encourage J. to maintain a normal routine as much as possible and to reward J. with stickers and other positive reinforcers when she completed meals and her chores. J.'s mother was also encouraged to not disrupt her social activities in response to J.'s headache complaints. By the fourth treatment session, J.'s mother reported that J. was experiencing only one headache per week and was no longer avoiding meals or her chores. She reported, however, that this decrease in headache activity was accompanied by an increase in J.'s general oppositional behavior. Four additional treatment sessions were spent implementing a more general behavioral program that involved the use of a time-out procedure as well as rewards for positive behavior in several other areas. At termination, J.'s mother reported that her daughter was no longer complaining of any head pain and was earning stickers and other privileges 75% of the time.

Case Study 2: School Age

D., a 10-year-old male, was referred by his oral surgeon and neurologist for behavioral evaluation of facial pain and headache. He initially presented to the oral surgeon with bilateral ear pain without any specific ear pathology. The pain was described as sharp and continuous, worse in the morning upon awakening, and sometimes accompanied by stiffness in the jaw. He had tenderness over the temporomandibular joint (TMJ) and prominent masseter muscles with mild tenderness over both masseter and lateral pterygoid muscles. There was no noise from the TMJ and he had a normal jaw opening pattern. Standard radiographs were negative. He was fitted with a night guard to reduce masticatory muscle hyperactivity, which was felt to be caused by clenching his teeth during sleep. The night guard resulted in complete remission of symptoms within 2 months.

Approximately 8 months later he developed a bilateral frontal headache occurring three to four times a week. He described the pain as throbbing, exacerbated by movement, and occasionally accompanied by dizziness and nausea. Neurological evaluation, including CT scan and cerebrospinal fluid (CSF) analysis, was negative. Propranolol, hydantoin, and Fiorinal had no effect on the headache. He continued to wear the night guard, but again began to experience facial pain approximately 2 months after the headache began. His mother and maternal aunt had suffered from migraine since childhood.

D.'s headache and facial pain were believed to be triggered by skeletal muscle hyperactivity; the result of clenching his teeth, but now during the day as well. Clenching was a response he learned in association with self-imposed and parental pressure to excel in school, religion class, and playing trumpet. Treatment consisted of (a) self-monitoring of headache and other pain symptoms, looking for patterns and precipitants; (b) EMG biofeedback training to reduce facial muscle hyperactivity; and (c) instruction in several relaxation techniques that was tape-recorded for use at home. After seven treatment sessions, D.'s headaches subsided to the level of mild pain once every 3 or 4 weeks. Facial pain continued to occur at a mild level for brief intervals every few days, most often in school. Correspondingly, he learned to use relaxation techniques to reduce muscular tension and as distraction from pain. Facial muscle activity returned to normal levels following EMG biofeedback training with the exception of masseteric activity, which remained mildly elevated. Follow-up 6 months after treatment ended showed D. to be maintaining the improvement, and he was no longer wearing the night guard.

Case Study 3: Adolescent

K. is a 15-year-old female, referred by her neurologist for treatment of migraine. Neurological evaluation, including an EEG and CT scan, was normal. K. and her mother reported that she had had severe infrequent headaches since early childhood, but that at around the age of 12 they increased in frequency and intensity. Pain was described as unilateral, located behind the eye, down the side of the neck, and in the temple area, and was described as jabbing in quality. K. stated that she had six or seven such headaches a month. Headaches usually lasted 4 to 6 hours, frequently occurred in the middle of the night and on weekends, but also occurred in school, and occurred less frequently in the summer months. The headaches were preceded by a prodromal phase of blurry vision and hand numbness. Nausea and vomiting frequently accompanied a headache. She reported light, sound, and odor sensitivity. She also stated that it frequently became difficult to "understand what other people or what I am saying." When a headache occurred, K. reported that she laid in bed and attempted to sleep. If a headache occurred in school, her mother picked her up at "the first sign of one coming on." At the time of referral, K. was taking 125 mg of pro-pranolol daily in divided doses. Family history was positive for migraine on both maternal and paternal sides.

K. is the second youngest of 10 children in an Irish Catholic family. She reported a good deal of conflict with her family, and in particular her sister M., with whom she shared a room. She reported that she was not close to either of her parents, whom she described as quite strict, particularly about dating. Per mother's report, K. had a quick and violent temper, which alienated the rest of the family. She reportedly was discourteous to her parents, and "picks with a sharp knife" at her siblings. Mother stated that the rest of the family "tries to be nice to her" because they "know that when she gets like that she's going to have a migraine." However, mother stated that she was very frustrated with K.'s behavior, since "it disrupts the entire family."

On clinical interview, K. appeared to be fairly depressed, exhibiting some sad affect, depressed mood, and restricted social activities, and appeared to harbor a good deal of anger. She was quite distrustful of the therapist and skeptical about the role of stress in her pain, and was thus very guarded about her feelings. It was hypothesized that academic and social difficulties at school, as well as an apparently difficult relationship with her parents and siblings, were contributing to her pain presentation. It appeared that K.'s anger manifested itself in outbursts at home, which triggered migraine activity. She appeared to be "an outsider" within her family, and headaches appeared be providing her with otherwise absent support and empathy.

Treatment was initially devoted to teaching K. a variety of self-regulation strategies to help her assume greater control over her headache symptoms. K. was instructed to monitor her headache periods, patterns, and precipitants. A progressive muscle relaxation tape was made with guided imagery sequences involving relaxing mental images. Biofeedback was introduced, and, over the course of six sessions, K. demonstrated increasing ability to lower her EMG and heart rate and to increase her skin temperature. Concurrently, she reported increasingly fewer headache periods. Work was done to assist in the generalization of these skills and in their application in stressful situations in school and at home.

Despite these improvements, K. remained skeptical about the value of these techniques, challenged and repeatedly questioned the connection between stress and physiological response, and practiced these skills only sporadically. It was decided that headache-maintaining factors, including family discord, depression, and anger, needed to be more directly addressed. K.'s feelings of rejection by her family and her mother in particular were explored. She spoke frequently about feeling like an outsider and a "black sheep" in the family, because she was the only one (of 10 children) who "fought back" or rebelled in any way. K. explored the relative contributions of her family's actions and her own behaviors in escalating cycles of antagonism at home. She described many instances of disagreements about rules with her parents and frustration with their rigid approach to her desires, and problem solved about alternative solutions to these conflicts. Many of the qualities found objectionable by her family were reframed as positive but as a "bad fit" with the situation. For example, what her family viewed as a "mean streak" could also be viewed as "feistiness" or "spirit" with friends if used in certain situations. Also discussed were issues of how she appeared to her peers, and of integrating the "quiet" K. of school with the "mean streak, Irish temper" K. of home.

K. was quite distrustful of meetings between her mother and the therapist, so only limited contact was made with mother, and the issues to be discussed were first reviewed with K. Some work was done with mother on normalizing K.'s rebellion in the context of adolescent development and on drawing mother's attention to K.'s depression and need for support and understanding. Ignoring of pain behavior was encouraged, with an increase in positive attention to healthy behaviors.

At termination, after 10 sessions, K. was experiencing approximately one headache per month. She stated that her attitude toward her headaches had changed; she no longer "spazzed out" when she got a migraine and realized that events that she hadn't "taken seriously" before were related to migraine attacks. At 8-week telephone follow-up, K. continued to experience fewer than one headache per month and had discontinued her medication. Mother reported that she and her husband were allowing K. more freedom to go places with her friends and more privacy at home.

References

Andrasik, F., Blake, D. D., & McCarran, M. S. (1986). A biobehavioral analysis of pediatric headache. In N. Krasnegor, J. Aresteh, & M. Cataldo (Eds.), *Child health behavior: A behavioral pediatrics perspective* (pp. 394–432). New York: Wiley.

Apley, J. (1975). *The child with abdominal pain*. Oxford: Blackwell.

Bandura, A. (1977). *Social learning theory*. Englewood Cliffs, NJ: Prentice-Hall.

Barlow, C. F. (1984). *Headaches and migraine in childhood*. London: Spastics International Medical Publications.

Benson, H. (1975). *The relaxation response*. New York: Morrow.

Bibace, R., & Walsh, M. E. (1980). Development of children's concepts of illness. *Pediatrics, 66*, 912–917.

Bille, B. O. (1962). Migraine in school children. *Acta Paediatrica Scandinavica, 51*(Suppl. 136), 1–151.

Bille, B. O. (1981). Migraine in childhood and its prognosis. *Cephalalgia, 1*, 71–75.

Brown, J. M., O'Keeffe, J., Sanders, S. H., & Baker, B. (1986). Developmental changes in children's cognition to stressful and painful situations. *Journal of Pediatric Psychology, 11*, 343–357.

Christensen, M. F., & Mortensen, O. (1975). Long term prognosis in children with recurrent abdominal pain. *Archives of Diseases of Childhood, 50*, 110–114.

Craig, K. (1983). Modeling and social learning factors in chronic pain. In J. J. Bonica, U. Lindblom, & A. Iggo (Eds.), *Advances in pain research and therapy* (Vol. 5, pp. 813–827). New York: Raven Press.

Edmeads, J. (1979). Vascular headache and the cranial circulation—Another look. *Headache, 19*, 127–131.

Edwards, P. W., Zeichner, A., Kuczmierczyk, A. R., & Boczkowski, J. (1985). Familial pain models: The relationship between family history of pain and current pain experience. *Pain, 21*, 379–384.

Fentress, D. W., Masek, B. J., Mehegan, J. E., & Benson, H. (1986). Biofeedback and relaxation-response training in the treatment of pediatric migraine. *Developmental Medicine and Child Neurology, 28*, 139–146.

Fordyce, W. E. (1976). *Behavioral methods for chronic pain and illness.* St. Louis: C. V. Mosby.

Forsythe, W. I., Gillies, D., & Sills, M. A. (1984). Propranolol in the treatment of childhood migraine. *Developmental Medicine and Child Neurology, 26*, 737–741.

Gaffney, A., & Dunne, E. A. (1986). Developmental aspects of children's definitions of pain. *Pain, 26*, 105–117.

Gaffney, A., & Dunne, E. A. (1987). Children's understanding of the causality of pain. *Pain, 29*, 91–104.

Ginsberg, H., & Opper, S. (1969). *Piaget's theory of intellectual development: An introduction.* Englewood Cliffs, NJ: Prentice-Hall.

Guidetti, V., Ottaviano, S., Pagliarini, M., Paolella A., & Seri, S. (1983). Psychological peculiarities in children with recurrent primary headache. *Cephalalgia, 3*(Suppl. 1), 215–217.

Hannington, E. (1986). Viewpoint: The platelet and migraine. *Headache, 26*, 411–415.

Hoag, N. L., & Masek, B. J. (in review). A test of specific and nonspecific effects in biobehavioral treatment of pediatric migraine. Manuscript submitted for publication.

Hockaday, J. M. (1978). Late outcome of childhood onset migraine and factors affecting treatment outcome, with particular reference to early and late EEG findings. In R. Green (Ed.), *Current concepts in migraine research* (pp. 41–48). New York: Raven Press.

Hoelscher, T. J., & Lichstein, K. L. (1984). Behavioral assessment and treatment of child migraine: Implications for clinical research and practice. *Headache, 24*, 94–103.

Holzman, A. D., Turk, D. C., & Kerns, R. D. (1986). The cognitive-behavioral approach to the management of chronic pain. In A. Holzman & D. Turk (Eds.), *Pain management: A handbook of psychological treatment approaches* (pp. 31–50). New York: Pergamon.

Jacobson, E. (1938). *Progressive relaxation.* Chicago: University of Chicago Press.

Kohlberg, L. (1969). Stage and sequence: The cognitive developmental approach to socialization. In D. Goslin (Ed.), *Handbook of socialization: Theory and research* (pp. 347–480). Chicago: Rand McNally.

Labbe, E. L., & Williamson, D. A. (1984). Treatment of childhood migraine using autogenic feedback training. *Journal of Consulting and Clinical Psychology, 52,* 968–976.

Lake, A. E. (1981). Behavioral assessment considerations in the management of headache. *Headache, 21,* 170–178.

Langford, W. S. (1948). Physical illness and convalescence: Their meaning to the child. *Journal of Pediatrics, 33,* 242–250.

Larsson, B., & Melin, L. (1986). Chronic headaches in adolescents: Treatment in a school setting with relaxation training as compared with information, contact, and self-registration. *Pain, 25,* 325–336.

Lord, G. D., Duckworth, J. W., & Charlesworth, J. A. (1972). Complement activation in migraine. *Lancet, i,* 781–782.

Ludvigsson, J. (1974). Propranolol used in prophylaxis of migraine in children. *Acta Neurologica Scandinavica, 50,* 109–115.

Masek, B. J., & Hoag, N. L. (1990). Headache. In A. M. Gross & R. S. Drabman (Eds.), *Handbook of clinical behavioral pediatrics* (pp. 99–109). New York: Plenum.

Masek, B. J., Russo, D. C., & Varni, J. W. (1984). Behavioral approaches to the management of chronic pain in children. *Pediatric Clinics of North America, 31,* 1113–1131.

McGrath, P. J., Humphreys, P., Goodman, J. T., Keene, D., Firestone, P., Jacob, P., & Cunningham, S. J. (1988). Relaxation prophylaxis for childhood migraine: A randomized placebo-controlled trial. *Developmental Medicine and Child Neurology, 30,* 626–631.

McGrath, P. J., & Unruh, A. M. (1987). *Pain in children and adolescents.* Amsterdam: Elsevier.

Mehegan, J. E., Masek, B. J., Harrison, R., Russo, D., & Leviton, A. (1987). A multicomponent behavioral treatment for pediatric migraine. *Clinical Journal of Pain, 2,* 191–196.

Moskowitz, M. A. (1984). The neurobiology of vascular head pain. *Annals of Neurology, 16,* 157.

Noronha, M. J. (1985). Double blind randomized cross-over trial of timolol in migraine prophylaxis in children. *Cephalalgia, 5*(Suppl. 3), 174–175.

Perrin, E. C., & Gerrity, S. (1981). There's a demon in your belly: Children's understanding of illness. *Pediatrics, 67,* 841–849.

Piaget, J. (1977). *The moral judgement of the child.* Middlesex: Penguin Education.

Pickoff, H. (1984). Is the muscular model of headache still viable? A review of conflicting data. *Headache, 24,* 186–198.

Prensky, A. L., & Sommer, D. (1979). Diagnosis and treatment of migraine in children. *Neurology, 29,* 506–510.

Ramsden, R., Friedman, B., & Williamson, D. (1983). Treatment of childhood headache reports with contingency management procedures. *Journal of Clinical Child Psychiatry, 12,* 202–206.

Rapoff, M., Walsh, D., & Engel, J. M. (1988). Assessment and management of chronic pediatric headaches. *Comprehensive Pediatric Nursing, 11,* 159–178.

Richter, I. L., McGrath, P. J., Humphreys, P. J., Goodman, J. T., Firestone, P., & Keene, D. (1986). Cognitive and relaxation treatment of pediatric migraine. *Pain, 25,* 195–203.

Ross, D. M., & Ross, S. A. (1984). Childhood pain: The school-aged child's viewpoint. *Pain, 20*, 179–191.

Schultz, J. H., & Luthe, W. (1969). *Autogenic training* (Vol. 1). New York: Grune & Stratton.

Sillanpaa, M. (1976). Prevalence of migraine and other headache in Finnish children starting school. *Headache, 16*, 288–290.

Sillanpaa, M. (1983). Changes in the prevalence of migraine and other headaches during the first seven school years. *Headache, 23*, 15–19.

Spielberger, C. D. (1970). *Manual for the State-Trait Anxiety Inventory for Children*. Palo Alto: Consulting Psychologists Press.

Spierings, E. L. (1988). Clinical and experimental evidence for a role of calcium entry blockers in the treatment of migraine. *Annals of New York Academy of Science, 522*, 676–689.

Spirito, A., Stark, L., & Williams, C. (1988). Development of a brief coping checklist for use with pediatric populations. *Journal of Pediatric Psychology, 13*, 555–574.

Stark, L., Spirito, A., Williams, C., & Guevremont, D., (1989). Common problems and coping strategies. I: Findings with normal adolescents. *Journal of Abnormal Child Psychology, 17*, 203–212.

Vahlquist, B., & Hackzell, G. (1949). Migraine of early onset: A study of thirty-one cases in which the disease first appeared between one and four years of age. *Acta Paediatrica, 38*, 622–636.

Varni, J. W., Jay, S. M., Masek, B. J., & Thompson, K. L. (1986). Cognitive-behavioral assessment and management of pediatric pain. In A. Holzman & D. Turk (Eds.), *Pain management: A handbook of psychological treatment approaches* (pp. 168–192). New York: Pergamon.

Varni, J. W., Katz, E. R., & Dash, J. (1982). Behavioral and neurochemical aspects of pediatric pain. In D. C. Russo & J. W. Varni (Eds.), *Behavioral pediatrics: Research and practice* (pp. 177–224). New York: Plenum.

Whitt, J. K. (1982). Children's understanding of illness: Developmental considerations and pediatric intervention. In M. Craich, D. K. Routh, & M. Woolraich (Eds.), *Advances in developmental and behavioral pediatrics* (Vol. 3, pp. 163–201). Greenwich: JAI Press.

Yen, S., & McIntire, R. W. (1971). Operant therapy for constant headache complaints: A simple response-cost approach. *Psychological Reports, 28*, 267–270.

15
Helping Children Cope With Painful Medical Procedures

Donald K. Routh and Marjorie D. Sanfilippo

Pain has been defined as "an unpleasant sensory and emotional experience associated with actual or potential tissue damage, or described in terms of such damage" (International Association for the Study of Pain, Subcommittee on Taxonomy, 1979). This definition clearly fits the situation discussed in this chapter, pain caused to children by various types of intrusive medical and dental procedures.

The biological function of pain seems to be to impel one to flee from danger, to take protective action when something is wrong with the body, or to fight off a predator. When young individuals experience pain, they often emit distress signals that cause their parents to come to their assistance. When a child's pain results from a medical procedure (such as an injection), none of the above "natural" reactions is considered to be socially appropriate. Children are not supposed to run away, to try to prevent the needle from piercing their skin, or to fight with the nurse who is administering the injection. The parents when aroused by the child's crying are not supposed to assist in such actions, either. Our social norms instead encourage the child and the family to cooperate with the "predator." This chapter concerns the search for the most helpful way of reconciling these somewhat incompatible biological and social demands on the child and family.

The Question of Procedural Pain in Infancy

The traditional view was that infants and children do not suffer as much pain as older individuals. Swafford and Allan (1968), for example, advised that "pediatric patients seldom need medication for the relief of pain after general surgery. They tolerate discomfort well" (p. 133). Fitzgerald (1988), in reviewing a recent medical textbook on the newborn, remarked on its total lack of coverage of the topic of pain. The volume discussed the exact details of many procedures such as catheterization, intracardiac injections, and lumbar punctures without mentioning the use of any analgesic. The otherwise comprehensive list of drugs at the end of the book did not include any analgesics or anesthetics.

Heel Lance

Pain is usually defined as a subjective state. The most convincing way in which people communicate such experiences is by describing them verbally. Obviously, infants will never be able to provide verbal statements about any inner distress they have, so we must depend upon inferences from their nonverbal behavior. Infants definitely show crying and facial grimacing to stimuli that an older person would describe as painful. Owens and Todt (1984) compared the effects of a heel lance (this procedure is typically used to obtain blood to screen for the inborn error of metabolism, phenylketonuria) with those of tactile stimulation in 20 infants on the 2nd day of life. Heart rate and the percentage of those who cried were significantly increased by the heel lance. Grunau and Craig (1987) studied 140 2-day-old infants responding to heel lance. They found that infants who were awake and alert responded to the lance with the most facial activity. Infants who were in a state of quiet sleep at the time had the least facial reactions and the longest latency to cry.

Harpin and Rutter (1983) demonstrated that a device called an "autolet" could be used to make heel lances less stressful for infants, as indicated by a significant decrease in emotional sweating.

Circumcision

Talbert, Kraybill, and Potter (1975) studied five male newborn infants' responses to circumcision during the first 6 hours of life. In each baby, serum cortisol and cortisone rose from baseline to a time 20 minutes after the procedure, presumably reflecting the "stress" component of the pain response. Gunnar, Fisch, and Malone (1984) examined the effects of giving a pacifier to infants undergoing circumcision. They studied 18 infants 2 to 5 days old, randomly assigning half of them to a group given a pacifier and the others to a group not given a pacifier. The pacifier reduced crying about 40% but did not have any apparent effect on adrenocortical response. Kirya and Werthmann (1978) administered a local anesthetic (penile dorsal nerve block) to newborn infants undergoing circumcision. They judged this to make the circumcision a relatively painless procedure to the infants. Williamson and Williamson (1983) followed this up with a controlled study of 30 healthy full-term newborns. Those who received a penile nerve block showed significantly reduced crying time, heart rate, and stress compared with the group without anesthetic. Transcutaneous oxygen pressure was also significantly affected. These authors remarked that the level of pain apparent in control group infants "would not be tolerated by older patients" (p.

40). It is worth noting that when circumcision is carried out on older children, for example on boys 5 to 6 years old (Martin, 1982), it is done with the same careful attention to analgesic medication that one would see with any other kind of surgery with that age group. Owens (1984) made the reasonable argument that the effectiveness of a penile nerve block in reducing crying and autonomic measures of distress is evidence that infants do, in fact, experience pain. In any case, Owens judged that the burden of proof should now be on those who do not believe that infants experience pain.

Injections in Infants

According to Eland's (1981) clear description, in an intramuscular injection "a needle penetrating intact skin mechanically irritates small fibers. A second source of pain originates from pressure exerted by the injected solution on small fibers" (p. 362). Johnston and Strada (1986) described the acute response of 14 infants 2 to 4 months old to routine DPT (diphtheria-pertussis-typhoid) immunization by injection. There was a drop in heart rate, a long high-pitched cry, a period of apnea, rigidity of the torso and limbs, and (the most constant feature) a facial expression of pain. There were, however, large individual differences in response. For example, one infant in the sample did not cry at all. The degree of behavioral distress shown by infants receiving injections appears to decline with age. Craig, McMahon, Morison, and Zaskow (1984) found that infants over 12 months old cried less than younger infants when they received their injections. Izard, Hembree, Dougherty, and Spizzirri (1983) carried out two studies of the facial expressions of infants 2 to 19 months old receiving DPT immunizations. The younger subjects reacted mostly to the injections as such, and their faces expressed pain uncontaminated by other emotions, whereas older ones showed more anticipatory crying and a greater admixture of distress and anger in their facial expressions. These developmental changes seem to be in line with what we said at the beginning of this chapter about the biological function of pain.

Current Opinions Regarding Pain in Infants

Purcell-Jones, Dormon, and Sumner (1988) surveyed a group of 60 pediatric anesthetists and found that 80% of them believed that even neonates perceived pain, although most were reluctant to prescribe anesthesia to this age group, because they saw the objective signs of pain as potentially misleading. Also, the dosages of such medications that might be used with young infants have in many cases not been worked out. Every anesthetist in the group believed that by the age of 1 to 3 months, infants perceived pain.

Common Sources of Procedural Pain in Preschool and School-Age Children

Unlike infants, even young children can speak for themselves and can to some extent "say where it hurts" if they are in pain. For example, Eland and Anderson (1977) found that 168 of 172 child patients, ages 4 to 10 years old, could correctly make an X on a body outline to indicate where they hurt. Young children can also provide at least limited information concerning the subjective aspects of their experience. Using a series of pictures of hypothetical pain stimuli, Belter, McIntosh, Finch, and Saylor (1988) found that children 3 to 6 years old were consistently able to differentiate situations connoting the absence of pain from low pain, and moderate from high pain. Nevertheless, we have to supplement such children's reports with objective observations of their behavior and physiological indices to judge their reactions to medical procedures and the efficacy of strategies intended to relieve pain. In contrast, older children are able to use more demanding assessment methods for reporting both the intensity and quality of their pain experiences.

Many intervention studies carried out with children receiving intrusive medical procedures are similar to research with adults (see review by Ludwick-Rosenthal & Neufeld, 1988) in that they often involve the presentation of information, training in relaxation, or cognitive-behavioral coping strategies. Interventions involving the use of peer models may include any or all of these approaches. The presentation of information seems fundamental to most interventions in that it "enables the individual to form accurate cognitive expectations about the procedures and thereby increases his or her sense of control" (Ludwick-Rosenthal & Neufeld, 1988, p. 327).

Injections

Injections remain the most common painful medical procedure experienced by children. Young children have typically had experience with injections before and may have come to fear them. Broome and Endsley (1989) studied 83 children ages 4 to 6 years and found that those rated by their mothers as highly anxious prior to their immunizations were the most likely to be distressed during the procedure. Among the sample of 28 third- and fourth-grade children studied by Ross and Ross (1985), over a third "expressed strong negative feelings about their ability to cope with 'shots.' Some children even became physically agitated if shots were mentioned" (p. 61).

In a unique intervention study, Eland (1981) randomly divided her sample of 40 prekindergarten children into four groups. Half of the children had a skin coolant sprayed on the injection site (the leg) immediately prior to the intramuscular DPT injection, whereas the others had a noncooling aerosol sprayed on the same area. Half were led to expect less pain, and the other half were not so instructed. The skin coolant reduced the children's report of pain significantly more than did aerosol spray; suggestion had no additional effect.

In another intervention aimed at managing injection pain, Fowler-Kerry and Lander (1987) studied 200 children ages 4 to 6 years. Subjects were assigned to a distraction condition (in which they listened to music over earphones), or to other conditions involving either distraction plus suggestion, suggestion only, or no treatment. Musical distraction significantly reduced the children's ratings of injection-related pain. As in Eland's (1981) study, suggestion had no additional effect.

Medical procedures take place in a social context, and it is important to examine the effects of this. In studies with two different age groups (18-month-olds and 5-year-olds), Shaw and Routh (1982) looked at the effect of the presence of the mother on children's reactions to immunization injections. Children were randomly assigned to receive the injections with mother either present or absent. Somewhat surprisingly, in both of these studies, these authors found that the children cried significantly more if the mother was there. In follow-up research, Gonzalez et al. (1989) also found that children 5 years, 6 months to 7 years, 9 months showed more behavioral distress if their parent was present. Despite the fact that they showed more distress, however, these children expressed a preference to have the parent with them during the injection. Thus, the parent (who would presumably provide effective comforting of the child if present) may serve as a discriminative stimulus for expressing distress. In other words, why cry if there is no one there to respond?

Other studies concerned with the issue of parental behavior and children's coping with procedural pain are reviewed under the heading of dental treatment below.

A current research project underway at the University of Miami by the authors involves the development of a questionnaire on children's strategies for coping with medical procedures, i.e., behaviors they might engage in when receiving an injection to try to make it hurt less. At present the questionnaire consists of 55 items (see Table 15.1). A large pool of items was initially written by the authors and compiled from several existing child, adolescent, and adult scales, adapted so as to be applicable to the medical situation. Items fit the broad definition of coping put forward by Lazarus and Folkman (1984) as "constantly changing cognitive and behavioral efforts to manage specific external and/or internal demands that are appraised as taxing or exceeding the resources of the person" (p. 141). Potential items were first evaluated by several psychologists to assure that they fit this definition. A pilot study with 28 children in grades 3, 4, 5, and 6 was carried out to make sure that the items were easily understood by the children and were checked with reasonable frequency. This pilot study also contained two initial open-ended items asking children to indicate what they would do or say to themselves to relieve anxiety in this situation. Then a revised list of 66

TABLE 15.1. Pediatric coping strategies scale.

Overall Instructions

Pretend that you are going to the doctor's office, and you know they have to do something to you that will hurt (like giving you a shot). I am going to tell you some things that some children either do or say to themselves to make themselves feel better. I want you to tell me which of these things you think you might say or do to make yourself feel better. There are no right or wrong answers. Would you:

Item	Test-retest phi coefficient[a]	Item-scale correlation
1. Pray to God and ask Him to not let it hurt?	.67*	.60*
2. Pray to God and ask Him to make you brave and strong?	.72*	.56*
3. Tell yourself it's not that bad?	.47*	.29
4. Tell yourself that the nurse is doing it to make you feel better?	.44*	.50*
5. Tell yourself that you'll feel better when it's over?	.53*	.49*
6. Remember times in the past when you were at the doctor's office and you did something to make yourself feel better?	.43*	.63*
7. Try to understand why the nurse has to do it?	.45*	.63*
8. Tell yourself that everything will be OK next time you have to go to the doctor's?	.39*	.44*
9. Tell yourself that it will never happen again?	.46*	.44*
10. Try to behave when the nurse gives you the shot, just so she won't do it again?	.37*	.48*
11. Make a fist or tense some other part of your body?	.78*	.20
12. Talk to your parents about it?	.43*	.55*
13. Want your parents there to make you feel better?	.49*	.19
14. Talk to a friend about it?	.48*	.42*
15. Talk to the nurse about it?	.57*	.62*
16. Do some things so you don't think about it (like counting things or talking to someone else while it's happening)?	.43*	.38*
17. Think about other things to take your mind off of the hurt (like good times you've had)?	.60*	.55*
18. Tell yourself that it won't hurt at all?	.60*	.43*
19. Pretend you are somewhere else?	.52*	.53*
20. Try to go somewhere else and hide?	.56*	.15
21. Let everyone know how you feel?	.53*	.49*
22. Talk to other kids who had the same thing happen to see what they did?	.53*	.58*
23. Make a promise to someone else (like your parents or the nurse) that you'd be good so it doesn't happen again?	.45*	.64*
24. Make a deal with the nurse or your parents so it won't hurt?	.46*	.58*

TABLE 15.1. *Continued*

Item	Test-retest phi coefficient[a]	Item-scale correlation
25. Try to feel better by exercising or playing after getting the shot?	.45*	.20
26. Tell yourself that it could be worse?	.57*	.09
27. Hold your breath?	.53*	.43*
28. Try to feel better by eating?	.62*	.41*
29. Try to be calm?	.41*	.34
30. Shut your eyes?	.41*	.42*
31. Get angry and fight the nurse to keep her from doing it?	.88*	.17
32. Look away?	.43*	.28
33. Try to think of things that would make you relax?	.50*	.53*
34. Think about something nice that's going to happen after you get the shot (like going to get ice cream or a toy)?	.46*	.51*
35. Tell yourself that everything will be OK?	.46*	.61*
36. Try to think of something good that will happen because you got the shot?	.68*	.57*
37. Try to learn something from getting the shot?	.51*	.61*
38. Ask your parents what to do?	.65*	.76*
39. Ask the nurse what to do?	.60*	.67*
40. Ask your friends what to do?	.51*	.49*
41. Ask the nurse to stop, to not do it?	.50*	.32
42. Try to think of ways to deal with the shot?	.43*	.56*
43. Try to daydream?	.55*	.53*
44. Pretend it just isn't happening?	.40*	.59*
45. Laugh about it?	.58*	.55*
46. Make jokes about it?	.52*	.51*
47. Ask the nurse why she has to do it?	.63*	.67*
48. Ask the nurse what is wrong with you?	.58*	.71*
49. Ask your parents why the nurse has to do it?	.64*	.76*
50. Ask your parents what is wrong with you?	.64*	.71*
51. Cry?	.51*	.21
52. Hit or mess up something other than a person?	.76*	.10
53. Try to move around a lot so the nurse can't get to you?	.80*	.19
54. Ask a lot of people (like your parents, the doctor, or the nurse) to tell you everything that is going to happen?	.54*	.60*
55. Tell yourself that you won't die from it?	.53*	.54*

[a]A phi coefficient is a Pearson product-moment correlation coefficient between two dichotomous variables. Its range may be restricted somewhat by lopsided marginal distributions.
*$p < .001$.

items was given to 72 additional children, with equal numbers from grades 3, 4, 5, and 6. These children's mean age was 10 years, 6 months (SD, 13.5 months). There were 38 males and 34 females in the sample. The same items were administered once again 1 to 2 weeks later to obtain information on test-retest reliability. Table 15.1 shows the final 55 items in the *Pediatric Coping Strategies Scale* (PCSS), together with their test-retest reliabilities and item-scale correlations (only items with test-retest reliabilities significant at the .001 level were retained). Given the retention criterion, the 55-item scale of course had high test-retest reliability over a 1 to 2 week interval — its overall test-retest correlation was .82. It also had high internal consistency, as indicated by a Cronbach's alpha of .94. The correlation between children's overall scores and age was not statistically significant, and there were no significant sex differences in the overall scores. The next step in the project will be to see which of these coping items predict children's level of distress when receiving an immunization injection (or having blood drawn).

Dental Treatment

As Siegel (1988) says, visits to the dentist constitute one of the certainties in life. In the dental chair, young children typically show more distress than older ones, are less cooperative, and require more of the dentist's time to treat them (Green, Meilman, Routh, & McIver, 1977). Compared to heel lances and immunizations, dental examination and treatment are more complex, involving a number of different activities and sources of stress. From the standpoint of distress, the most salient experiences of children during dental restorative treatment are choking, injections, and the use of the dental drill (Cuthbert & Melamed, 1982). In the Green et al. (1977) study, a peer modeling film failed to have any significant effect compared to control conditions, probably because the procedures observed included only an examination and prophylaxis, not the administration of anesthetic or any restoration. In other words, if children do not show much distress as a result of a particular medical or dental procedure, there is a "floor effect" in which it is more difficult for interventions to appear effective in reducing distress.

Children's reactions to dentistry typically change over time as they experience repeated visits. For example, they learn which procedures are painless and which ones are painful (Venham, Bengston, & Cipes, 1977; Venham, Murray, & Gaulin-Kremer, 1979). Kleinknecht, Klepac, and Alexander (1973) present evidence that adult dental fears in many cases may have been learned in childhood. Follow-up studies assessing the long-term effects of interventions that decrease children's dental pain and distress will therefore be of interest in the future.

According to Siegel (1988), the three basic strategies that have been used in attempting to treat children's dental distress are providing procedural and sensory information, teaching coping skills, and the use of modeling. One of the earliest controlled intervention studies (Ghose, Giddon, Shiere, & Fogels, 1969) demonstrated the effectiveness of older siblings as models for children 3 to 5 years old undergoing their first experience of dental treatment. Children who went into the dental operatory and watched their older sibling during the administration of anesthetic and amalgam restoration were subsequently more cooperative during a similar procedure than a control group who stayed in the waiting room while their older sibling was treated.

In another intervention study, Machen and Johnson (1974) compared the effects of desensitization with those of a filmed model and a no-treatment control condition on the behavior of 31 children (36 to 65 months of age) receiving dental restorative treatment. Both of the interventions studied were effective in comparison to the control, but they did not differ significantly from each other. The dependent measure in this study was distress rated by observers.

Melamed, Hawes, Heiby, and Glick (1975) compared the effects of a filmed model of a cooperative child in the dental chair with those of a nondental control film. The subjects in the modeling condition showed significantly fewer disruptive behaviors. They were also rated as significantly less fearful than children in the control condition. The findings of the study by Melamed, Weinstein, Hawes, and Katin-Borland (1975) with children in the age group 5 to 9 years, were essentially similar. They found significant effects of a peer model film on disruptive behaviors and on a behavior profile. The children's subjective reports were not influenced by this intervention, however.

An important study by Melamed, Yurcheson, Fleece, Hutcherson, and Hawes (1978) showed that the effects of modeling films are not always beneficial. They observed children 4 to 11 years old during three dental sessions and reported that those with previous dental experience benefited most from the film, whereas those with no previous experience were actually *sensitized* by the film and showed more distress after watching it.

Siegel and Peterson (1980) compared (a) a self-control coping skills procedure, (b) a procedure presenting sensory information, and (c) a contact-control condition. Subjects were 42 preschool children. Both of the treatments were superior to the control condition in terms of behavioral, physiological, and self-report measures but did not differ from each other. Siegel and Peterson (1981) restudied 26 of these children 1 week later during a second dental treatment session and found that the treatment effects were maintained.

Nocella and Kaplan (1982), studying a group of 30 children, compared (a) a stress inoculation procedure (actually a "package" of cognitive-behavioral treatments), (b) an attention-placebo procedure, and (c) a no treatment control group. The stress inoculation group made significantly fewer body movements during the dental treatment procedure than the other two groups. This should be considered a favorable outcome in view of the fact that many body movements (such as putting one's hand in front of the mouth) are quite disruptive of dental treatment.

Schwartz, Albino, and Tedesco (1983) studied a group of 3- to 4-year-old children who had to be hospitalized for dental restorations or extractions under general anesthesia, a more threatening set of circumstances than the child's usual dental experience. None of these children had been hospitalized previously. The 45 children were randomly assigned to either a play therapy group involving the presentation of extensive information about what was going to occur, an unrelated play therapy group, or a no-treatment control group. The main play therapy intervention significantly decreased how upset the children were and led to more cooperative behavior at seven different stress points during their hospital stay.

In summary, there have been far more studies of psychological interventions on children's response to dental treatments than to the other procedures reviewed so far. It is clear that a number of psychological interventions are effective in comparison to placebo or no-treatment controls. What is still uncertain is exactly what elements make for an effective psychological intervention. Most studies comparing different interventions to each other find them equally effective and so are nonspecific.

A promising exception to this nonspecificity is the research of Klingman, Melamed, Cuthbert, and Hermecz (1984). These investigators studied children 8 to 13 years old who were highly fearful of dentists. Two groups watched modeling videotapes, but one group was encouraged to rehearse the behaviors of the model actively, whereas the other (the so-called symbolic modeling group) was not. The children who participated more actively with the model obtained significantly more information from the videotape, reported less dental anxiety, and displayed fewer disruptive behaviors during dental treatment than those who merely watched the tape passively.

In a study in agreement with the statement of Gonzalez et al. (1989) mentioned above that children prefer to have their parent present in a stressful situation, Frankl, Shiere, and Fogels (1962) found that children 41 to 49 months old were more cooperative and less fearful in the dental operatory if their mother was present than if she was absent. However, many dentists make a regular practice of excluding parents from the operatory (Association of Pedodontic Diplomates, 1972). Siegel (1988), in reviewing this issue, cites the work of Venham, Bengston, and Cipes (1978) and others in support of the conclusion that it is the mother's specific behavior in the dental operatory and the quality of the mother-child relationship that are critical, not simply her presence or absence. Although it is not concerned with dentistry, the research of Bush, Melamed, Sheras, and Greenbaum (1986) addresses mother-child interaction patterns in relation to coping with procedural stress. Bush et al. observed 50 children in a diagnostic medical examination situation, using their Dyadic Prestressor Interaction Scale (DPIS). They found that maternal use of distraction and low rates of ignoring the child were associated with better stress tolerance. Maternal reassurance or agitation on the other hand were associated with behavioral distress in the child. More research like this is needed in relation to procedural pain of all kinds.

Hospitalization

Most children have to undergo hospitalization at one time or another. The most common types of surgery that are necessary for them include the removal of tonsils, adenoids, and the vermiform appendix, insertion of myringotomy tubes in the eardrum, and inguinal hernia repair. Obviously, the particular procedures involved in hospitalization are more diverse than those involved in dental treatment. Hospitalization does usually involve certain common experiences: separation from parents, diagnostic tests (e.g., venipuncture), presurgical sedation, induction of anesthesia, the surgery itself, time in the recovery room, and coping with postoperative pain in an unfamiliar environment. Some research encompasses the entire experience of hospitalization, whereas other studies focus on only one aspect of it. We will deal with each of these subtopics in turn.

Hospitalization in General

Reissland (1983) interviewed a group of 58 children 4 to 13 years old in St. Charles Hospital, London for tonsillectomy or adenoidectomy. The younger children in the group seemed to understand going into the hospital mostly in terms of their family relationships. They indicated that they would have to depend on their parents to help them cope with their fear and pain. The older children in contrast could generally come up with strategies of their own for dealing with their experiences. Indeed, research strongly supports the younger children's view that they need their parents to help them cope with hospitalization. Douglas (1975) studied over 1,000 children born in 1946 and admitted to the hospital before age 5, at a time when hospitals greatly restricted parental visits. These children, especially those hospitalized for over 2 weeks, had behavior problems at home after returning from the hospital and continued to have various difficulties still detectable at an adolescent follow-up. Hospitals have responded to strong evidence like this by greatly liberalizing their policy on parental visitation. It is now common for hospitals to permit parents to "room in" with young children in order to minimize the stress of parental separation.

For older children who are able to comprehend the nature of their illness and the rationale for hospitalization, the overall meaning of their experience to them may turn out to be very important. After all, dogs trained in a Pavlovian procedure may learn to salivate to a noxious stimulus if it always signals food. In a classic study of soldiers on the Anzio beachhead during World War II, Beecher (1956) found that only 32% of those with battlefield wounds required narcotics, compared to 83% of a group of civilians with comparable injuries. In fact, 66% of the wounded soldiers said that they did not feel pain. Beecher's explanation was that for these soldiers the wounds had a very positive meaning, namely an honorable release from the horrors of war and a ticket home. Price, Harkins, and Baker (1987) presented data collected from adults using visual analogue scales. These investigators were able to elicit direct comparisons between the intensity of sensory and affective components of people's experiences of pain. (It has not yet been possible to do this in research with children.) Interestingly, they found that patients with cancer or chronic pain gave affective pain ratings that were higher than their sensory ones. In contrast, women in labor or individuals exposed to experimental pain gave affective pain ratings that were lower than their sensory ones. It would be interesting to try to identify a similar phenomenon in children. One piece of information that might make procedural pain more tolerable to children is that it is generally quite temporary.

According to the theory of Janis (1958), there is a certain "work of worry" that needs to be carried out by the patient in preparing for a surgical procedure. He found that adult patients with a moderate level of anxiety before surgery adjusted better than those with either high or low levels of anxiety. Unfortunately, little research with children has attempted to test hypotheses from this theory.

Zabin and Melamed (1980) developed a questionnaire to try to predict how children would respond to hospitalization. The predictors they found were aspects of parental discipline. Parents who reported that they used positive reinforcement, modeling, and persuasion tended to have children with low anxiety and fear. Those who reported that they used punishment, force, and reinforcement of dependency in contrast tended to have highly anxious children.

Psychological procedures to prepare children for hospitalization have gone far beyond the experimental stage. They are used every day. Surveys indicate that about 75% of children's hospitals use formal preparation procedures (Peterson & Ridley-Johnson, 1980), as do about a third of pediatric wards in regular hospitals (Azarnoff & Woody, 1981). However, as Peterson and Mori (1988) point out, there is not a very close linkage between the preparation hospitals offer and what the research literature indicates to be effective.

What is the best time for preparation for hospitalization? Peterson and Mori (1988) point out that to help children cope with emergency medical events, preparation would have to be made a routine event of childhood, perhaps in the school classroom. Ross and Ross (1985) have in fact developed a curriculum of "pain instruction" for elementary school students that might serve as a model for what is needed. At present this needs to be validated in terms of its effects on children's reactions during actual painful experiences including hospitalization.

In an intervention with 40 children ages 3 to 11 hospitalized for cardiac catheterization, Cassel and Paul (1967) examined the effects of puppet therapy: two 30-minute sessions involving the presentation of information about the procedure and role play with the children. The children in the treatment group were rated as significantly less disturbed during their hospital stay than those in the control group. A subsequent parent questionnaire also indicated that children in the treatment group were more willing to return to the hospital for further treatment if need be.

Johnson and Stockdale (1975) assigned 43 hospitalized children ages 5 to 8 years to puppet therapy or control conditions. The puppet therapy familiarized the children with hospital routines and procedures as well as with the surgery that they were to undergo. This treatment reduced anxiety (as indicated by palmar sweating) both subsequent to the puppet show and after surgery compared to the control group.

In their well-known research on the effects of filmed modeling ("Ethan has an Operation"), Melamed and Siegel (1975) studied 60 children 4 to 12 years old randomly assigned to treatment and control groups. They did not assess children's pain during specific invasive procedures. They did find that pre- and postoperative fear and behavior problems as indicated by the Behavior Problem Checklist were significantly decreased by the intervention. Peterson and Mori (1988) conclude that modeling films of this type are the best researched procedure for preparing children for hospitalization. Although the exact mechanisms through which these films work has yet to be demonstrated clearly, they are now regarded as the standard preparation procedures against which new ones may be compared.

Peterson and Shigetomi (1981) studied 63 children ages 2 to 10 years who were hospitalized for elective tonsillectomies. They compared the following experimental conditions: information only, coping, filmed modeling, and coping plus filmed modeling. Using behavioral, physiological, and self-report measures, these investigators found some evidence that the combined condition (coping plus modeling) was superior to either of its components alone. This study is interesting because it goes beyond nonspecific treatment effects.

Blood Drawing

Fernald and Corry (1981) contrasted two different procedures for preparing children for either a finger stick or venipuncture. One was described as empathetic ("I'll bet the alcohol feels cold. In a moment I'm going to stick you. You're probably feeling scared . . . "). The other was called directive ("Act big and brave. Remain very still."). The empathetic method was superior: it led to fewer distress behaviors and more positive self-reports. Many of the directively prepared children felt angry and thought that the technician had actually tried to hurt them. Very few of the children prepared empathetically reacted in this way.

Gross, Stern, Levin, Dale, and Wojnilower (1983) studied children's response to blood drawing in the presence or absence of their mothers, and found that more fear was expressed immediately before the procedure if the mother was there. These results resemble those of Shaw and Routh (1982) with children receiving injections and are equally ambiguous of interpretation. As already noted, Gonzalez et al. (1989) found that children prefer their parent to be present even though they may appear more upset under these conditions.

Induction of Anesthesia

The study of Vernon and Bailey (1974) was one of the first using a filmed modeling condition and featured the child models each receiving anesthesia through a mask and then appearing to go to sleep. Children who watched the modeling film were rated as significantly less anxious when entering the operating room themselves and being given anesthesia than children who had spent an equivalent amount of time with their parents.

Postoperative Pain

There is considerable evidence that both adults and children (but especially children) receive inadequate analgesic medication after surgery. For example, Marks and Sachar (1973) carried out structured interviews with 37 adult medical inpatients being treated with narcotic analgesics for postsurgical pain. Of these, 41% were in moderate distress and 32% in severe distress. Beyer, DeGood, Ashley, and Russell (1983) studied 50 children and 50 adults following open heart surgery. Seventy percent of the adults were given postoperative analgesics, versus only 30% of the children. Children were given significantly fewer potent narcotics than were adults, and six of the children did not even have orders for postoperative analgesics written in their charts. Mather and Mackie (1983) studied 170 children recovering from surgery in two major teaching hospitals. Of these, 16% had no orders for analgesics at all. Regardless of what was prescribed, only 25% of these children were pain free on the day of surgery, and 13% reported severe pain. Most pro re nata (p.r.n.) orders for analgesics were interpreted by nurses to mean "as little as possible." The nurses seemed to view children who were withdrawn as coping effectively. Research underway at the University of Miami by Juan Gonzalez and Donald K. Routh with standardized vignettes describing postsurgical patients of different ages confirms that children are especially at risk for undermedication. This study also aims to identify factors in nurses' backgrounds that might explain this. Angell (1982) in an editorial in the *New England Journal of Medicine*, describing pain as "soul destroying," agreed that there is a general need for more postsurgical analgesia and suggested the following remedy: "A prn order for a range of doses could be written, but the patient asked at each specified interval whether he needs relief from pain and, if so, whether he needs a relatively small or large dose" (p. 99).

In research at the University of Miami by Frances Johnson and Donald K. Routh, children and adolescents with postoperative pain are being observed under three conditions: playing video games, watching television, or with no intervention. The expectation is that the video game condition, as an active distraction condition, will provide the greatest relief from pain. The idea behind this study is an old one. According to Blitz and Dinnerstein (1971), the philosopher Pascal found a challenging problem to be a helpful way of distracting his attention from his neuralgia, and Kant used a similar strategy in dealing with his pain from gout. McCaul and Malott (1984) reviewed the literature on distraction and coping with pain. They defined distraction as "any strategy whose purpose is to block awareness of the painful stimulus or its effects" (p. 517) and hypothesized that distraction techniques that required more attentional capacity would be more effective. In a study with adult patients, Corah, Gale, and Illig (1979) found that playing video ping pong was successful in relieving anxiety during dental restoration. A relaxation procedure was equally effective in relieving anxiety, but the patients liked the ping pong better.

The Role of Previous Medical Experience

Most research on preparation of children for hospitalization has avoided those with previous surgical experiences. Indeed, research summarized by Peterson and Mori (1988) confirms that children with previous experience in the hospital may not benefit from the usual preparation procedure or may need something more specifically tailored to their needs.

Timing of Preparation

It is also somewhat unclear from present research what the optimum timing of preparation for hospitalization should be in different age groups. Further research is needed on this question.

Procedural Pain in Particular Medical Populations of Children

It is hardly possible for a child to grow up without dealing with heel lances, injections, dental treatment, and an occasional hospitalization. However, some medical conditions require procedures that are out of the ordinary. The ones that have received the most study from the standpoint of procedural pain are burns and cancer. A group that has been the subject of research at the University of Miami is sexually abused children requiring forensic gynecological examinations. Let us discuss these groups in turn.

Children With Burns

Burns are painful in themselves, both immediately and during the long period of time it takes for healing to take place. In fact, thermal sources can differentially stimulate unmyelinated C nerve fibers and open the pain "gate" (Melzack & Wall, 1965; Wall, 1978), temporarily increasing the pain sensitivity of the skin (Fields, 1987; Price, Hu, Dubner, & Gracely, 1977). (Pain sensations from the skin are transmitted mainly by two types of fibers, the A-delta or faster, myelinated ones, and the slower C fibers. This arrangement is responsible for the well established phenomenon of double pain responses of the human skin to a single stimulus, e.g., Lewis & Pochin, 1937.)

Serious burns also require special, painful medical procedures: removal of the dressings, immersing the body in water, and especially the debridement of the wound or removal of necrotic tissue to prevent infection and promote healing. As Miller, Elliott, Funk, and Pruitt (1988) state, "this procedure is generally acknowledged to represent one of the most painful medical procedures children undergo, and it is frequently associated with high levels of patient protest and distress" (p. 430). According to Miller et al., some children's resistance to the tanking and debridement procedures may be extreme and involve not only crying and screaming but also biting, kicking, swearing, running away, refusal to follow instructions, and even urinating or defecating in the hydrotherapy tank (which requires the child's immediate removal from the tank because of the possibility of infection). Nor does the situation get better with time, for children seem to become *less* tolerant of hydrotherapy as their experience with it increases. Kavanaugh (1983a, 1983b) has discussed some parallels between the situation of these burned children and the phenomenon of "learned helplessness" studied in the animal laboratory. This hypothesis would explain the development of chronic anxiety, eating disturbances, and various depressive symptoms seen in some children undergoing burn treatment. Children with burns also frequently have to undergo skin grafting and other painful surgical procedures (see chapter 11).

Although children in hospital burn units in the United States have levels of pain rated as moderate by the staff and severe by the patients themselves, the usual treatment regimen involves the use of no narcotic analgesics or (in many cases) no analgesics at all (Perry & Heidrich, 1982). Thus, one high-priority question for researchers is whether effective analgesic protocols can be developed for children undergoing burn treatment.

One of the earliest controlled studies of a psychological intervention with burn patients was that of Wakeman and Kaplan (1978). In this research, a group of adult and child patients given both hypnosis and medication requested significantly less ad lib analgesic medication than a group given medication alone. It was also reported that children requested a significantly lower percentage of the maximum allowable medication than did adults. Commenting on the use of hypnosis in general, Hilgard (1975) has stated that "its success in completely suppressing severe pain requires highly hypnotizable patients, who are in the minority" (p. 213). Further research on the efficacy of hypnotic interventions thus would probably benefit from the use of standardized hypnotic susceptibility scales of the kind developed by Hilgard and others.

Kelley, Jarvie, Middlebrook, McNeer, and Drabman (1984) used a reversal design to study the effects of cartoon viewing and reinforcement of low levels of distress behaviors on two young girls undergoing debridement procedures for their burn injuries. The children's observed scores on the Procedure Behavior Rating Scale went down during the intervention and rose once more with a return to baseline conditions. Perhaps with studies like this in mind, Lavigne, Schulein, and Hahn (1986b) stated that in pain treatment research, single subject designs may be impractical or even unethical. Having once successfully removed severe pain, what humane person would wish to allow it to return? Would well-informed parents consent to such a procedure for their children? However, the absence of any subjective measures in the Kelley et al. (1984) study leave open the question of whether the intervention really reduced pain or whether it simply increased the children's stoic acceptance of their situation.

Elliott and Olson (1983) studied the efficacy of an intervention package including distraction, breathing exercises designed to promote relaxation, and the use of emotive imagery for four children undergoing burn treatment (hydrotherapy, debridement, and dressing changes). Using a multiple baseline and reversal experimental design, they found that these procedures decreased observed behavioral distress (the study did not include subjective or physiological measures). They also found that coaching during the actual burn treatment process was essential for their intervention to be effective.

As Miller et al. (1988) note, other descriptions of psychological interventions for pain in child burn patients in the literature are generally uncontrolled studies or at best are case reports with single-subject experimental designs. Much more research is needed in this area before firm conclusions will be possible concerning optimum interventions. At this point the suffering of children being treated for burns is highly stressful, not only to the children themselves but also to their parents and to the hospital staff who care for the children.

Children With Cancer

The most common type of cancer in childhood is acute lymphoblastic leukemia (ALL), a disease that originates in the bone marrow where blood cells are produced (Stehbens, 1988). Almost all psychological research on procedural pain in children with cancer concerns children with ALL. For diagnostic purposes, children with leukemia are required to undergo repeatedly a very painful medical procedure, bone marrow aspiration. The prophylaxis of the central nervous system that is part of the treatment of ALL usually involves intrathecal medication, requiring another painful procedure, lumbar puncture. Young children subjected to repeated procedures such as these often come to exhibit negative behaviors such as kicking, screaming, and so much resistance that they have to be physically carried into the treatment room. In the absence of psychological intervention, it may take them as long as 2 or 3 years before they learn to cooperate with the procedures (Jay, 1988). The heightened negative affective quality of the children's pain from such procedures could very well be intensified by the meaning of cancer as a life-threatening disease. As a part of one of her intervention packages, Jay awards children trophies for doing their best to cope with procedural pain. She explains that

the purpose of the trophies is to try and transform the meaning of pain for the child. Rather than perceiving the bone marrow aspiration or lumbar puncture as an aversive, punitive event, the idea is to try to get children to perceive it as a challange and an opportunity to master a difficult situation, hence resulting in positive feelings of self-efficacy and increased self-esteem. (p. 408)

Katz, Kellerman, and Siegel (1980) developed a Procedure Behavior Rating Scale and used it to study 115 children with cancer who received bone marrow aspirations. They found no habituation over time in the amount of distress shown in response to these procedures. Age was a significant predictor of distress (with young children showing more distress), and females were significantly more distressed than males. Katz et al. (1982) found that children's beta-endorphin immunoreactivity as measured from samples of cerebrospinal fluid was significantly correlated with acute behavioral distress in children with leukemia. This is an especially interesting finding. It links research on children's procedural pain with basic research on opiate receptors in the brain (Pert & Snyder, 1973) and endogenous opioid substances that stimulate them (Hughes, 1975).

Jay, Ozolins, Elliott, and Caldwell (1983) studied 42 child cancer patients, ages 2 to 20, who received bone marrow aspirations, using the Observation Scale of Behavioral Distress (OSBD). They were able to find predictors accounting for 86% of the variance in the OSBD ($R^2 = .86$), namely age ($r = -.76$), number of previous procedures of the same kind ($r = .48$), and parental trait anxiety ($r = .46$). In other words, younger children showed more overt distress; there was an apparent sensitizing effect of an increasing number of bone marrow aspirations; and children with anxious parents showed heightened distress.

LeBaron and Zeltzer (1984) studied 50 cancer patients ranging from 6 to 18 years of age using self-reports as well as observer reports and a behavior checklist. They confirmed the findings of other investigators that the observed behavioral distress of their subjects during bone marrow aspirations declined significantly with age. However, patient self-reports showed no age differences, implying that the age changes might be in pain behaviors rather than in subjective pain itself. This agrees with the opinion of Lavigne, Schulein, and Hahn (1986a) that in general emotional outbursts associated with pain decline with age, whereas self-control and muscular rigidity increase with age.

Jay (1988), going somewhat beyond children with cancer in her discussion, classifies the types of psychological interventions used with children undergoing invasive medical procedures into (a) preparation, (b) hypnosis, (c) behavior therapy, and (d) cognitive-behavioral interventions, although as is already apparent from the material in this chapter, there is considerable overlap among these. As she states, the major component of most attempts at preparation is information, commonly divided into *sensory* information (a description of the sensations a patient will experience) and *procedural* information (a description of what will be done). For example, under the heading of sensory information, a child being prepared for a bone marrow aspiration "might be told that the cleansing of his or her back would feel 'cold,' whereas the numbing medicine would feel like a 'pinch' or a 'prick'" (Jay, p. 402). The procedural information might convey in simple language such technical details as that bone marrow aspirations "involve the insertion of a needle into the child's hip bone (posterior ileac crest); marrow is suctioned out with a syringe to be examined for presence or absence of cancer cells" (p. 406). Jay points out that the term *hypnosis* as applied to children most often includes imaginative involvement and other types of distraction and thus may be difficult to distinguish from so-called cognitive-behavioral procedures. Formal hypnotic induction procedures are rarely used with preadolescent children (for further information concerning the types of hypnosis used with children, see Gardner & Olness, 1981). Behavior therapy is described as including procedures such as desensitization, modeling, contingency management, and relaxation. The distinction between *mastery* and *coping* models is made: a mastery model undergoes the invasive procedure with apparent ease, whereas the coping model shows some anxiety or other difficulty but then overcomes it. Coping models are generally thought to be more effective (e.g., Meichenbaum, 1971).

Jay, Elliott, Ozolins, Olson, and Pruitt (1985) carried out a pilot intervention study on five children with cancer, ages 3 to 7 years who underwent bone marrow aspirations and lumbar punctures. Using a multiple baseline across subjects, they obtained some evidence of the efficacy in reducing behavioral distress of a package of cognitive behavioral treatments including emotive imagery (utilizing Wonder Woman or the Incredible Hulk), breathing patterns, reinforcement, behavioral rehearsal, and a filmed model.

Zeltzer and LeBaron (1982) carried out an intervention study of 33 children and adolescents with cancer who received either bone marrow aspirations or lumbar punctures or both. They compared hypnotic (individualized imagery and fantasy) and nonhypnotic (supportive counseling and environmental distraction) procedures and found the hypnotic ones significantly more effective at relieving both pain and anxiety. Dependent measures included both self-reports and observer ratings. Just as in the case of interventions with burn patients, hypnotic interventions appear promising as a way of dealing with acute procedural pain in children with cancer. Hilgard and LeBaron (1982) found that scores on the Stanford Hypnotic Clinical Scale for Children predicted 24 children's self-reported reductions in pain from bone marrow aspirations resulting from hypnotic treatment. Further research using standardized measures of hypnotic susceptibility will be useful.

As in other areas of procedural pain, parent-child interaction has been a focus of research on children with cancer receiving bone marrow aspirations and lumbar punctures. Blount et al. (1989) made transcriptions of audio-tapes of interactions among children, parents, and various health professionals and scored these on the Child-Adult Medical Procedure Interaction Scale (CAMPIS). They found that reassuring comments, apologies, statements giving control to the child, or criticism by adults tended to precede the child's distress. On the other hand, adult commands to the child to engage in coping procedures, nonprocedural (distracting?) talk, and humor directed to the child tended to precede and follow coping by the child. It will be important to follow up these descriptive findings with experimental manipulations to find out what is causing what, here.

Children With Suspected Sexual Abuse

A recently completed doctoral dissertation at the University of Miami by Thevenin (1989) concerned an intervention with prepubertal children suspected of sexual abuse who received a gynecological examination for forensic purposes. This particular type of examination involved the insertion of a long Q-tip into the child's vagina to check for bacteria representing a sexually transmitted disease. Unlike most of the other procedures discussed in this chapter, this examination did not involve penetration of the surface of the skin or any tissue damage. Nevertheless, the procedure is associated with a clinically significant amount of physical discomfort, not to mention the embarrassment or social discomfort that might be involved. Thevenin (1989) randomly assigned the 30 children in her study to one of two groups: information plus coping or attention placebo. Those in the information plus coping condition received detailed sensory and procedural information concerning the pelvic examination, including a demonstration using the identical medical equipment and an anatomically correct doll. They were also instructed in using an imagined trip to the beach to distract themselves from any discomfort the procedure involved. The attention placebo group spent an identical time in nonprocedure-related play with the therapist. The intervention produced a significant reduction in the children's distress compared with the control condition, both in terms of self-reported fear and behavioral distress as rated by observers blind to the subjects' group assignment. The effect of the intervention even reduced the distress of a subgroup of these children who later underwent blood drawing (which, incidentally, was rated as a significantly more distressing procedure than the pelvic examinations).

Balk, Dreyfus, and Harris (1982) observed 123 routine physical examinations of children by pediatric house staff. In these examinations, the ears, heart, and abdomen were examined 97% of the time. However, male genitalia were examined 84% of the time and female genitalia only 39% of the time. The neglect of gynecological examinations of infants and children possibly because of lingering sexual taboos, has clearly prevented the discovery of many congenital defects (such as an absent vagina), and has hindered the early identification of childhood gynecological cancer and vaginal infections (Routh & Andersen, 1988). Millstein, Adler, and Irwin (1984) investigated anxiety related to pelvic examinations reported by 84 teenagers. The main concern of these adolescent females was about how painful the procedure would be, with fear concerning the discovery of pathology or embarrassment being secondary issues. Thus, interventions reducing the discomfort associated with gynecological examinations seem well worth exploring further.

Discussion

Procedural pain is a fact of life for children, just as it is for the rest of us. The specific experiences of heel lance, immunization injections, dental restoration, and various painful experiences associated with hospitalization seem to be universal among children. In addition, children with particular medical conditions such as burns or cancer are subjected to painful procedures that other children will not have to experience. There are other such conditions not discussed in detail here because of the lack of information in the literature about them. For example, children with insulin-dependent (Type I) diabetes mellitus have to learn to give themselves repeated insulin injections, and it would be interesting to know what useful strategies they devise for minimizing the discomfort involved in these. We do not know of any research on this question. Similarly, some children with allergies or asthma must learn to tolerate repeated injections, and it would be of interest to know how they learn to cope with these.

The measurement of procedural pain is frequently confounded by the fear that is also part of the child's experience. As much as purists may wish to separate these two negative processes, in practice it is frequently impossible. In fact, pain and fear may even be confounded at a neurophysiological level. Duncan, Bushnell, Bates, and Dubner (1987) trained monkeys to press a lever after a light cue came on, signaling intense heat to the skin. It was found that after a time the animal's dorsal horn cells, which are supposedly "pain transmission neurons," fired when the light cue began, *before the onset of the noxious stimulus.* Somehow, this kind of research finding makes one feel better about measuring nonspecific "behavioral distress" in humans, whether by observer ratings, self-reports, or physiological indices. Nevertheless, it must be admitted that these behavioral distress measures are sensitive to many kinds of events beyond pain. For example, Gonzalez et al. (1989) found that Jay's Observation Scale of Behavior Distress was sensitive to young children's protest at the departure of their parent, an event not thought to involve any physical pain.

Can one conclude anything from the procedural pain literature about the relationship of pain to age? The research does appear to be consistent with the view that even infants feel pain. One implication of this is that infants should not be exposed to intrusive procedures such as cardiac catheterization or other surgical operations without proper attention to anesthetic or analgesic medication. Beyond these statements, it is difficult to make a generalization. The most frequently cited study in the literature addressing the relationship of age and pain is one by Haslam (1969) in which 115 children ages 5 to 18 years had their lower leg (tibia) stimulated by a plunger powered by a spring and protruding from a metal box. There was a .66 rank order correlation between pain thresholds and age; i.e., the younger children reported pain at lower plunger intensities. This parallels Jay et al.'s (1983) finding of a −.76 correlation between age and observed behavioral distress during bone marrow aspirations (younger children showed considerably more distress). One must remember, though, that LeBaron and Zeltzer (1984) observing a similar procedure found a relationship only between age and behavioral distress, not age and self-reported pain. In a sense, behavioral distress is a measure of how much pain a person is willing to tolerate. In another context, Hilgard (1975) remarked that "tolerance measures are measures of heroism as much as they are measures of pain" (p. 214). If this is true, what may be happening with age is an increase in bravery (or perhaps in the use of effective coping strategies), not just a decrease in pain. Much more research on the relationship between age and pain needs to be done before secure conclusions are possible.

Although it is natural for psychologists to focus on behavioral and psychological interventions for dealing with pain, we should not let our professional biases blind us to the value of analgesic medications. Unnecessarily severe pain and suffering are now endured by burned children receiving hydrotherapy and wound debridement, by leukemic children undergoing bone marrow aspirations and lumbar punctures, and by many children experiencing postsurgical pain. The long-term solutions to many of these problems could lie as much in the domain of pharmacology as in psychology. One role of behavioral scientists at this point may be to investigate factors causing physicians and nurses to undermedicate such children as well as to help evaluate new pharmacologic agents.

Finally, the various controlled studies reviewed in this chapter provide convincing evidence that a number of psychological interventions are significantly effective in relieving pain and helping children cooperate in necessary medical procedures. A major research challenge is to ask more refined questions about what particular components of these interventions are necessary to their effectiveness.

Acknowledgments. Marion W. Routh served as a helpful editor of an initial draft.

References

Angell, M. (1982). The quality of mercy. *New England Journal of Medicine, 306,* 98–99.

Association of Pedodontic Diplomates. (1972). Techniques for behavior management: A survey. *Journal of Dentistry for Children, 34,* 368–372.

Azarnoff, P., & Woody, P. D. (1981). Preparation of children for hospitalization in acute care hospitals in the United States. *Pediatrics, 68,* 361–368.

Balk, S., Dreyfus, N., & Harris, P. (1982). Examination of genitalia in children: "The remaining taboo." *Pediatrics, 70,* 751–753.

Beecher, H. K. (1956). Relationship of significance of wound to pain experienced. *Journal of the American Medical Association, 161,* 1609–1613.

Belter, R. W., McIntosh, J. A., Finch, A. J., Jr., & Saylor, C. F. (1988). Preschoolers' ability to differentiate levels of pain: Relative efficacy of three self-report measures. *Journal of Clinical Child Psychology, 17,* 329–335.

Beyer, J. E., DeGood, D. E., Ashley, L. C., & Russell, G. A. (1983). Patterns of postoperative analgesic use with adults and children following cardiac surgery. *Pain, 17,* 71–81.

Blitz, B., & Dinnerstein, A. J. (1971). Role of attentional focus in pain perception: Manipulation of response to noxious stimulation by instructions. *Journal of Abnormal Psychology, 77,* 42–45.

Blount, R. L., Corbin, S. M., Sturges, J. W., Wolfe, V. V., Prater, J. M., & James, L. D. (1989). The relationship between adults' behavior and child coping and distress during BMA/LP procedures: A sequential analysis. *Behavior Therapy, 20,* 585–601.

Broome, M. E., & Endsley, R. (1989). Parent and child behavior during immunization. *Pain, 37,* 85–92.

Bush, J. P., Melamed, B. G., Sheras, P. L., & Greenbaum, P. E. (1986). Mother-child patterns of coping with anticipatory medical stress. *Health Psychology, 5,* 137–157.

Cassel, S., & Paul, M. H. (1967). The role of puppet therapy on the emotional responses of children hospitalized for cardiac catheterization. *Journal of Pediatrics, 71,* 233–239.

Corah, N. L., Gale, E. N., & Illig, S. J. (1979). Psychological stress reduction during dental procedures. *Journal of Dental Research, 58,* 1347–1351.

Craig, K. D., McMahon, R. J., Morison, J. D., & Zaskow, C. (1984). Developmental changes in infant pain expression during immunization injections. *Social Science and Medicine, 19,* 1331–1337.

Cuthbert, M. I., & Melamed, B. G. (1982). A screening device: Children at risk for dental fears and management problems. *Journal of Dentistry for Children, 61,* 432–435.

Douglas, J. W. B. (1975). Early hospital admissions and later disturbances of behaviour and learning. *Developmental Medicine and Child Neurology, 17,* 456–480.

Duncan, G. H., Bushnell, M. C., Bates, R., & Dubner, R. (1987). Task related responses of monkey medullary dorsal horn neurons. *Journal of Neurophysiology, 57,* 289–310.

Eland, J. M. (1981). Minimizing pain associated with prekindergarten intramuscular injections. *Issues in Comprehensive Pediatric Nursing, 5,* 361–365.

Eland, J. M., & Anderson, J. E. (1977). The experience of pain in children. In A. K. Jacox (Ed.), *Pain: A sourcebook for nurses and other health professionals* (pp. 453–471). Boston: Little, Brown.

Elliott, C. H., & Olson, R. A. (1983). The management of children's distress in response to painful medical treatment for burn injuries. *Behaviour Research and Therapy, 21*, 675–683.

Fernald, B. F., & Corry, J. J. (1981). Empathetic versus directive preparation of children for needles. *Children's Health Care, 10*, 44–47.

Fields, H. L. (1987). *Pain*. New York: McGraw-Hill.

Fitzgerald, M. (1988). Review of Textbook of Neonatology, edited by N. R. C. Robertson. *Pain, 34*, 107–108.

Fowler-Kerry, S., & Lander, J. R. (1987). Management of injection pain in children. *Pain, 30*, 169–175.

Frankl, S., Shiere, F., & Fogels, H. (1962). Should the parent remain with the child in the dental operatory? *Journal of Dentistry for Children, 29*, 150–162.

Gardner, G. G., & Olness, K. (1981). *Hypnosis and hypnotherapy with children*. New York: Grune & Stratton.

Ghose, L. J., Giddon, D., Shiere, F. R., & Fogels, H. R. (1969). Evaluation of sibling support. *Journal of Dentistry for Children, 36*, 35–49.

Gonzalez, J. C., Routh, D. K., Saab, P. G., Armstrong, F. D., Shifman, L., Guerra, E., & Fawcett, N. (1989). Effects of parent presence on children's reactions to injections: Behavioral, physiological, and subjective aspects. *Journal of Pediatric Psychology, 14*, 449–462.

Green, R. V., Meilman, P., Routh, D. K., & McIver, F. T. (1977). Preparing the preschool child for a visit to the dentist. *Journal of Dentistry, 5*, 231–236.

Gross, A. M., Stern, R. M., Levin, R. B., Dale, J., & Wojnilower, D. A. (1983). The effect of mother-child separation on the behavior of children experiencing a diagnostic medical procedure. *Journal of Consulting and Clinical Psychology, 51*, 783–785.

Grunau, R. V. E., & Craig, K. D. (1987). Pain expression in neonates: Facial action and cry. *Pain, 28*, 395–410.

Gunnar, M. R., Fisch, R. O., & Malone, S. (1984). The effects of a pacifying stimulus on behavioral and adrenocortical responses to circumcision in the newborn. *Journal of the American Academy of Child Psychiatry, 23*, 34–38.

Harpin, V. A., & Rutter, N. (1983). Making heel pricks less painful. *Archives of Disease in Childhood, 8*, 226–228.

Haslam, D. R. (1969). Age and the perception of pain. *Psychonomic Science, 15*, 86–87.

Hilgard, E. R. (1975). The alleviation of pain by hypnosis. *Pain, 1*, 213–231.

Hilgard, J. R., & LeBaron, S. (1982). Relief of anxiety and pain in children and adolescents with cancer: Quantitative measures and clinical observations. *International Journal of Clinical and Experimental Hypnosis, 30*, 417–442.

Hughes, J. (1975). Isolation of an endogenous compound from the brain with pharmacological properties similar to morphine. *Brain Research, 88*, 295–308.

International Association for the Study of Pain, Subcommittee on Taxonomy (1979). Pain terms: A list with definitions and notes on usage. *Pain, 6*, 249.

Izard, C. E., Hembree, E. A., Dougherty, L. M., & Spizzirri, C. C. (1983). Changes in facial expressions of 2 to 19-month-old infants following acute pain. *Developmental Psychology, 19*, 418–426.

Janis, I. (1958). *Psychological stress*. New York: Wiley.

Jay, S. M. (1988). Invasive medical procedures: Psychological intervention and assessment. In D. K. Routh (Ed.), *Handbook of pediatric psychology* (pp. 401–425). New York: Guilford.

Jay, S. M., Elliott, C. H., Ozolins, M., Olson, R. A., & Pruitt, S. D. (1985). Behavioral management of children's distress during painful medical procedures. *Behaviour Research and Therapy*, *23*, 513–520.

Jay, S. M., Ozolins, M., Elliott, C. H., & Caldwell, S. (1983). Assessment of children's distress during painful medical procedures. *Health Psychology*, *2*, 133–147.

Johnson, P. A., & Stockdale, D. F. (1975). Effects of puppet therapy on palmar sweating of hospitalized children. *Johns Hopkins Medical Journal*, *137*, 1–5.

Johnston, C. C., & Strada, M. E. (1986). Acute pain response in infants: A multidimensional description. *Pain*, *24*, 373–382.

Katz, E. R., Kellerman, J., & Siegel, S. E. (1980). Behavioral distress in children with cancer undergoing medical procedures: Developmental considerations. *Journal of Consulting and Clinical Psychology*, *48*, 356–365.

Katz, E. R., Sharp, B., Kellerman, J., Marston, A. R., Hershman, J. M., & Siegel, S. E. (1982). Beta-endorphin immunoreactivity and acute behavioral distress in children with leukemia. *Journal of Nervous and Mental Disease*, *170*, 72–77.

Kavanaugh, C. (1983a). A new approach to dressing change in the severely burned child and its effect on burn-related psychopathology. *Heart and Lung*, *12*, 612–619.

Kavanaugh, C. (1983b). Psychological intervention with the severely burned child: Report of an experimental comparison of two approaches and their effects on psychological sequelae. *Journal of the American Academy of Child Psychiatry*, *22*, 145–156.

Kelley, M. L., Jarvie, G. J., Middlebrook, J. L., McNeer, M. F., & Drabman, R. S. (1984). Decreasing burned children's pain behavior: Impacting the trauma of hydrotherapy. *Journal of Applied Behavior Analysis*, *17*, 147–158.

Kirya, C., & Werthmann, M. W., Jr. (1978). Neonatal circumcision and penile dorsal block: A painless procedure. *Journal of Pediatrics*, *92*, 998–1000.

Kleinknecht, R., Klepac, R. K., & Alexander, L. D. (1973). Origins and characteristics of fear of dentistry. *Journal of the American Dental Association*, *86*, 842–848.

Klingman, A., Melamed, B. G., Cuthbert, M. I., & Hermecz, D. A. (1984). Effects of participant modeling on information acquisition and skill utilization. *Journal of Consulting and Clinical Psychology*, *52*, 414–422.

Lavigne, J. V., Schulein, M. J., & Hahn, Y. S. (1986a). Psychological aspects of painful medical conditions in children: I. Developmental aspects and assessment. *Pain*, *27*, 133–146.

Lavigne, J. V., Schulein, M. J., & Hahn, Y. S. (1986b). Psychological aspects of painful medical conditions in children: II. Personality factors, family characteristics and treatment. *Pain*, *27*, 147–169.

Lazarus, R. S., & Folkman, S. (1984). *Stress, appraisal, and coping*. New York: Springer.

LeBaron, S., & Zeltzer, L. (1984). Assessment of acute pain and anxiety in children and adolescents by self-reports, observer reports, and a behavior checklist. *Journal of Consulting and Clinical Psychology*, *52*, 729–738.

Lewis, T., & Pochin, E. E. (1937). The double pain responses of the human skin to a single stimulus. *Clinical Science*, *3*, 67–76.

Ludwick-Rosenthal, R., & Neufeld, R. W. J. (1988). Stress management during noxious medical procedures: An evaluative review of outcome studies. *Psychological Bulletin*, *104*, 326–342.

Machen, J. B., & Johnson, R. (1974). Desensitization, model learning, and the dental behavior of children. *Journal of Dental Research, 53,* 83–90.

Marks, R. M., & Sachar, E. J. (1973). Undertreatment of medical inpatients with narcotic analgesics. *Annals of Internal Medicine, 78,* 173–181.

Martin, L. V. H. (1982). Postoperative analgesia after circumcision in children. *British Journal of Anaesthesiology, 54,* 1263–1266.

Mather, L. E., & Mackie, J. (1983). The incidence of postoperative pain in children. *Pain, 15,* 271.

McCaul, K. D., & Malott, J. M. (1984). Distraction and coping with pain. *Psychological Bulletin, 95,* 516–533.

Meichenbaum, D. H. (1971). Examination of model characteristics in reducing avoidance behavior. *Journal of Personality and Social Psychology, 17,* 298–307.

Melamed, B. G., Hawes, R. R., Heiby, E., & Glick, J. (1975). Use of filmed modeling to reduce uncooperative behavior of children during dental treatment. *Journal of Dental Research, 54,* 797–801.

Melamed, B. G., & Siegel, L. (1975). Reduction of anxiety in children facing hospitalization and surgery by use of filmed modeling. *Journal of Consulting and Clinical Psychology, 43,* 511–521.

Melamed, B. G., Weinstein, D., Hawes, R., & Katin-Borland, M. (1975). Reduction of fear-related dental management problems with use of filmed modeling. *Journal of the American Dental Association, 90,* 822–826.

Melamed, B. G., Yurcheson, R., Fleece, L., Hutcherson, S., & Hawes, R. (1978). Effects of film modeling on the reduction of anxiety-related behaviors in individuals varying in level of previous experience in the stress situation. *Journal of Consulting and Clinical Psychology, 46,* 1357–1367.

Melzack, R., & Wall, P. D. (1965). Pain mechanisms: A new theory. *Science, 150,* 971–978.

Miller, M. D., Elliott, C. H., Funk, M., & Pruitt, S. D. (1988). Implications of children's burn injuries. In D. K. Routh (Ed.), *Handbook of pediatric psychology* (pp. 426–447). New York: Guilford.

Millstein, S., Adler, N., & Irwin, C. (1984). Sources of anxiety about pelvic examinations among adolescent females. *Journal of Adolescent Health Care, 5,* 105–111.

Nocella, J., & Kaplan, R. M. (1982). Training children to cope with dental treatment. *Journal of Pediatric Psychology, 7,* 175–178.

Owens, M. E. (1984). Pain in infancy: Conceptual and methodological issues. *Pain, 20,* 213–230.

Owens, M. E., & Todt, E. H. (1984). Pain in infancy: Neonatal reaction to a heel lance. *Pain, 20,* 77–86.

Perry, S., & Heidrich, G. (1982). Management of pain during debridement: A survey of U.S. burn units. *Pain, 13,* 267–280.

Pert, C. B., & Snyder, S. H. (1973). Opiate receptors: Demonstration in nervous tissue. *Science, 179,* 1011–1014.

Peterson, L., & Mori, L. (1988). Preparation for hospitalization. In D. K. Routh (Ed.), *Handbook of pediatric psychology* (pp. 460–491). New York: Guilford.

Peterson, L., & Ridley-Johnson, R. (1980). Pediatric hospital response to survey on prehospital preparation for children. *Journal of Pediatric Psychology, 5,* 1–7.

Peterson, L., & Shigetomi, C. (1981). The use of coping techniques to minimize anxiety in hospitalized children. *Behavior Therapy, 12,* 1-14.

Price, D. D., Harkins, S. W., & Baker, C. (1987). Sensory-affective relationships among different types of clinical and experimental pain. *Pain, 28,* 297-307.

Price, D. D., Hu, J. W., Dubner, R., & Gracely, R. H. (1977). Peripheral suppression of first pain and central summation of second pain evoked by noxious heat pulses. *Pain, 3,* 57-68.

Purcell-Jones, G., Dormon, F., & Sumner, E. (1988). Paediatric anaesthetists' perceptions of neonatal and infant pain. *Pain, 33,* 181-187.

Reissland, N. (1983). Cognitive maturity and the experience of fear and pain in hospital. *Social Science and Medicine, 17,* 1389-1395.

Ross, D. M., & Ross, S. A. (1985). Pain instruction with third- and fourth-grade children: A pilot study. *Journal of Pediatric Psychology, 10,* 55-62.

Routh, D. K., & Andersen, B. (1988). Infancy through childhood. In E. Blechman & K. Brownell (Eds.), *Handbook of behavioral medicine for women* (pp. 3-11). New York: Pergamon.

Schwartz, B. H., Albino, J. E., & Tedesco, L. A. (1983). Effects of psychological preparation on children hospitalized for dental operations. *Journal of Pediatrics, 102,* 634-638.

Shaw, E. G., & Routh, D. K. (1982). Effect of mother presence on children's reaction to aversive procedures. *Journal of Pediatric Psychology, 7,* 33-42.

Siegel, L. J. (1988). Dental treatment. In D. K. Routh (Ed.), *Handbook of pediatric psychology* (pp. 448-459). New York: Guilford.

Siegel, L. J., & Peterson, L. (1980). Stress reduction in young dental patients through coping skills and sensory information. *Journal of Consulting and Clinical Psychology, 48,* 785-787.

Siegel, L. J., & Peterson, L. (1981). Maintenance effects of coping skills and sensory information on young children's responses to repeated dental procedures. *Behavior Therapy, 12,* 530-535.

Stehbens, J. A. (1988). Childhood cancer. In D. K. Routh (Ed.), *Handbook of pediatric psychology* (pp. 135-161). New York: Guilford.

Swafford, L. I., & Allan, D. (1968). Pain relief in the pediatric patient. *Medical Clinics of North America, 52*(1), 131-136.

Talbert, L. M., Kraybill, E. N., & Potter, H. D. (1975). Adrenal cortical response to circumcision in the neonate. *Obstetrics and Gynecology, 48,* 208-210.

Thevenin, D. M. (1989). *Effects of information and coping instructions on prepubertal children's reactions to gynecological exams.* Unpublished Ph.D. dissertation, University of Miami.

Venham, L. L., Bengston, D., & Cipes, M. (1977). Children's response to sequential dental visits. *Journal of Dental Research, 56,* 454-459.

Venham, L. L., Bengston, D., & Cipes, M. (1978). Parent's presence and the child's response to dental stress. *Journal of Dentistry for Children, 45,* 213-217.

Venham, L. L., Murray, P., & Gaulin-Kremer, E. (1979). Child-rearing variables affecting the preschool child's response to dental stress. *Journal of Dental Research, 58,* 2042-2045.

Vernon, D. T. A., & Bailey, W. C. (1974). The use of motion pictures in the psychological preparation of children for induction of anesthesia. *Anesthesiology, 40,* 68-74.

Wakeman, R. J., & Kaplan, J. Z. (1978). An experimental study of hypnosis in painful burns. *American Journal of Clinical Hypnosis, 21*, 3–12.

Wall, P. (1978). The gate control theory of pain mechanisms: A re-examination and re-statement. *Brain, 101*, 1–18.

Williamson, P. S., & Williamson, M. L. (1983). Physiologic stress reduction by a local anesthetic during newborn circumcision. *Pediatrics, 71*, 36–40.

Zabin, M. A., & Melamed, B. G. (1980). Relationship between parental discipline and children's ability to cope with stress. *Journal of Behavioral Assessment, 2*, 17–38.

Zeltzer, L., & LeBaron, S. (1982). Hypnosis and non-hypnotic techniques for reduction of pain and anxiety during painful procedures in children and adolescents with cancer. *Journal of Pediatrics, 101*, 1032–1035.

Afterword
Future Pain Horizons:
The Other Side of Pain

. . . a merry heart doeth good like a medicine . . .

A life-span perspective is the main thread that ties the chapters of this volume together and directs future research efforts. The authors view pain and pain behaviors as changing aspects of individuals' abilities to communicate their experiences. Pain is not simply a precursor or by-product of illness or injury, it is a phenomenon guided by the capacities of individuals and modified by the life experiences and support systems provided by their environment, their culture, and other human beings. Pain is both a percept and a drive. It is an active process directing the actions of the sufferer and the caregiver, both those paid professionals and those parents for whom the option of "cutting off their own right arms" unfortunately does not exist.

In the following thoughts I would like to reemphasize many of the illuminating points made in the contributions and tie them together within a framework for future research into understanding the complexity and the positive side of pain. I propose some preposterous thoughts, including: *pain farms*, for families to learn how to manage and milk their concerns into healthier responses; *pain profiles*, to pinpoint those at risk for injury, psychopathology, or serious neglect of themselves and their offspring; *profiles in courage*, to describe those who suffer quietly or cry loudly enough to enable providers to react differentially to their needs (within the limits of our medical and psychological knowledge; the importance of individual coping styles in reaction to pain is just beginning to be studied); the philosophy and religion of pain receive inadequate attention, thus, finally, the *church of pain* is added to the brew. The words of Norman Cousins proselytizing in *Head First* (1989) on the importance of laughter and positive feelings in overcoming illness and pain will be briefly discussed. Within this context we understand the limits of our knowledge, we understand the sense of our helplessness at loss, and hopefully we learn how to limit the suffering of those whom we cannot save but can merely sedate and comfort on their journey home. The ethical dilemmas provided by medical advances are dealt with both within a humanistic tradition and with respect to the religious and

425

cultural differences of the families in which illness, catastrophe, or chronic pain reside.

It is a family systems approach that I am postulating as the integrating feature of the contributions to this volume. This is developed by assuming that due to the interrelationship of all members of the family, the illness and pain of one member will affect the entire system and thus illness cannot and should not be viewed as separate.

Let us so begin our journey.

Pain was viewed in 1644 by Descartes as the bell that signals the body to respond. He suggested that the system is like the bell-ringing mechanism in a church: a man pulls the rope at the bottom of the tower and the bell rings in the belfry; a flame sets particles in the foot into activity and the motion is transmitted up the leg and back into the head, where, presumably, something like an alarm system is set off. The person feels pain and is motivated to respond to it.

Pain has in fact been found to be coded in the human organism, as it is in other species, by the capacity of the nervous system to signal the brain to withdraw or to respond to it with the appropriate chemical release and healing actions. It is also seen in this volume as a product of disease. It is seen as a dependent variable in research to be measured and eliminated; yet, from a theoretical perspective, pain is a multitude of experiences from which we learn to change our behavior.

This book would be incomplete if it did not attempt to set forth a model of the construct of pain with testable hypotheses. Some of these apply directly in the chapters herein and some, if linked together, would be relevant to other critical areas such as compliance with medical regimens (e.g., juvenile rheumatoid arthritis) in which medication and exacerbations may not be clearly linked in time. The model not only should include the self-regulatory theories applauded by Karoly (Chapter 3) and others, but also should extend to the application of preventive or computerized methods to assure compliance with healthy behaviors that reduce the likelihood of pain. It is important to understand how pain serves to heighten our awareness of human social functioning, both within and across cultures. Without pain we might not develop empathy, altruism, and the motive to pursue happiness. In some cultures, such as that of the "firewalker" sect in Greece, the tolerance of pain is a sign of higher commitment to religious beliefs. However, this conceptual belief area will prove fruitful for another volume perhaps jointly undertaken by anthropologists, psychologists, historians, and clergy.

The developmental approach of Piaget is an excellent model that has received primary emphasis throughout the contributions of the authors. When dealing with children across a broad enough age range, we are forced to view pain within an understanding of maturation, sex role differences, conceptual abilities, and hormonal influences. However, we should not lose sight of the guidance of more dynamically oriented approaches, such as Lois Murphy's (1982) insight that coping behavior is prompted by frustration and discomfort. Thus, the goal is not found in the entire elimination of pain, but in its value as a guide to signal, motivate, and lead to a pleasurable outcome, one of mastery.

Pain Model

The theoretical perspective of this book is weighted toward Piagetian stage theory in which the maturation of a child's physical capacities, coupled with his/her growing conceptual understanding, is viewed as the decoder of the capacity to cope with pain related to illness, injury, and acute medical experiences that are likely to recur across time. The emphasis on understanding pain within the framework of the child's wisdom and previous experience is well taken. Age-related abilities are a useful guide but not an infallible predictor. Adolescence is viewed as a unique period in which hormonal, social, and self-regulatory changes become paramount. The reciprocal influences of parents and peers also serve as the focus of several contributors.

There are many paradoxes involved in our interpretation and evaluation of effective pain responses. At a time when children are most uncomfortable, scared with the uncertainty of illness, and separated from those they love and depend on to take care of and protect them, they are also admonished to "be a good patient," "be a brave young man," "don't be a sissy," or "don't cry." Reassurances such as "this will hurt me more than it hurts you" or "it will only hurt for a minute" often heighten their anticipation of painful events. The research literature reminds us that often the anticipation of pain is greater than the actual acute pain experience. We also know that arousal does accelerate our response to acute pain. But in dealing with the chronic and sometimes severely restricting pain experiences of the child with juvenile rheumatoid arthritis, sickle cell anemia, or the nausea of chemotherapy and radiation side effects, a different model might need to be invoked. A longitudinal perspective is recommended, one that takes into account the patterning or lack of consistency of pain episodes and the youngsters' experiences in dealing with these in the context of their families' support.

The paradox of the independence struggle of a teenager saddled with a chronic illness, which limits his/her ability to regulate diet, play, and commerce within the subculture, is raised by P. J. McGrath and Pisterman (Chapter 9). Although typical teenage-onset illness or discomfort such as migraines or dysmenorrhea may well be due to hormonal alterations, self-esteem issues caused by physical development or lack of it in chronically ill cystic fibrosis or renal adolescent patients who need to pay constant attention to compliance may require a more vigorous intervention given their life threat value. In contrast to their parents and physicians, these youngsters are often more concerned with the immediate limitations of their quality of life than with the shortened expectancy of life span. With these disease-related somatic problems, the age, incidence, and sex of the child may be important aspects of both tolerance and expression. Measures of quality of life are now being defined for chronically ill children (Boggs & Goodman, 1991).

Measurement of Pain

It is often heard that you should always believe the individual's subjective experience of pain as true; yet in trying to ameliorate it we need to examine a way of determining its expression, promote consensual validation, and provide quantitative measurement.

Age differences require different assessment tools not only because of differences in understandability but also because of cultural expectations. A young child is freer to cry and more likely to move about when worried or in pain, whereas an older child may grin and bear it. The pleading grimace of the adult dental phobic is an example of pain behavior that may not hamper the immediate procedure but can put strains on future cooperation. I can remember as a 14-year-old being in the midst of a pool party at the Ping-Pong table and having the first menstrual pain of my life. Before I cringed, the warm feeling of reinterpreting those cramps as my induction into womanhood brought, instead, a smile to my lips. I stood proudly aside as the others followed the match with a swim, explaining merely that it was "my time of the month."

Theory and Research

The theories that have served us well in understanding much of human development (those of innate reflexes, operant and classical conditioning, self-regulation, and social learning) must be given appropriate attention in elaborating the schemata by which we should understand the pain experience. Thus, chief among the interventions that are taught to those who must live with pain are cognitive-behavioral approaches that have components derived from each of the aforementioned theories. Developmental stage theories need to be integrated with these other powerful approaches.

The pain memory as a prototype on which concurrent influences modify the expression of pain receives mention in this volume but needs elaboration. The importance of memories in anticipation, preparation, and forgetting of painful experiences must be reemphasized and reviewed within that which has been presented to us through this voluptuous volume of information that calls forth our creative future efforts, not to eliminate pain but to use it better. Ross and Ross (1988) set forth a model of how to interview children. Walco and Varni (Chapter 12) use self-report as a valid indicator of children's pain through the visual analogue scale (VAS). Children with chronic recurrent pain (juvenile rheumatoid arthritis and sickle cell anemia) had lower pain thresholds. Cognitive-behavioral treatment must take into account both perception of pain regulation and pain behavior regulation. Applying an acute pain model of intervention (which assumes that as the condition resolves, pain will dissipate) may be accurate for those who have sickle cell disease, except for those (especially adolescents) whose lifestyles are marked by maladaptive coping patterns, poor psychological adjustment and inadequate family and social support, and school absenteeism and failure. There still exists the myth of real versus in-head pain.

The research perspective needed and acknowledged by all is a longitudinal approach, by which the child's growing awareness of separateness and competence can be tracked throughout the life span as it develops, is imposed upon and shaped by environmental events, and is influenced by the reactions of others. This obviously is difficult in a mobile society in which the wealthy often move their families during acute medical crises closer to the best centers. I feel that we need to combine the research on children's mood-dependent memory, which is sparse, with the data we are collecting regarding pain schemata. We are already forced to face the fact that children too young to verbalize forced sexual abuse or incest are later scarred by these experiences.

Karoly (Chapter 3) in his psychosocial elaboration model (PEM) views a symptom such as pain as the product of interactive forces within the person and in the external world. It produces one or more of six reactions: (1) autonomic arousal; (2) emotional response; (3) communicative or expressive reaction; (4) motor activity; (5) efforts at understanding or justification; and (6) efforts toward symptom management.

This theoretical overview should be specifically applied to generate hypotheses to be tested by much of the data presented. Thus, in setting the guidelines for future research, I briefly name each of the ingredients to be considered (see Table A.1), although the more accurate model will involve feedback loops and more selective measurement for evaluating causal models and directional predictions.

Responses of Others

Peterson and her colleagues (Chapter 2) choose a specific focus for their interactive systems analysis that perhaps is most efficient in looking at our youngest children. Child–parent attachment may modulate internal emotional responses to pain and familial models can influence a child's cognition and beliefs about pain. They conclude clearly that children's cognition about pain independent from their beliefs about illness has not been well studied.

TABLE A.1. Variables to be considered in a pediatric pain model.

Input	Mediators	Outcome
Medical	Individual	Behavior
Disease status	Age, race, sex	Affect
Prognosis	Coping style preference	Cognition
Treatment requirements	Temperament	Response of others
	Family	
	Size	
	Heredity	
	Pain model	
	Caregiver	
	Reinforcer	
	Punisher	
	Religion	
	Belief system	
	Sacrifice	
	Time (experience)	
	Acute	
	Chronic	
	Acute but recurrent	

Cognition

Looking more closely at cognition, Peterson and her colleagues' categories of pain (Chapter 2) vary along a complexity dimension. Understanding progresses from external causes to physiological or psychological causes. First we develop the theory, then the tool, then perhaps a better understanding of pain schemata for individual analysis.

Affect

Physiological indices must be used. Pain is more than the sum of its parts. The Melzack and Wall (1983) Gate Theory of pain emphasizes the role of cognitive and arousal interaction in interpreting incoming stimuli that may be reacted to as "painful." We remember the Grinker and Spiegel (1945) stories of soldiers in battle who seemed completely unaware that shrapnel was hanging out over a bleeding surface and remained in battle. And how many of us have had the universal toe-stubbing experience in which no one present so our cry is suppressed? We know that the infant brain is capable of supporting pain experience. The tactile system is well-developed at birth. Intrauterine nociception appears to be demonstrated by invasive methods of fetal assessment. Biological maturation proceeds at a rapid rate, thus prospects for pain having a long-lasting impact are considerable. There is now little doubt that infants experience pain; only their expression of it may be diffuse or difficult to interpret, not their sense of discomfort. Most mothers can distinguish their infants' expressions of the emotion of pain from those signaling hunger, wetness, or anger. Developmental process in pain comprises a complex reciprocal relationship between caregiver and infant with survival features.

Behavior

It is less clear how the severity of pain expression is modulated by ongoing variations in the state of the central nervous system. A tired child will be less responsive to pressure pain than an alert, orienting one. The newborn has the self-quieting response. In the second 6 months of life we note the emergence of anticipatory pain responses. The immediate response to pain is a display of anger. At this stage distraction could intervene. The capacity to anticipate pain clearly signals memory and can only support the notion of perceptual schemata with earlier origins. Few studies exist of the persisting behavioral effects of pain in the newborn and infant.

Gedaly-Duff (Chapter 8) presents a wonderful developmental analysis of the preschooler, postulating the idea of a socialized person with a capacity to communicate to others his/her personal needs and desires as well as the skills necessary to respond to the demands of others and to interact with them with some skill and effectiveness. The child learns familial and cultural patterns of pain expression. Thus a less than one-to-one correspondence between experience of discomfort and pain expression should be predicted. As the child grows older and experiences the bumps and scrapes of childhood without serious injury or enduring damage, his/her parents become relatively inured to minor crises and are likely to require that children withhold demands unless there are genuinely serious problems. In this manner, parents also promote the process of self-management and personal independence.

In developing our understanding of central nervous system processes, we also need to look to the biology of hope and, as Cousins puts it, "the healing power of the human spirit." He cites Josh Billings, "There ain't much fun in medicine, but there's a heck of a lot of medicine in fun" (p. 25). His ideas have been borne out by many *New England Journal of Medicine* citations showing that laughter is useful in combatting chronic disease. Investigations into the mechanisms by which endorphins are released and through which the immune system is supported are just now beginning to yield interesting results.

Experience

Siegel and Smith describe research methods for evaluating children's coping with pain (Chapter 6). A specific coping response is not inherently adaptive or maladaptive. They postulate the importance of not only knowing coping strategies, but also having experience in the successful use of them. The relationship between coping style and temperament may be interactive. Preferred style may be determined by children's experience with techniques and the particular time during the illness. What works for nausea control might not work during a lumbar puncture. It is equally important to define task difficulty in terms of the stage of disease. Early oncology patients prefer avoidance.

Peterson and Toler (1986) have shown the important differences in coping success when considering a child's typical preference for information-seeking in the face of painful medical procedures. Lumley, Abeles, Melamed, Pistone, and Johnson (1990) found that the interaction of maternal style of dealing with the difficult-temperament child influenced adaptive coping when the child was alone in face of anesthesia induction. Thus, withdrawn children who had been managed with distraction did better than those whose mothers attempted to provide information in the face of a medical presurgical examination.

Medical Problems

Pain Profile as Predictor

Hodges and Burbach's recurrent abdominal pain (RAP) research (Chapter 10) revealed that the ratio of stress to personal resources or coping skills may be more important than absolute amount of life stress. RAP children have frequent school absences and poor social skills.

Maron and Bush (Chapter 11) cite a remarkable statistic: 25% of all children admitted for burns may be abuse victims. Burn victims may have to endure separation and physical disfigurement. Some caregiving behaviors that are usually soothing, such as physical stroking, cannot be used. Painful treatments are often seen by the child as harmful or as punishment for misbehavior. High rates of depression and posttraumatic stress disorder occur in parents of children who have been burned. Pretraumatic adjustment problems have also been found to be more common among burn victims than in the general population. The caveat about pain within the system is further supported by their finding that social support, especially within the family, is considered to be the most important predictor of post-burn adjustment. These children often come from chaotic families.

Manne and Andersen (Chapter 13) report that pain in head or stomach tissues often signals possible cancer. Variability among different pain ratings may provide an opportunity to understand different perspectives on the child's pain experience. The use of observational coding with inclusion of parents or practitioners is similar to marital coding procedures and allows for the systems influence to be evaluated (Blount, Landolf-Fritsche, Powers, & Sturges, in press; Bush, Melamed, Sheras, & Greenbaum, 1986).

Members of medical staff often assess psychological problems rather than pain or disease-related problems. It is difficult for them to face that they must inflict pain in order to assist in the cure.

Collaborative Treatment Approaches

Gillman and Mullins (Chapter 5) raise a most important point that is too often neglected, that is, How may we get into the system as pediatric psychologists prior to the last ditch effort? The collaborative team model addresses this role of the psychologist as pain manager. The authors offer a number of practical tips based on satisfaction with consultation, emphasizing the importance of congruence of perceived goals by the pediatrician and the psychological consultant.

Intervention strategies need to be matched to the patient's capacity to use them and to the procedure during which they need to be employed. Vieyra, Hoag, and Masek (Chapter 14) found that children who suffer migraines that do not remit within 6 months usually continue to have them during adulthood. They say that 7 years is the minimally effective age for a biobehavioral approach to migraines.

Summary and Conclusions

This volume has succeeded in its aim to describe the childhood conditions accompanied by pain, to point out the developmental perspective in order to define the individual's concepts of pain in causality and expression, and to define the treatment interventions being used singly or in multimodal packages to control pain.

References

Blount, R., Landolf-Fritsche, B., Powers, J., & Sturges, J. (in press). Differences between high and low coping children and between parent and staff behaviors during painful medical procedures. *Journal of Pediatric Psychology*.

Boggs, S. R., & Goodwin, D. (1991, April). Development and Validation of a Quality of Life Measure with Pediatric Oncology Patients. Florida Child Health Conference, Gainesville, FL.

Bush, J. P., Melamed, B. G., Sheras, P. L., & Greenbaum, P. (1986). Mother–child patterns of coping with anticipatory medical stress. *Health Psychology, 5*, 137–157.

Cousins, N. (1989). *Head first: The biology of hope.* New York: Dutton.

Grinker, R. R., & Spiegel, J. P. (1945). *Men under stress.* Philadelphia: Blakiston.

Lumley, M., Abeles, L., Melamed, B. G., Pistone, L., & Johnson, J. H. (1990). Coping outcomes in children undergoing stressful medical procedures: The role of child-environment variables. *Behavioral Assessment, 12*, 223–238.

Melzack, R., & Wall, P. D. (1983). *The challenge of pain*. New York: Basic Books.

Murphy, L. (1982). *The home hospital*. New York: Basic Books.

Peterson, L., & Toler, S. (1986). An information seeking disposition in child surgery patients. *Health Psychology, 5*, 343–358.

Ross, D. M., & Ross, S. A. (1988). Assessment of pediatric pain: An overview. *Issues in Comprehensive Pediatric Nursing, 11*, 73–91.

Author Index

Subject Index